INTRODUCTION TO CARDIOLOGY

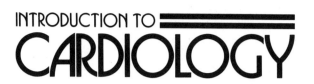

INTRODUCTION TO

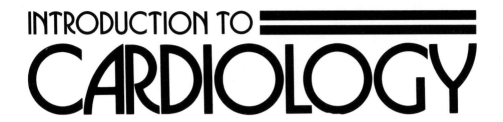

CARDIOLOGY

EDITED BY **ROBERT H. EICH**, M.D.

Professor
Chief, Cardiology Section
Department of Medicine
State University of New York
Upstate Medical Center
Syracuse, New York

9 Contributors

HARPER & ROW, PUBLISHERS
HAGERSTOWN

Cambridge		London
New York		Mexico City
Philadelphia		São Paulo
San Francisco		Sydney

1817

6 5 4 3 2 1

Library of Congress Cataloging in Publication Data
Main entry under title:
Introduction to cardiology.
   Bibliography
   Includes index.
   1. Heart—Diseases.   2. Cardiology.   I.   Eich,
Robert H.   [DNLM: 1.   Heart diseases.   WG200 I64]
RC681.I57   616.1'2   80-14841
ISBN 0-06-140770-4

CONTENTS

CONTRIBUTORS

ROBERT H. EICH, M.D.

Professor of Medicine
Chief, Cardiology Section
State University of New York
Upstate Medical Center
Syracuse, New York

C. THOMAS FRUEHAN, M.D.

Associate Professor of Medicine
Director, EKG Department
State University of New York
Upstate Medical Center
Syracuse, New York

DANIEL S. FULEIHAN, M.D., F.A.C.C.

Clinical Assistant Professor of Medicine
State University of New York
Upstate Medical Center
Syracuse, New York

SAKTIPADA MOOKHERJEE, M.D., M.R.C.P.

Associate Professor of Medicine
State University of New York
Upstate Medical Center
Syracuse, New York

Staff Cardiologist
Syracuse Veterans Administration Medical Center
Syracuse, New York

ANIS I. OBEID, M.D.

Clinical Associate Professor
State University of New York
Upstate Medical Center
Syracuse, New York

JAMES L. POTTS, M.D.

Associate Professor of Medicine
Director, Cardiac Catheterization Laboratory
State University of New York
Upstate Medical Center
Syracuse, New York

HAROLD SMULYAN, M.D.

Professor of Medicine
State University of New York
Upstate Medical Center
Syracuse, New York

Chief, Cardiology Section
Syracuse Veterans Administration Medical Center
Syracuse, New York

F. DEAVER THOMAS, M.D.

Professor of Radiology
Director, Division of Nuclear Medicine
State University of New York
Upstate Medical Center
Syracuse, New York

ROBERT A. WARNER, M.D.

Assistant Professor of Medicine
State University of New York
Upstate Medical Center
Syracuse, New York

Staff Cardiologist
Syracuse Veterans Administration Medical Center
Syracuse, New York

PREFACE

This book is written expressly to meet the need for a textbook in clinical cardiology designed for medical students and junior house officers. Since 1968, the
majority of our seniors at the State University of New York Upstate Medical
Center at Syracuse has chosen our elective in clinical cardiology. In order to
provide a basic fund of information to these students, we have given each group
a series of lectures; this textbook is based on the lectures prepared for these
series.

The book is not designed to be an exhaustive review of the topics that are
covered. For more detail, the reader may turn to one of several standard textbooks of cardiology, including those by Drs. J. Willis Hurst and Noble O.
Fowler. A few key references are provided at the end of each chapter for students who wish to investigate the subjects in greater depth. There is no chapter
specifically devoted to physiology and pathology, since these topics are covered
in each chapter where pertinent. The first six chapters follow the sequence that
the physician uses in his approach to the patient. Chapter 1 concerns the history; Chapter 2, the physical examination; Chapter 3, the chest roentgenograph;
Chapter 4, the electrocardiogram; Chapter 5, the echocardiogram; and Chapter
6, cardiac catheterization. For the sake of convenience, masculine pronouns are
used in referring to patients.

The authors are all members of the Cardiology Section of the State University of New York at the Upstate Medical Center in Syracuse. We recognize that
many aspects of cardiology are controversial; on such matters, the members
have expressed their own opinions.

ROBERT H. EICH

HISTORY

Robert H. Eich

1

BASIC EVALUATIVE TECHNIQUES

In evaluating a patient with suspected heart disease, the physician tries to determine: 1) whether the patient does have heart disease; 2) if so, what type—coronary artery disease, valvular heart disease, hypertensive cardiovascular disease, congenital heart disease, or cardiomyopathy; 3) how severe the disease is; and 4) how to further evaluate and treat the patient. Whether the patient seeks help for symptoms of cardiac disease or is found incidentally to have such symptoms when being considered for elective surgery, the basic steps of the evaluation are the same. They are the subject of the opening chapters of this volume. The first step is the obtaining of a complete medical history. Second is the physical examination. Third, if the physician feels that he still needs more information, he will order a chest film, possibly with cardiac fluoroscopy, and an electrocardiogram.

Fourth, if the history, physical examination, chest film, and electrocardiogram are not sufficient to establish the presence and type of heart disease, special tests may be ordered. Some, such as the widely used echocardiogram and treadmill stress tests, are noninvasive. Other extremely helpful noninvasive tests include radionuclear studies and vector cardiograms. Less commonly used now is the phonocardiogram, although it still has a place in timing cardiac events.

Finally, the physician may decide that cardiac catheterization is indicated. This is an invasive procedure, of course, and the risk of the test must be weighed against the yield. If the patient's disease has been diagnosed with certainty and has responded to therapy, cardiac catheterization would not normally be indicated. Catheterization is useful for both diagnosis and management, but

1

the physician must always ask himself how much information can be obtained in this way and how much it will help the patient.

THE HISTORY

As mentioned earlier, the history is the most important of these techniques. It is also the most difficult to learn. The physician's major mistakes will almost invariably be due to failure to obtain the proper information, either because he or she has not asked the right questions or because the patient is unable to respond to them adequately. The history serves two functions. First, it provides information which can be used to establish the diagnosis, pathological anatomy, functional classification, and treatment of the disease. Second, and equally important, it establishes the physician's relationship with the patient. The physician must demonstrate that he can be trusted and is concerned about the patient. I find it very useful to start off the history with a few simple questions about occupation, hometown, referring physician, and age, which helps to establish rapport and often will give considerable insight into the patient's feelings. Rapport is usually not a problem for a senior physician because the patient is there specifically to see him. It may be more difficult for students and house staff to establish a good relationship with the patient, but the secret is to show genuine concern about him.

Students, when they first start obtaining the history from a patient, should use a check list. Excellent lists are available in texts of physical diagnosis. With experience, the list will no longer be necessary. Likewise, with better understanding of the disease that the patient presents with, one will be aware that certain symptoms should be explored in greater detail. It is extremely important in taking the history, to continually try to organize the information into a diagnosis. Although students are taught to ask first about the chief complaint, then the present illness, next the past medical history, and finally to make the system review, questions may well be asked out of this order, and, depending on the patient and the disease, different components of the history will be emphasized. For example, if a patient appears to have a myocardial infarction, one would not dwell on the system review nearly as much as in a patient with an undetermined diagnosis. The standard format is really most useful in writing down the information after the history and physical examination are done.

An excellent method to use in organizing the information obtained from the history, physical examination, and laboratory tests is the problem-oriented medical record of Dr. Lawrence Weed.

In taking the history, it is important to sit and interview the patient in a quiet room without distraction. Unfortunately, interviews usually will be attempted in a hospital room where there are a number of distractions, and the examiner must be patient as well. Often the spouse will accompany the patient. This may be an advantage, enabling the examiner to verify points in the history. However, there is the risk of unproductive discussions between the patient and spouse regarding exact dates or other things that are not particularly germane, and it may be better to ask the spouse to leave and question him or her later. The time needed to obtain the history and perform the physical examination will decrease with experience, but a careful evaluation certainly takes time, particularly if the diagnostic problem is complex.

Obviously the most important item in the history for patients with suspected heart disease is the investigation of the patient's symptoms. Other key items include the history of past illnesses, family history of heart disease, and the assessment of other risk factors for coronary artery disease (age, sex, smoking, or conditions such as hypertension, diabetes mellitus, and hyperlipidemia); these will be discussed subsequently. When taking the history, one should be sure to ascertain the results of any previous evaluations of the present illness, including diagnosis and current therapy.

SYMPTOMS OF HEART DISEASE

The cardinal symptoms of heart disease are chest pain, dyspnea, fatigue, and syncope. Less frequent but still important are cough, hemoptysis, orthopnea, paroxysmal nocturnal dyspnea, edema, palpitations, and dizziness. Cyanosis is infrequently reported in the history.

CHEST PAIN

The most frightening symptom of heart disease is chest pain. Patients often equate any chest pain with heart disease, invalidism, and death, so that this symptom will bring them to seek medical attention sooner than any other. Chest pain, of course, can be caused by disease in any structure in the chest, including ribs, sternum, pleura, lungs, pericardium, thoracic spine, and esophagus. Gallbladder disease, peptic ulcer, and cervical spine disease may also cause chest pain. In my experience and that of my colleagues, neither gallbladder disease nor peptic ulcer truly mimic cardiac pain.

The most important cardiac diseases associated with chest pain are angina pectoris and myocardial infarction. Both in angina pectoris and early in the course of a myocardial infarction, the history may be the only positive clue to the disease; physical examination, and EKG are often normal. The types of pain associated with these two diseases are distinct, and the "history" of the pain can often establish the diagnosis.

Angina Pectoris

Angina pectoris is chest discomfort brought on when the oxygen needs of the myocardium are increased beyond the ability of the coronary circulation to provide adequate blood flow. (The pathophysiology of angina pectoris is discussed further in Chapter 10.) Basically, the oxygen needs of the myocardium depend on blood pressure, heart rate, myocardial contractility, and diastolic fiber length. When needs increase, the coronary arteries dilate, and blood flow increases. However, if coronary artery disease is present, flow may be limited, and angina then occurs. Classically, the sensation of angina is substernal and brought on by exertion. It is important to emphasize that most patients do not refer to it as "pain." It is described as a sensation of burning, pressure, or tightness. Patients will occasionally tell the physician that the feeling is not unpleasant, and their best efforts to describe it will often be vague. Beware of dramatic expressions, such as, "It felt like an elephant was sitting on my chest!"; such patients may be suffering from anxiety, rather than heart disease. An occasional patient will say that the sensation is similar to the burning in the chest that he used to get when he was a young child and had run hard for a long time. The pain is almost never sharp or knifelike. The patient may even refer to the sensation as "gas."

As already noted, the sensation is typically substernal and may radiate to the shoulders, arms, back, or neck. Radiation to the jaw or teeth is an extremely helpful, but uncommon, point in the history and is highly suggestive of coronary artery disease. Angina is classically brought on by exertion, excitement, or anything that increases the myocardial oxygen needs. It is worse in cold weather and after eating. However, it is important to emphasize that patients have good days and bad days, and that when walking, they don't always get angina at the same crack in the sidewalk. There may be days when they can do almost anything. Patients will frequently have angina in the morning and not get it again all day.

There are several special features of the pain or discomfort of angina. It should have some exertional component; it tends to get worse if the exertion is continued; and once the patient stops the exertion, with or without taking nitroglycerin, the discomfort subsides in 1 to 3 min.

In our cardiac catheterization laboratory, as in most, about 15% of patients admitted for catheterization with chest pain resembling angina pectoris will be found to have normal coronary arteries. This syndrome of chest pain with normal coronary arteries is complicated; it probably has a complex etiology and its history may at times be hard to separate from that of anyone due to coronary artery disease. However, most people with chest pain and normal coronary arteries have something unusual in their history. For example, the pain is not burning; it is often sharp; it is not exertional; they can keep going with it; it doesn't go away when they stop; or it is not promptly relieved by nitroglycerin. If the patient is under 35, has no family history of heart disease, and is not affected by any other risk factors, the physician can be much more confident that the atypical chest pain is not the result of coronary artery disease. With a careful history, he can correctly diagnose most of his patients as having angina due to coronary artery disease, although in a small percentage of cases, he will be wrong.

Myocardial Infarction

The pain of myocardial infarction is clearly pain. Patients seldom describe it as pressure. However, it can be mild and sometimes can be ignored. Approximately 20% of myocardial infarctions discovered on a routine electrocardiogram will not be associated with any history suggestive of a myocardial infarction in the past. It is important to emphasize that the electrocardiograph and cardiac injury enzymes may be normal for several hours after the onset of an infarction, and the decision regarding admission to the coronary care unit will have to be made on the basis of the history alone.

Classically, patients with an acute myocardial infarction give an extremely reproducible and typical history, compared to the variability observed in the history of patients with angina. Frequently, the patient with an acute myocardial infarction will have had premonitory symptoms in the 2 weeks prior to the infarction. These may be the new onset of either angina or fatigue. Obviously, fatigue is a nonspecific and common complaint. However, if the patient has had angina, the pattern may change: the episodes may become more frequent and be set off by less exertion. The pain of the classical infarction will then develop and persist, although it may wax and wane at first. The pain will be much more severe than the anginal pain and usually will have a substernal component. The patient will almost always sweat with it and often will be nauseated. Other associated symptoms may occur, including dyspnea and apprehension, but these are not necessary for the diagnosis. The pain may or may not radiate down the arms, into the shoulder or jaws. It is not related to breathing or to position and is usually not relieved by moving around, so that the patient tends to stay still. Typically, the patient has had pain for about 2 hours before deciding to seek medical aid.

While the history of chest pain is crucial for the diagnosis of acute myocardial infarction, only about one-half of the patients admitted to a coronary care unit with suspected myocardial infarction will actually have one demonstrated. Some will be found to have unstable angina with severe pain, only partially relieved by nitroglycerin, but EKG and cardiac injury enzymes will indicate no myocardial necrosis. Other diseases to be considered in the case of acute chest pain include acute pericarditis, aortic dissection, pulmonary embolus, and pneumothorax. Acute pericarditis can mimic an acute myocardial infarction with an abrupt onset of severe chest pain. The pain, however, is more positional, is relieved by sitting up and leaning forward, and is worse with respiration. It is important to remember that acute myocardial infarction can be complicated by pericarditis, but this does not usually occur until several days after the infarction. The pain of aortic dissection is classically extremely severe, going into the back and unrelenting. It generally occurs in patients who are hypertensive or who have Marfan's syndrome. The EKG usually will not show evidence of an acute infarction. The chest pain of pulmonary embolus is more often pleuritic, and associated with shortness of breath. Pneumothorax can also present with rather severe chest pain and is associated with shortness of breath. Pneumothorax usually appears after severe exertion and most often occurs in young people. Obviously, the physical examination and chest film are diagnostic for these conditions.

SHORTNESS OF BREATH

The second major symptom of heart disease is shortness of breath. This is clearly related to decreased lung compliance and is usually asssociated with an increase in airway resistance which increases the work of breathing. The left-ventricular end diastolic pressure and the left-atrial pressure both rise, or, as in mitral stenosis, the left-atrial pressure alone rises. This results in pulmonary vascular congestion and a fall in lung compliance, which produces dyspnea, or shortness of breath. (The term **dyspnea** is more precise for medical usage, but in talking with patients I prefer to call it "shortness of breath," because this is more easily understood.)

The sensation of dyspnea must be different from, and more unpleasant than, the shortness of breath experienced by normal people during exercise, where the shortness of breath is due to a metabolic change rather than a physical change. However, qualitative differences are difficult, if not impossible, to measure. It is therefore essential to quantitate the exertion necessary to cause shortness of breath, in order to separate the dyspnea of heart disease from normal shortness of breath. Normal subjects can walk on the level ground without trouble, keep up with others of their own age, climb a single flight of stairs without getting short of breath, and two flights without stopping. People with shortness of breath due to heart disease cannot do these things. The quantitative difference is the basis of the New York Heart Association's functional classification of patients according to the severity of their heart disease:

> **Class I.** Patients with cardiac disease, but without resulting limitation of physical activity. Ordinary physical activity does not cause undue fatigue, palpitation, dyspnea, or anginal pain.
>
> **Class II.** Patients with cardiac disease resulting in slight limitation of physical activity. They are comfortable at rest. Ordinary physical activity results in fatigue, palpitation, dyspnea, or anginal pain.
>
> **Class III.** Patients with cardiac disease resulting in marked limitation of physical activity. They are comfortable at rest. Less than ordinary physical activity causes fatigue, palpitation, dyspnea, or anginal pain.
>
> **Class IV.** Patients with cardiac disease resulting in inability to carry on any physical activity without discomfort. Symptoms of cardiac insufficiency or of the anginal syndrome may be present even at rest. If any physical activity is undertaken, discomfort is increased.

It is important to remember that patients with shortness of breath on exertion tend to limit their physical activity. If you ask a patient whether he gets short of breath, he may very well say no. Then you learn that he lives in a trailer with no stairs, and no longer is able to walk out and get the mail. It is true that he doesn't get short of breath—since he no longer exerts himself.

Another symptom due to pulmonary vascular engorgement is orthopnea, a condition in which the patient becomes short of breath with recumbency and uses more than one pillow to sleep. This is a difficult symptom to evaluate because sleeping habits are variable and many people normally sleep on two pillows. However, the new onset of orthopnea is a useful symptom of heart disease. Likewise, paroxysmal nocturnal dyspnea which awakens the patient from a sound sleep is an extremely useful symptom, especially of hypertensive and aortic valve disease. But, again, people may wake up from bad dreams with premature ventricular contractions and interpret this as dyspnea.

Patients with chronic lung disease also complain bitterly of shortness of breath. It may be difficult to separate heart disease from lung disease, and at times, of course, they may be combined. Shortness of breath caused by lung disease is usually seen in patients with a long history of smoking and chronic cough. The shortness of breath is of gradual onset, often becoming more severe than in patients with heart disease. Patients with lung disease are less likely to have orthopnea or paroxysmal nocturnal dyspnea, but many do. Probably the most useful feature identifying severe lung disease is the very gradual onset, after years of heavy smoking, and the eventual extreme dyspnea which is associated with it.

FATIGUE

Fatigue is the third cardinal symptom of heart disease and is a reflection of a decreased or limited cardiac output. Patients with heart disease will often complain bitterly of fatigue. Interestingly, many patients with significant heart disease, especially valvular disease, stop walking, not because of shortness of breath, but because of fatigue, especially in the legs. In patients with postmyocardial infarction, fatigue may be the major symptom. Obviously, however, fatigue can be due to many causes, including insomnia, depression, overwork, and disease other than heart disease.

SYNCOPE

The fourth major symptom of heart disease is syncope, or loss of consciousness. This may be caused either by abnormalities of the circulation or by abnormalities of neurophysiology. Abnormalities of the circulation include tachyarrhythmias, bradyarrhythmias, the common faint or vasodepressor syncope in which blood pools on the venous side, and intracardiac obstruction to flow with a fixed cardiac output, such as occurs in aortic stenosis. These are discussed further in Chapter 21. The neurological causes include seizure disorders caused by epilepsy or brain tumor and cerebrovascular occlusive disease, primarily vertebral and basilar artery disease. With the tachyarrhythmias and bradyarrhythmias the patient may faint with no premonitory symptoms. However, with fixed output in aortic stenosis the patients will often report a history of lightheadedness with exertion leading, with continued exertion, to loss of consciousness. The mechanism is: exertion causes peripheral vasodilatation in the skeletal muscles; then, because of the obstruction to flow across the aortic valve, cardiac output cannot be increased, blood pressure falls, and the patient either becomes lightheaded or actually faints.

DIZZINESS AND VERTIGO

True dizziness and vertigo (the sensation that the room is spinning around one) are almost never the result of cardiac disease. However, lightheadedness may be called "dizziness" by patients with either arrhythmias or aortic valve disease. The differential diagnosis for dizziness should include consideration of labryinthitis, cerebrovascular disease, and cervical arthritis. Very often the lightheadedness which accompanies cerebrovascular disease and cervical arthritis and labyrinthitis is related to turning the head.

Transient ischemic attacks and strokes due to cardiovascular disease usually do not present with syncope. In older patients without evidence of cerebrovascular disease, syncope should be evaluated by ambulatory EKG monitoring.

OTHER SYMPTOMS

Other, less definitive symptoms of heart disease include cough, hemoptysis, and recurrent respiratory infection, all related to pulmonary congestion. None of these symptoms is essential for the diagnosis of congestive heart failure. Cough may be the presenting symptom in elderly patients who have congestive failure. Hemoptysis can be caused by bronchitis, pulmonary embolus and infarction, or rupture of bronchial veins which drain into the left atrium. In severe mitral stenosis, hemoptysis may be a major symptom, but again, it is not necessary for the diagnosis of significant mitral stenosis.

Other useful symptoms include palpitations, edema, claudication, and cyanosis. Palpitations, the sensation of irregular heart beat, is often described as a fluttery feeling in the chest. Tachyarrhythmias or bradyarrhythmias may cause palpitations, but the commonest specific cause is premature ventricular contractions. In patients with rheumatic heart disease, this is an important symptom, since it is often associated with the development of atrial fibrillation, which represents a milestone in the course of the disease. Occasionally, however, patients will have atrial fibrillation and be unaware of it.

Edema is a late symptom of heart disease. This is usually dependent, developing in the feet and ankles after the patient has been upright for several hours. Typically, it disappears during sleep and recurs with dependency. Again, it should be emphasized that the edema occurs late in the course of heart disease, while shortness of breath occurs early, so that one should be able to make the diagnosis of significant heart disease long before the onset of edema. The differential diagnosis of edema should include consideration of venous disease of the lower extremities, hypoproteinemia, prolonged dependency of the legs, and renal and hepatic disease.

Cyanosis is not particularly common. It occurs in complicated congenital heart disease in infancy. New cyanosis in the adult is much more often acrocyanosis caused by reduced peripheral flow. Cyanosis is more commonly seen in severe lung disease. Certainly it is a manifestation of serious disease, but it is not a particularly useful diagnostic sign in the adult with heart disease.

Claudication is a valuable symptom of peripheral vascular disease, which is frequently associated with coronary artery disease. With claudication, the patient complains of burning or tightness in the leg, usually the calf muscles, occurring with exertion, increasing if the exertion continues, and promptly disappearing with rest.

HISTORY OF PAST ILLNESSES, FAMILY HISTORY, AND RISK FACTORS

In addition to the present illness, the history should include a careful history of past illnesses, a family history, and a consideration of significant risk factors for coronary artery disease. The history of past illnesses should include questions about general health in the past, particularly any previous history suggesting heart disease, such as a heart murmur or a history of rheumatic fever. Most patients with essential hypertension will have had labile blood pressure earlier. They may have had trouble with physical examinations in school, difficulty obtaining life insurance, or problems with military enlistment, and may be able to document prior episodes of elevated blood pressure. If the patient has essential hypertension, there should be not only his own history of labile blood pressure but also a positive family history. If neither of these are present, then one would certainly look for curable forms of hypertension, including renal artery stenosis.

The family history is extremely valuable in evaluating patients for possible heart disease. Both hypertension and diabetes mellitus (conditions often associated with heart disease) have a familial incidence. The history of a myocardial infarction or stroke in a parent before age 55 is indicative of accelerated vascular disease, which seems to be familial in many patients. Congenital heart disease and rheumatic heart disease may have a familial incidence. Other diseases which probably have familial incidence include the mitral-valve prolapse syndrome and idiopathic hypertrophic subaortic stenosis. Cardiomyopathy occasionally has a familial incidence, and Marfan's syndrome clearly does.

My colleagues and I have found the risk factors for coronary artery disease to be extremely important in evaluating a patient for the presence of heart disease. If the patient has atypical chest pain and is not affected by any of the risk factors, we would be much less likely to diagnose coronary artery disease. The risk factors include:

1. Age: coronary artery disease increases with age into the 50s.
2. Sex: coronary artery disease is more common in men than in women until age 55 to 60.
3. Hypertension and diabetes mellitus in either the patient or the family.
4. Smoking one package of cigarettes per day for 10 years—a major risk factor. We seldom see a patient under 45 with a myocardial infarction who has not smoked; if the patient stops smoking, he will still be at an increased risk for another 10 years.
5. Hyperlipidemia—either elevated cholesterol or triglyceride levels, or both—clearly represents an important risk factor.
6. A family history of cardiac disease.
7. Minor risk factors, including obesity, stressful occupation, and personality, none of which we feel are particularly important.

Gout, in our experience, has not been a risk factor.

PHYSICAL EXAMINATION

2

Robert H. Eich, Anis Obeid,
and Saktipada Mookherjee

Nowhere in medicine is the physical examination more exciting and challenging than in the field of cardiology. Students and house staff truly enjoy examining the cardiovascular system, and the most frequently asked questions directed at the cardiology section almost always involve arguments over heart murmurs or sounds. In teaching the physical examination, while lectures and demonstrations are helpful, they will not replace the student's actually examining the patient himself. While often only a single patient will be necessary to enable students to identify a mitral or aortic systolic murmur, on the other hand, the student may not be able to hear the murmur of mitral stenosis until his or her senior year in medical school.

This chapter is not intended as a comprehensive textbook on the physical examination, and students are referred to several books on the subject, including Tavel, *Clinical Phonocardiography and External Pulse Recording*, Fowler, *Cardiac Diagnosis and Treatment*, Constant, *Bedside Cardiology*, and a very excellent series of pamphlets by the American Heart Association which covers the history and physical examination of the heart.

The physical examination should follow a standard format, so that essential points are not omitted. Obviously, if the examiner forgets something or something is in doubt, he should go back and check it again. While we teach that the physical examination involves inspection, palpation, percussion, and auscultation, these steps need not be rigidly followed one after the other. We seldom use percussion, and inspection starts the minute the physician sees the patient. Before even taking the history, the examiner has already looked at the patient and drawn certain conclusions.

For the examination, the patient should be comfortable, in a warm, quiet

11

room. These conditions are not available to the student who has to examine a patient in a noisy hospital room, but usually one can at least briefly turn off the neighboring television set while listening to the heart. The patient will have had at least two other examiners, so one should be considerate. Sometimes one can break up the physical examination into two parts and let the patient rest in between. If the physician lets the patient know that he is interested and concerned, the patient usually is most cooperative. To examine the heart, the chest has to be uncovered, which may be embarrassing for some women, but by providing covering with a towel or the front of the pajamas one can help such patients to feel comfortable.

INSPECTION

Inspection initially helps the examiner to make major decisions about the patient's condition and the directions to take with the history. Does the patient appear to be acutely or chronically ill, is he short of breath, in pain, confused, or hostile? If the patient answers yes when asked if he has ankle edema, it is a good idea to check that at once and actually look at the ankles. Points such as this are simply matters of common sense and hardly require a detailed listing. The important point is for the examiner to look closely at the patient both when he first sees him and when taking the history.

Some specific points to be included in inspection are to check for the presence of skin abnormalities, cyanosis, skeletal abnormalities, and clubbing of the nail beds. Skin abnormalities include jaundice, pallor from anemia or peripheral vasoconstriction, and various rashes associated with drugs and disease. Usually the rashes are obvious, and the patient will complain of them. Some are less obvious, however; for example, petechiae associated with endocarditis may have to be carefully searched for. Cyanosis, although uncommon, is an important physical finding. Acrocyanosis, involving the fingertips, ear lobes, and occasionally the tip of the nose, is related to poor peripheral blood flow and is associated with a normal arterial oxygen saturation. This is the type of acrocyanosis which everyone has seen in children whose fingernails turn blue after they have stayed in swimming in cold water for too long. Central cyanosis (a far more serious sign) is recognized in the mucous membrane and is associated with an arterial saturation under 80%. It occurs with lung disease, congenital heart disease, and certain hemoglobinopathies. Only mucous membrane cyanosis accurately reflects arterial oxygen saturation.

Skeletal abnormalities are useful findings and may suggest certain types of heart disease. Severe kyphoscoliosis may be associated with cor pulmonale. Rheumatoid arthritis and ankylosing spondylitis may be associated with aortic valve disease and myocardial conduction defects. Marfan's syndrome, characterized by tall, lanky extremities, high arched palate, lenticular abnormalities, and pectus excavatum, is associated with a significant incidence of aortic dissection. One of the most common cardiac abnormalities, the mitral-valve prolapse syndrome, which may occur in up to 6% of the population, has a very high incidence of associated skeletal abnormalities, including pectus excavatum, straight back with loss of the normal anterior and posterior curves of the spine, and scoliosis of the spine.

Clubbing of the fingers and toes may occur in a number of clinical conditions, including cardiovascular disease. New clubbing is most often associated with cancer of the lung, but clubbing occurs in congenital heart disease and endocarditis as well.

PERIPHERAL EXAMINATION

The physical examination itself begins with the determination of blood pressure, pulse, respiration, and temperature. The examiner should be sure that the patient's temperature has been taken and recorded. Many patients will have a slight elevation of temperature caused by the anxiety of coming into the hospital and consequent vasoconstriction, but any elevation should be carefully noted. The respiratory rate is counted and the pattern of respiration observed. Respiration may be labored in patients with congestive failure. Dyspnea in congestive failure is usually inspiratory in contrast to dyspnea caused by chronic obstructive pulmonary disease, which, at least in the early stages, is more often expiratory. In congestive failure with a low cardiac output, especially in elderly patients, periodic breathing with Cheyne-Stokes respiration may be observed. The patient may be somnolent during the apneic phase and agitated during the phase of hyperpnea.

Patients usually are apprehensive about being examined, so that starting with the routine, familiar taking of blood pressure and pulse is reassuring. The blood pressure should be taken first in both arms, with the patient either sitting or lying. The record should show whether the blood pressure was taken in the right arm or the left, and whether the patient was supine or sitting. When the patient is in a sitting position, the arms should be on a table at heart level.

Hospital blood-pressure cuffs are usually the aneroid type, which can vary widely in their accuracy. If possible, the examiner should use his own cuff, or, if he is using the hospital cuff and the blood pressure measured seems out of line, he should check the cuff on himself or try another one. The cuff should fit well and be 20% wider than the limb diameter. A big arm combined with a small cuff can falsely elevate the blood pressure to a significant degree. The 12 to 14 cm width of the usual cuff is satisfactory for only the "standard" arm, and many patients don't fit this standard.

A deflated cuff should be applied with the lower margin 2 ½ cm above the antecubital fossa. The arrow on the cuff should be placed over the brachial artery. Blood pressure is first taken by palpation, inflating the cuff until the radial pulse disappears and then slowly releasing the cuff, the pressure being recorded when the pulse is first felt. This will give at least a general range for the systolic blood pressure. The cuff is then deflated completely and a stethoscope applied to the antecubital fossa over the previously palpated brachial artery. The stethoscope head should be applied firmly, but not with heavy pressure. With the stethoscope in place, the pressure is raised by inflating the cuff to 20 to 30 torr above the point at which the radial pulse disappeared and then released at a rate of 2 to 3 torr per second. It is well for the student to practice this on himself. Two to three torr per sec is much slower than one may think, and if one releases the cuff faster or slower, there will be errors.

As the pressure falls, the Korotkoff sounds become audible over the artery below the cuff and pass through four phases: phase 1, the period in which the sounds first appear; phase 2, the period in which there is a swishing quality; phase 3, when the sounds are crisp; phase 4, there is an abrupt, distinct muffling of the sound; and, phase 5, the point at which the sounds disappear. Determining the systolic pressure is easy; there is general agreement that it is measured at the point at which the initial tapping is first heard. When to measure the diastolic pressure remains somewhat controversial. Some people recommend phase 4, some phase 5. In my experience, phase 5 is better. If there is a large discrepancy between the readings taken in these two phases, then both should be recorded as 140/80/70, meaning that the fourth phase was 80 and the fifth phase was 70.

If the blood pressure is elevated in both arms, then it certainly should be checked in the legs. For this, a larger cuff, 18 to 20 cm wide, is used. The cuff is placed around the thigh, the stethoscope is placed in the popliteal space, and the same general technique is used to determine the pressure.

When the examiner has determined the blood pressure in both of the arms and, if necessary, in the legs, he will take the pulse, noting the rate and regularity. If irregular, it is very useful to record the rate of the pulse and compare that to the apical rate obtained with the stethoscope. In atrial fibrillation, the pulse will be considerably less in the peripheral pulse than in the apex. This is because the rapid beats fail to open the aortic valve and thus produce no pulse, although they will produce heart sound. A difference between the peripheral and apical pulse is known as a **pulse deficit.**

The pulse has been examined since antiquity, and considerable information about the cardiovascular system can be obtained from it. The pulse should be examined for amplitude or volume, tension, and condition of the arterial wall. The quality may be strong or bounding; weak; collapsing (as in aortic insufficiency); slowly rising (as in aortic stenosis); bisferiens or biphasic (as in idiopathic hypertropic subaortic stenosis); alternating in strength, or **alternans** (as seen in severe heart disease); or finally, paradoxical (as seen in cardiac tamponade). While not quantifiable, a bounding pulse indicates a large stroke volume or an inelastic vessel. A thready pulse implies a low stroke volume and intense vasoconstriction. The collapsing, or Corrigan's, pulse is seen in aortic insufficiency, with a rapid fall in diastolic pressure. Slowly rising pulse is seen in aortic-valvular stenosis, and the rate of rise is inversely related to the severity of the stenosis. A slower rise implies more severe stenosis. The bisferiens pulse is characterized by two waves, an initial soft wave, called a **percussion wave**, and a subsequent **tidal wave**, which give the bisferiens quality. This is seen in idiopathic hypertropic subaortic stenosis, in which the obstruction occurs later in systole, so that the first part of the pulse is rapid; then the pulse falls, and rises again slowly for the second part. Bisferiens pulse is also seen in pure aortic insufficiency, or in aortic stenosis and insufficiency combined. Pulsus alternans, in which a strong beat is followed by a weaker one, is a valuable sign of severe left-ventricular failure. Finally, paradoxical pulse is an invaluable sign of cardiac tamponade with resultant restriction to cardiac filling. While the name is a misnomer, since blood pressure normally falls slightly with respiration, if the systolic blood pressure falls more than 10 torr during inspiration, the paradoxical pulse is abnormal and is evidence of either tamponade, severe congestive failure, or chronic obstructive pulmonary disease with severe dyspnea.

All the peripheral pulses should be checked—the radial, brachial, and femoral pulses, and the two pulses in the feet, the dorsalis pedis and the posterior tibial. The popliteal pulse is extremely difficult to feel, and, in general, we do not examine it routinely. One would examine it, however, if there were no dorsalis pedis or posterior tibial pulse. The posterior tibial pulse is felt just below the medial malleolus of the ankle and the dorsalis pedis pulse is felt on top of the foot in the medial area. The student should practice taking these two pulses on himself. Femoral pulses are very easy to feel, just below the inguinal ligament in the femoral triangle. In addition, one should listen for a bruit over the femoral artery. This is done with a stethoscope; the bruit will sound like a murmur. Similarly, in patients who are hypertensive, auscultation should be carried out over the abdomen to detect a possible bruit over a stenotic renal artery. The examiner will already have noted the blood pressure in both arms, so that he has information about the brachial and radial arteries.

Examination of the carotid artery is much more difficult. It is extremely important to become proficient in examining this pulse, since from it one might be able to detect arteriosclerosis in the carotid artery, which can be a prelude to a major stroke but is preventable if detected and treated early. In addition, we use the carotid artery to obtain information about the aortic valve.

The common carotid artery can be felt up to its bifurcation. This is best felt at the level of the thyroid cartilage with the patient's head elevated a little and turned just slightly away from the examiner. If carotid disease is suspected, it is wise to check the carotids for a bruit before pressing. The presence of a bruit in a carotid artery is extremely significant and suggests vascular disease. One should also be careful to press gently, on one side only, and for no more than 10 to 20 sec. One should never press both carotids at once.

As was said, the carotid can provide useful information about the character of the pulse, especially the slow upslope characteristic of aortic stenosis. Feeling this requires a good deal of practice, but it is a useful skill, and the student should develop it by feeling and evaluating the carotid in all of his patients.

Next, one will probably examine the neck for neck-vein pulsations and distension. The neck veins are enormously useful indicators, since they can function almost like a manometer to give a fairly accurate measurement of the right atrial pressure. If there is no tricuspid-valve disease, then the neck veins reflect not only right-atrial pressure but right-ventricular diastolic pressure as well. Thus we have bedside evidence of the competency of the right ventricle. In addition, the appearance of the neck veins provides important information about the pulmonary artery pressure and, indirectly, left-sided pressures.

For the examination of the neck veins, determination of the height of the right-atrial pressure, and inspection for pulsations the patient must be properly positioned. Usually the right-sided neck veins are examined; they should be well lit, using tangential light, if possible, in order to make the pulse stand out in relief. The patient should be relaxed, the head of the bed gradually elevated 30 to 45°, keeping the patient's neck and trunk straight until the uppermost level of venous pulsation can be seen. The elevation required may vary from 10 to 90°, but normally venous pulsations should disappear when the bed is elevated above 30°.

The veins in the neck are the internal and external jugular. The external jugular vein is usually easier to see, but it may be thrombosed, it has valves, and it is less reliable. One should not say that there is no neck vein distension just because he doesn't see the external jugular vein, since it may be thrombosed. The internal jugular vein, while more reliable, lies deep to the sternocleidomastoid muscle and the pulse in it may be difficult to identify and separate from the carotid pulse. However, some points of distinction are that the venous pulse is wavy rather than jerky and the pulsations are exaggerated during inspiration, while at the same time the level of the pulsation actually falls with inspiration. The pulsation can be easily obliterated by compression of the vein just above the clavicle, while obviously the pulsation in the carotid artery cannot. Finally, the neck veins have a hepatojugular reflux. If one compresses the abdomen in the right upper quadrant, the neck veins often will increase in distension.

Once the internal jugular vein is identified, the upper level of pulsation is measured as the distance from the meniscus of the venous pulse to the sternal angle, and by adding 5 to 6 cm to this distance, the right-atrial pressure can be estimated in centimeters of water. Right-atrial pressure is elevated in congestive failure, hypervolemia, constrictive pericarditis, and tricuspid-valve disease.

Next, somewhat more difficult but part of the fun of the physical examination, is to identify the waves in the neck veins. Practically, we see two crests and two troughs in the neck veins. The a-wave precedes the carotid pulse and the v-wave follows it. With the thrust of the carotid pulse, the x-descent occurs, and following the second crest of the v-wave there is a second trough, the y-descent. A c-wave may be seen at times on the downward descent of the x-trough. The a-wave corresponds to atrial systole, the c-wave is probably caused by the closure of the tricuspid valve and its bulging into the right atrium, and the v-wave is the result of atrial filling. The x-descent occurs when the base of the ventricle is drawn down with ventricular systole, and the y-descent follows the opening of the tricuspid valve.

With experience, several important abnormalities can be determined in the jugular venous pulse. In atrial fibrillation, there is a loss of atrial contraction, and the a-wave is absent. An increase in the a-wave (giant a-wave) occurs with pulmonary hypertension. This could be acute, as in a large pulmonary embolus, or chronic, as in rheumatic heart disease or congenital heart disease with pulmonary hypertension. Prominent a-waves, called cannon waves, occur in complete heart block or junctional rhythm, where the atrial and ventricular contractions are no longer sequential. The cannon wave is produced when the atrium contracts against a closed tricuspid valve.

The v-wave is actually a combination of the c and the v waves with the loss of the x-descent. An increase in the v-wave occurs with tricuspid insufficiency, which, again, may be acute or chronic. If the tricuspid regurgitation is severe enough, systolic hepatic pulsation may be seen or felt, and even the hand and arm veins will pulsate. Finally, following the v-wave there is a rapid fall in pressure caused by the opening of the tricuspid valve, which provides the y-descent. This will be exaggerated in tricuspid insufficiency, and in chronic constrictive pericarditis there is a sharp y-descent followed by an almost equally abrupt rise in diastolic pressure, producing the so-called square-root sign in the ventricular pressure. Normally the neck veins decrease with inspiration (inspiratory collapse), and there are various signs used for changes in the neck vein with respiration which we have not found particularly useful.

EXAMINATION OF THE HEART

INSPECTION

When the peripheral examination is over, we turn to examination of the heart, using inspection, palpation, and auscultation. Although certain physical findings can be emphasized by changes in position, we prefer to start the examination with the patient lying flat. Patients with significant orthopnea will have to have one or two pillows under their heads, or the head of the bed may be raised. In any case, the patient should be made as comfortable as possible before the examination is started. As mentioned before, with women it may be helpful to develop some technique to preserve the patient's modesty.

The areas to be inspected and palpated include the left precordium, left parasternal area, supraclavicular fossae, and epigastric and right upper quadrant of the abdomen. The left precordium is inspected first, and the most important thing to look for is the point of maximum impulse (the apical impulse, or **PMI**). This is delineated with the onset of ventricular systole, when the cardiac apex moves anteriorly. This anterior impulse is not normally well seen, unless the patient is thin. If seen at all, it will be inside the midclavicular line in the fifth interspace. It should not exceed an area of 2 cm in diameter, and it should not be visible for more than 80 msec. Although it is useful to measure the PMI from the midsternal line, because of differences in chest size most of us use the midclavicular and nipple line as estimations for the limits of the PMI. In men, the nipple line is obviously a more useful landmark than in women. If the PMI is lower down or is outside the left midclavicular line, this is impressive evidence of chamber enlargement, usually left-ventricular enlargement, although right-ventricular enlargement can push the left ventricle out.

In addition to inspection for the PMI, one should look for any kind of abnormal pulsations over the entire precordium. In aneurysms of the left ventricle, a diffuse heave will often be seen over much of the anterior wall of the left ventricle. The PMI may be seen outside the midclavicular line, with a separate precordial bulge inside the midclavicular line. One should look for evidence of a right-ventricular lift along the left sternal border in the third and fourth interspace, just to the left of the sternum. In some patients pulsation of the pulmonary outflow tract can be seen in the second left interspace.

PALPATION

Palpation is an invaluable tool. It is easily learned, dependable, and does not require a quiet room. In the usual noisy hospital room, the grade-I aortic insufficiency murmur may be heard only by the professor and chief of cardiology, but the presence of a heaving PMI can be demonstrated to even the crustiest senior physician with great certainty. Palpation is usually best carried out with the palm of the hand, but one uses both the palm and the fingertips. Also, it is important here to examine the patient in different positions, especially in the left-lateral position, which will bring the PMI out towards the chest wall. Palpation is carried out in both systole and diastole.

Besides being displaced, the cardiac impulse can be abnormal in other ways. The apical impulse may be felt over a wider area, or be more sustained than normal. This can occur in cases of ventricular hypertrophy and enlargement, as in hypertension, aortic stenosis, or diffuse myocardial disease. More than one impulse may be felt at the apex. In conditions in which left-ventricular compliance is abnormally reduced, a presystolic component (S_4) may be felt. At times this can be felt better than heard. It is an important sign of left-ventricular abnormality. Likewise, an abnormal impulse in early diastole (S_3) may be felt.

In feeling for both of these, it is often necessary to turn the patient with the left side down. The rest of the precordium should be palpated for ectopic areas of bulging, which occur with ventricular aneurysm. One should feel for the right-ventricular lift along the left sternal border and then for any abnormal pulsations in the aortic, pulmonic, and supraclavicular areas. Next one should feel in all of the areas of the heart, for a thrill. The four areas include the apex, which is at the point of maximal impulse (usually in the fifth interspace); the base, which includes the second left interspace, the pulmonic area to the left of the sternum, and the second right interspace; the aortic area, to the right of the sternum; and finally the tricuspid area, which is in the fourth interspace just to the left of the sternum. A thrill is the palpation equivalent of a loud murmur. Aortic stenosis will produce a thrill in the second left or right interspace or in the suprasternal notch. Pulmonic stenosis may produce a thrill in the second left interspace. Mitral insufficiency may produce a thrill at the apex, and at times a diastolic thrill can be felt at the apex in patients with mitral stenosis. To determine whether or not the patient has an aortic thrill, the examiner should have him sit up, lean forward, and expire; this provides optimum conditions for feeling a thrill, getting the aortic area as close as possible to the chest.

As already mentioned, my colleagues and I very seldom use percussion. Fundamentally, we get more valuable information about cardiac borders by inspection and palpation. However, the presence of a pericardial effusion can be suspected if the point of maximal impulse is felt inside the left border of cardiac dullness as determined by percussion.

AUSCULTATION

Auscultation is the part of the cardiovascular examination that probably leads to the most argument. One reason for these arguments is the fact that patients don't always sound the same. Physical signs elicted in the office may be different from those found when the patient is seen in the hospital. For example, in the office, murmurs are often accentuated, because the patients are more anxious when first seen. Because of this variability in the signs, if a student is convinced that he hears something but the resident does not, it is certainly worthwhile for the student to stick to his point and get everyone to listen again.

The stethoscope currently functions more or less as a status symbol, carried by all medical personnel, but seldom used. However, when properly used for auscultation of the heart it is a powerful tool. There are excellent discussions of the type of stethoscope that is best in the textbooks referred to previously, and clearly some are better than others. The Leatham, Sprague Rappaport, Harvey, and Hewlett-Packard are all good stethoscopes. Basically, the stethoscope should have a bell and a diaphragm. Two different diaphragms are useful; the stiffer diaphragm will help one to hear the very high-pitched sounds. The bell should have as large a diameter as possible, since if applied lightly to the skin, a large bell provides the least damping of the low-frequency sounds, especially the murmur of mitral stenosis and the S_3. The tubing should be rubber, and as short as possible (25–35 cm is generally ideal but may not be practical, depending on the physician's height and the height of the patient beds in the hospital). The inside diameter should be 0.32 cm. The ear pieces must be comfortable, and finding some that are will take considerable trial and error. All of us have finally discovered some stethoscope with comfortable ear pieces, and we clutch these forever.

For auscultation one follows the same rules as in giving the rest of the physical examination, striving to have: (*1*) a comfortable patient, (*2*) a quiet room, and (*3*) some kind of system, so that nothing is overlooked. The examiner listens systematically in all four areas of the heart, listening to each sound in both systole and diastole. He also listens over precordial bulges and abnormal areas. I personally have found it useful to listen with my eyes closed, since I think one can concentrate on the sound better.

Because timing is all-important, one may choose to listen first in the pulmonic area, because here the second sound is always the loudest; this loud sound is followed by diastole. Often, if the rate is slow, one can separate systole and diastole, because diastole lasts longer. However, with faster rates, one has to use the second sound for timing.

In listening to the heart, one should first establish the rate and rhythm. The examiner compares the counted heart rate at the apex with the radial-pulse heart rate and establishes whether the rhythm is regular or irregular. Most examiners then concentrate on the sounds, starting usually with the second sound.

Heart Sounds

In listening for sounds, the examiner tries to identify their timing, intensity, and variability, and to note any reduplication or splitting. Sounds are generally examined best with the patient supine. Either the bell or diaphragm can be used, although the sounds are heard somewhat better with the diaphragm.

The second sound in the pulmonic area has two distinct components—aortic and pulmonic—caused by closures of these semilunar valves. The aortic component is the first of the two components. Students must memorize this (a memory device—"A before P in the alphabet." "arterial pressure is higher so A closes sooner"—may be helpful). The aortic component of the second sound, referred to as A_2, is normally louder.

The second sound splits into its two components normally with inspiration. As the subject inspires, venous return increases, which prolongs right-ventricular systole and moves the pulmonic second sound out. The aortic second sound may stay the same or move slightly inward, due to pooling of blood in the pulmonary veins and decrease in left-ventricular output. Also, because of increased compliance of the pulmonary vasculature, there is a delay or "hangout" in closing the pulmonic valve, which plays a role in widening the split. Splitting in normal subjects with normal respiration is about 25 to 35 msec at the end of inspiration. This is about the closest split that the ear can distinguish. One will be able to hear this split in many normal subjects.

Wide splits are usually above 35 msec. The split can be prolonged in right bundle-branch block, left-ventricular pacing, left-ventricular pre-excitation, pulmonic stenosis, or an atrial septal defect where right-ventricular systole is prolonged. Likewise, the split may be wide if left-ventricular systole is shortened, as in mitral insufficiency and a ventricular septal defect. The split may be paradoxical—that is, decreasing with inspiration—in left-bundle-branch block, right-ventricular pacing, or severe left-ventricular dysfunction. In this case, the aortic component has become the second of the two components, because of the delay in emptying of the left ventricle. With inspiration, the pulmonic component moves out normally, which then brings it to the delayed aortic second sound, and the split seems to come together, on inspiration, and thus is paradoxical.

Splitting of the second sound—normal, wide, fixed, or paradoxical—is relatively easy to hear and an extremely valuable finding. If possible, splitting should also be evaluated with the patient sitting up. If one hears a fixed split which doesn't vary with respiration and is wide, then a left-to-right shunt at the atrial level is almost certainly a possibility. Thus one can diagnose, or at least suspect, an atrial septal defect on the basis of physical examination.

We also listen to the second sounds in the aortic area, but there the splits are less well heard. Older teaching held that the aortic sound was heard in the aortic area and the pulmonic sound in the pulmonic area, but that is not correct; both are heard well in the pulmonic area. At the apex, under normal conditions, only one component of the second sound, the aortic, is heard.

The first sound is complex, with probably four different componenets, two of which are closure of the mitral and tricuspid valves. Normally, the mitral closure slightly precedes the tricuspid, but this is variable, and the mitral sound is usually so much louder that it drowns out the tricuspid sound. Splitting of the first heart sound is best heard in the tricuspid area. Generally we don't pay attention to splitting of the first sound, although in some conditions, such as right-bundle-branch block, in which the tricuspid closure is very late, this split is easy to recognize.

The quality of the first heart sound, however, is valuable, and we listen for it at the apex. A loud first heart sound is suggestive of a high cardiac output, a thickened mitral valve with mitral stenosis, or a short P-R interval. Likewise, a decrease in the intensity of the first heart sound is heard in poor left-ventricular function from congestive failure or a myocardial infarction, or in conditions where the valves tend to float shut before systole, such as a long P-R interval or loss of the atrial contribution due to atrial fibrillation. However, many things besides cardiac output affect loudness of the first heart sound, especially the thickness of the chest wall. Variability in the sound is also useful in evaluating the first heart sound. This is seen with tachycardias and arrhythmias and with complete heart block, in which case the variability is related to the sequence of activation of the atrium and ventricle.

In addition to the first and second sounds, extra sounds, called **clicks**, occur in systole. They are relatively sharp and high-pitched, and are heard best with the diaphragm. If the click occurs early, with the onset of systole, it is called an **ejection click**, while the middle-to-late systolic clicks are called **systolic clicks.** Ejection clicks occur with pulmonary or systemic hypertension, which alters the distensibility of the vessels, so that the click is produced with the phase of the rapid rise in pressure. Ejection clicks can also occur when the aortic or pulmonic valve is thickened. Aortic ejection clicks are well heard over the entire heart, usually both at the apex and at the base, while pulmonic clicks are usually heard only over the pulmonic area, and vary in intensity, decreasing with inspiration.

The systolic clicks, mid-to-late systole, occur with the syndrome of mitral- or tricuspid-valve prolapse. They are often followed by a systolic murmur. The mitral-valve-prolapse syndrome is the result of a defect in the mitral-valve apparatus. The click is probably produced by the redundant cordi snapping tight; this is followed by mitral regurgitation and a systolic murmur. Systolic clicks are almost always heard at the apex. Maneuvers such as sitting in the upright posture, which tend to decrease heart size, will move the click toward the first sound and often increase the duration and intensity of the murmur.

Diastolic sounds are more difficult to hear and require considerably more practice. There are three diastolic sounds: the mitral or tricuspid opening snap, the S_3, and the S_4. The opening snap actually is a diastolic click and results when the mitral valve has been thickened by rheumatic heart disease. This is a fairly loud sound occurring after the second sound and is associated with a mitral-valve opening. It occurs 40 to 120 msec after the A_2. It is heard with the diaphragm or bell between the apex and the left sternal border. It is possible to confuse an opening snap with the S_2. However, careful examination will reveal three sounds in inspiration at the pulmonic area. The time between the A_2 and the opening snap (A_2-OS interval) interval is related to left-atrial pressure: the higher the pressure, the shorter the A_2-OS interval; this can be used for a rough estimation of the severity of mitral stenosis.

The other two diastolic sounds, S_3 and S_4, are filling sounds. These are very important physical findings. In young people an S_3 can be normal, but in older patients the presence of an S_3 is diagnostic of severe left-ventricular dysfunction. Initially these sounds were called **gallops**, and the S_3 was called a **ventricular gallop**. However, we much prefer the term S_3. The S_3 occurs with the rapid filling phase of diastole; it is a reflection of decreased compliance and is presumably related to sudden tensing of some component of the left ventricle. The S_3 is heard only with the bell, and is heard best with the patient lying on his left side. At times it can really be felt better than it can be heard. Right-sided S_3 sounds occur, and are heard, along the left sternal border in the third and fourth interspace, increasing with inspiration.

The S_4, or **atrial gallop**, is heard after atrial systole, before the first sound. The S_4 may represent a decreased ventricular compliance, but it is not diagnostic of congestive failure, and it can be heard in normal subjects with an elevated cardiac output. An S_4 is distinctly abnormal in younger people, but in the elderly its clinical significance decreases. Again, the S_4 is best heard with the bell at the apex. In the normal heart, a split first sound can easily be mistaken for an S_4; if the patient is young and generally healthy, one can assume that the sound is a split. The split first sound is heard with the diaphragm, while the S_4 is best heard with the bell and can be attenuated by pressure with the bell.

Extra cardiac sounds are most commonly heard with pericarditis. Pericardial friction rubs are easily observed now in most teaching hospitals because of the large number of patients who have undergone cardiopulmonary surgery or who have chronic renal disease. The pericardial rub has both a systolic and diastolic component and is characteristically high-pitched and scratchy, with a close-to-the-ear quality. A pericardial knock or an early diastolic filling sound is often indicative of constrictive pericarditis.

Murmurs

Finally, after listening in all of the cardiac areas for sounds, the examiner repeats the procedure, listening for murmurs. The exact mechanism of murmur production remains somewhat controversial. For years, murmurs were ascribed to turbulence, but more likely the vortex shedding theory of Aeolian tones is a better explanation. Murmurs may occur with high flow through normal or abnormal valves, forward flow through a constrictive or irregular valve or into a dilated vessel or chamber, or with backward or regurgitant flow through an incompetent valve, septal defect, or patent ductus arteriosus. Frequently a combination of these factors is operative.

Murmurs are classified by timing (systolic, diastolic, or continuous). Attention should also be paid to their pitch, intensity, location, and radiation. Timing, however, is the most crucial matter, and the area in which students are apt to make the greatest number of mistakes. It is important to time using the pulmonic second sound in the pulmonic area. Diastole follows this second sound. If the murmur is apical, one starts in the pulmonic area, identifies the second sound, and then inches down along the chest to the apex, continuing to follow the second sound until one reaches the apex and times the apical murmur.

Pitch is important and good cardiologists pay attention to it, but identifying variations in pitch requires considerable experience. Regurgitant murmurs are high-pitched, stenotic murmurs medium-pitched. The aortic-insufficiency diastolic murmur is high-pitched, and the mitral-stenosis murmur is low-pitched, with a rumbling quality. When auscultation is taught to students, pitch is described in many different ways. The various pitches of murmurs are best learned through experience, and each physician must develop his own concept of pitch, using the known pitch of the mitral-insufficiency and aortic-stenosis murmur.

Grading by intensity is not difficult, and students generally have no trouble grading loudness. Intensity is a useful indication, since it is known that most significant systolic murmurs are grade III in the system for classifying murmurs developed by Levine. Systolic murmurs are graded from I through VI. A grade I murmur is audible only after the listener has spent time listening. A grade II systolic murmur is the faintest murmur which is audible immediately upon placing the stethoscope on the chest. A grade V murmur is a loud murmur which cannot be heard with the stethoscope removed from the chest, but can be heard with the stethoscope just touching the chest. A grade VI murmur is audible with the stethoscope actually off the chest. Grade III and IV murmurs are intermediate.

Diastolic murmurs are not graded, as they are almost never loud. If they are, there is usually some unusual condition.

Radiation of murmurs is related to both loudness and anatomy. The aortic-ejection murmur classically radiates to the neck and carotid artery, while the mitral-regurgitation murmur classically goes to the axillae. However, in some cases, the mitral-regurgitation murmur may radiate towards the aortic area, and occasionally the aortic-stenosis murmur may be very well transmitted to the apex, unfortunately changing pitch as it goes, making it much harder to tell from the mitral-regurgitation murmur.

Systolic murmurs were classified by Leatham as either ejection or regurgitant murmurs, and while there are exceptions, the classification is useful. Systolic ejection murmurs are caused by a forward flow across the aortic or pulmonic valve or ventricular outflow tract. Many of these murmurs are not necessarily the result of an abnormal valve but can also occur with a normal valve and high flow or a normal valve and normal flow into a dilated aorta or pulmonary artery. An older person with a dilated aorta will have an aortic ejection murmur. The ejection murmur starts after the first heart sound with the opening of the aortic and pulmonic valve, and it stops before the second sound. The murmur of aortic-valve stenosis is best heard in the second right and left interspaces; medium-pitched, and quite loud, it is transmitted into the carotid artery. The murmur is somewhat diamond-shaped, increasing or louder in mid-systole and while it stops before the aortic second sound, if it goes through the pulmonic component (the aortic being delayed), it may be mistaken for a regurgitant murmur. A late-peaking murmur tends to be associated with more severe stenosis, while shorter murmurs are associated with a milder form of stenosis. As stated, the murmur of aortic stenosis may be transmitted to the apex, becoming higher pitched and at times being difficult or impossible to distinguish from the murmur of mitral insufficiency. The most useful sign distinguishing the two is that when a change in cycle length occurs as with premature ventricular contraction or a long cycle in atrial fibrillation, with aortic stenosis the beat following the pause will be more forceful, and the murmur will get louder, while the murmur of mitral insufficiency will not be affected.

The pulmonic-stenosis murmur is also an ejection murmur, best heard in the second left interspace. Again, it may go through the aortic component of the second sound, making it seemingly a regurgitant murmur.

Regurgitant systolic murmurs are classified by Leatham as pansystolic or holosystolic; they start with the first sound and end with the second. However, the murmur of mitral-valve prolapse or of a papillary-muscle dysfunction starts in the middle of systole and is still the result of regurgitation. The murmur of mitral insufficiency is high-pitched, heard well with the diaphragm and bell, and transmitted usually to the apex, although it may go to the base and be heard best at the apex. The murmur of tricuspid insufficiency is a regurgitant murmur best heard along the left sternal border in the fourth interspace. Classically, this murmur increases with inspiration—a valuable finding, although it may be absent in the presence of severe right-ventricular failure.

There are two significant diastolic murmurs: the murmur of mitral- or tricuspid-stenosis and the murmur of aortic or pulmonic insufficiency. The mitral-stenosis murmur is probably the most difficult murmur to hear. This is low-pitched, rumbling, heard at the apex, and heard only with the bell. It can be brought out by having the patient exercise a bit and then turn on his left side. It starts after the opening snap, if one is present, and will have a presystolic accentuation due to atrial contraction if the patient is in sinus rhythm, or occasionally this accentuation can be heard even with the patient in atrial fibrillation. My teachers told me that the murmur was almost *felt* in the ear rather than heard, which sounds strange, but is true. It is a very difficult murmur to appreciate. Usually the loud S_1 on the opening snap will alert one to the possibility of mitral stenosis. The murmur of tricuspid stenosis is again a very difficult murmur to identify, heard along the left sternal border in the fourth interspace, and much more high-pitched than the mitral-stenosis murmur. It may resemble the murmur of aortic insufficiency.

The murmur of aortic insufficiency would be suspected from a wide pulse pressure and a low diastolic pressure taken with the cuff. However, minimal aortic insufficiency would not affect the blood pressure. Again, it is a difficult murmur to hear—high-pitched, heard with the diaphragm, and beginning after the second sound. The patient should sit up, expire, hold his breath in expiration, and lean forward. This will get the aortic area as close to the examiner as possible. If there are two degrees of stiffness in the diaphragm, one should use the stiffest. This murmur is never loud, or, if it is, some unusual condition must be present. My colleagues and I have had countless patients in whom no one could detect a murmur, but who at catheterization were shown to have some aortic insufficiency.

The murmur of pulmonic insufficiency is similar and is heard in the pulmonic second left interspace. This murmur will often follow a loud P_2. Separating aortic insufficiency from pulmonic insufficiency is difficult and may require cardiac catheterization.

Aortic insufficiency from rheumatic heart disease is always heard best to the left of the sternum, beneath the pulmonic area. As a rule, if one hears the aortic-insufficiency murmur in the aortic area, there is something unusual about it, suggesting luetic aortic insufficiency, a prolapsing semi-lunar cusp, or some other condition.

The only other diastolic murmur of great importance is the so-called machinery murmur, heard with a patent ductus arteriosus. This is a continuous murmur heard with the bell in the pulmonic area, a little further away from the sternum than the ordinary pulmonic second sound. It is not quite a continuous murmur: often there will be a faint pause in it before the start of systole. The important feature is that this murmur continues through the second sound into diastole.

The major problem in cardiology in the auscultation of the heart is the functional murmur. A high percentage of children have murmurs, especially when they have a fever or are excited. If one were to listen very carefully, in a sound-proof room, one would probably find murmurs in 70% of healthy children. These are at times difficult to evaluate. The first major rule is that any diastolic murmur is significant, so that diastolic murmurs should be treated with great respect. There is a diastolic murmur called the Carey Coombs murmur which is caused by very high flow across the normal mitral valve in children with fevers; obviously, if one hears that murmur, one would certainly want to wait and see what it sounded like when the patient was afebrile. The major problem in deciding which murmurs are significant is with systolic murmurs. My experience has been in general that the so-called functional murmurs are less loud, more vaiable from time to time and even from moment to moment, tend to be in the first half of systole, and tend to disappear as the child grows up. The so-called Still's murmur will tend to disappear in the late teens or early 20s. There is a useful adage which says that a good cardiologist should be a little bit deaf, meaning that he won't hear these faint murmurs, and therefore won't concern either himself or the patient about them. The physician may take his time, of course, to be sure; if in doubt, it is better not to call the murmur significant, and to listen again in 6 months. One should remember that patients may become very frightened by discussion about murmurs, so that it is wise to play down discussion of such a finding in front of the patient.

Obviously, other parts of the physical examination are important supplements to the cardiac examination. Percussion and auscultation of the lungs for a pleural effusion or inspiratory rales will help in the diagnosis of congestive failure. Findings of peripheral or presacral dependent edema are important in the same diagnosis. Hepatomegaly is seen in right-sided congestive failure and splenomegaly is valuable in diagnosing endocarditis.

We have now discussed the salient points of the physical examination. It should be emphasized again that the student can learn best by doing, by listening to and examining patients with known lesions and known disease, so that he can develop his own knowledge of what aortic stenosis, aortic insufficiency, mitral stenosis, and mitral insufficiency sound like. One should also remember that physical findings tend to change. If the examiner has been careful and has found an S_3 that is not there when somebody else listens, that does not mean that the first examiner was wrong; it may just mean that the sound is gone. The student should stick to his original conclusion, but also bear in mind that learning to do the physical examination does take experience.

CARDIAC ROENTGENOLOGY

Daniel Fuleihan

3

The cornerstone of the cardiovascular evaluation of a patient is a careful and complete history and physical examination. Once these have been completed and initial impressions have been formulated, a number of important laboratory aids may be utilized to support or alter the working diagnosis. The plain roentgenograph of the chest and the electrocardiogram are the two initial studies which should be obtained and evaluated.

As with any study, a basic understanding of the technique, uses, and limitations of the chest roentgenographic examination is essential for proper interpretation. In the ambulatory patient, a standard frontal and lateral view of the chest is taken. The frontal view, by convention, is the posterior-anterior (PA), which refers to the direction of the x-ray beam as it traverses the chest from back to front. The anterior chest wall is positioned against the film holder so as to minimize magnification of the silhouette of the heart, which is an anterior structure. Also by convention, the lateral view is a left-lateral projection in which the left side of the chest is placed adjacent to the film cassette, the x-ray beam traversing the thorax from right to left. The standard tube-to-film distance is 6 feet; a distance chosen to minimize magnification and distortion. All films are taken in the inspiratory phase of respiration. Whether the film is exposed during systole or diastole is usually of little importance, since the variation in heart size in these two phases is not significant.

A chest film taken with a portable machine, which may be made with the patient in the supine or sitting position, cannot be compared to the standard frontal film of the chest. When this machine is used, the film cassette is placed adjacent to the posterior chest wall and the x-ray beam traversees the thorax from the anterior to the posterior wall (AP), resulting in magnification of the anterior chest structures such as the heart. Also, the tube-to-film distance is much less than 6 feet, resulting in further magnification and some distortion.

The relative radiodensities of the various structures and tissues in the chest permit the identification and differentiation of the images on the chest film. Air, fat, water, and bone (metal) are the four basic radiodensities. The heart, containing muscle and blood within its chambers, has a water density, and the cardiac silhouette is therefore defined by its differentiation from the adjacent lungs, with a predominant air density. The same principle is applied in the recognition of a pericardial effusion or a thickened pericardium on the lateral chest film, because of the presence of fat densities outlining the water density of the pericardium or pericardial effusion.

The evaluation of the routine chest film should entail a systematic examination of all structures. Therefore, the cardiac silhouette, the pulmonary vascular system, lung fields, diaphragms, bony structures, pleura, soft tissues, and upper air passages should be individually evaluated. The cardiac silhouette represents a composite of the various cardiac chambers and walls. Since the advent of cardiac angiography, the structures making up the borders of the cardiac silhouette in the chest film have been firmly established. Before an abnormality of the cardiovascular system can be identified, an appreciation of the normal cardiac silhouette and vascular system must exist.

NORMAL CARDIAC SILHOUETTE AND
VASCULAR STRUCTURES

STANDARD POSTERIOR-ANTERIOR PROJECTION

In the standard frontal chest film, the right cardiac border is formed by the right atrium (Fig. 3-1). The boundary between the right atrium and the right ventricle lies medial to the right heart border and is not visible. The right atrium forms a well-rounded convex shadow and merges superiorly with a slightly convex or perpendicular shadow which represents the right edge of the superior vena cava. The upper portion of the superior vena cava shadow merges with the right border of the right inominate vein, which bends concavely towards the clavicle.

The left cardiac silhouette is composed of a convex arc which represents the anterior wall of the left ventricle and the left-ventricular apex. The left-ventricular silhouette merges superiorly, almost imperceptibly, with the left-atrial appendage. The distinctly convex left border of the main trunk of the pulmonary artery merges with the atrial appendage. Just below the left-clavicular shadow is the aortic knob, formed by the distal portion of the aortic arch; this distinctly rounded, convex shadow merges inferiorly with the pulmonary trunk.

The pulmonary trunk arises superiorly, anteriorly, and to the left of the aorta and curves upward from the pulmonic valve to form, as stated earlier, a segment of the left heart border. Slightly to the left of the midline and approxi-

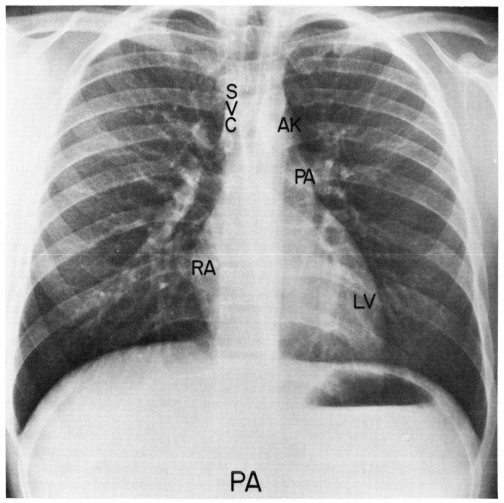

FIG. 3-1.
Chest film showing normal anatomy in the posterior anterior projection. **PA,** posterior
anterior projection; **RA,** right atrium; **SVC,** superior vena cava; **AK,** aortic knob; **PA,**
pulmonary artery; **LV,** left ventricle.

mately at the level of the carina, the pulmonary artery bifurcates into its two main divisions, the right and left branches. It has been noted in normal subjects that the left hilum is almost universally higher or, in a small percentage of cases, at the level of the right hilum, due to the fact that the left main branch of the pulmonary artery curves sharply upwards and backwards, while the right branch remains almost horizontal in position.

LEFT LATERAL PROJECTION

The ability to properly interpret the left lateral roentgenograph carries the same importance as understanding the posterior-anterior film. In this view, the heart is projected between the shadow of the sternum and the spine (Fig. 3-2). The anterior margin of the cardiac silhouette is formed by the right ventricle and more superiorly by the outflow tract of the right ventricle, which merges superiorly with the anterior wall of the ascending aorta. Normally the anterior cardiac silhouette is in close proximity to the lower third of the anterior chest wall. The upper two-thirds of the chest wall are separated from the right-ventricular outflow tract and the aortic arch by radiolucent lung. The posterior border of the heart is composed mainly of the posterior wall of the left atrium, which merges inferiorly with the posterior wall of the left ventricle. These appear as a convex shadow which, in the most inferior portion, may be joined by a concave shadow which represents the inferior vena cava. The tracheal air shadow can be identified running vertically down the midline and then bifurcating into the right and left main bronchi. The left main bronchus is identified as a radiolucent circular structure, superior to which runs a branch of the left main pulmonary artery. Above this is the arch of the aorta. The right main bronchus continues inferiorly and slightly posteriorly from the point of bifurcation of the trachea. The right main pulmonary artery is identified as an oval structure, slightly anterior and inferior to the left main bronchus and posterior to the aorta. Identification of these structures is more than of academic interest, as may be seen from the localization of calcium in either the aortic or the mitral valve. A line drawn from the anterior costophrenic sulcus to the bifurcation of the trachea will identify the aortic valve as superior and anterior to this line, while the mitral valve will be below and posterior to it.

RIGHT ANTERIOR OBLIQUE (RAO) VIEW

A complete cardiac series includes in addition to films made in the frontal and left lateral projections, as already described, films with right and left anterior oblique projections, taken with rotations of approximately 45° (Fig. 3-3). These four views, with the esophagus opacified by barium, allow the various chambers and great vessels to be brought into profile.

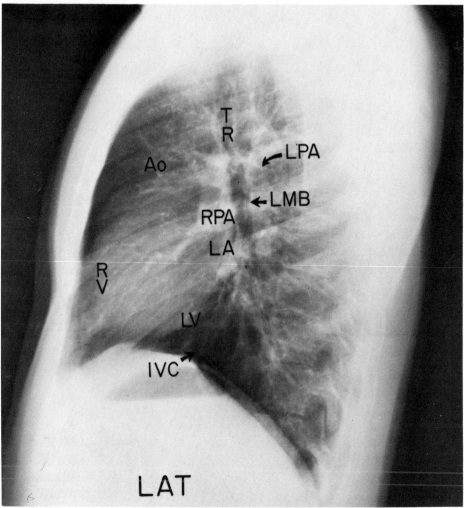

FIG. 3-2.
Chest film showing normal anatomy in the left lateral projection. **LAT,** left lateral projection; **Ao,** aorta; **IVC,** inferior vena cava; **LA,** left atrium; **LMB,** left main bronchus; **LPA,** left main pulmonary artery; **LV,** left ventricle; **RV,** right ventricle; **RPA,** right main pulmonary artery; **TR,** tracheal air shadow.

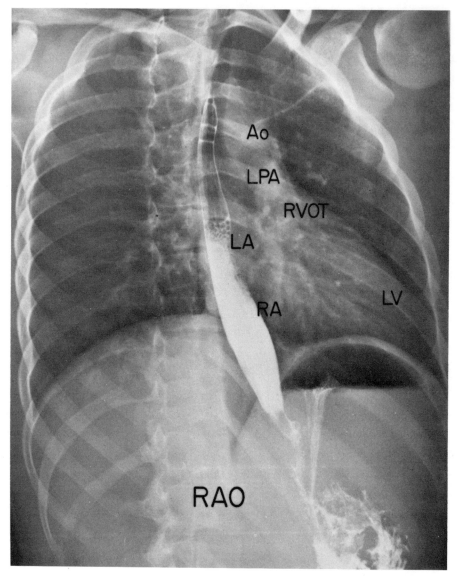

FIG. 3-3.
Chest film showing normal anatomy in the right anterior oblique projection. **RAO,**
right anterior oblique view; **Ao,** aorta; **LPA,** left main pulmonary artery; **RVOT,**
right-ventricular outflow tract; **LA,** left atrium; **RA,** right atrium; **LV,** left ventricle.

In the right anterior oblique view, the right chest wall abuts the film cassette, with rotation of the left chest wall away from the film cassette to approximately a 45° angle. In this projection, the spine is projected out of the cardiac shadow to the right, and clear lung field is noted between the spine and the cardiac silhouette. With barium in the esophagus, the utility of this view for defining the left atrium can be appreciated, since the posterior wall of the left atrium can be appreciated, since the posterior wall of the left atrium forms the cardiac shadow adjacent to the esophagus. The right border of the heart is formed by the posterior aspect of the left atrium above and by the posterior border of the right atrium below. The left border of the cardiac silhouette is formed by the ascending aorta, pulmonary trunk and the right-ventricular outflow tract, and the anterior wall of the left ventricle. The plane of the interventricular septum is perpendicular to the x-ray beam, with resultant superimposition of the right- and left-ventricular chambers. A helpful hint for the novice in determining which oblique view is being visualized is, as stated previously, to remember that in the right anterior oblique view, the spine is to the right of the cardiac silhouette and the gastric shadow, filled with barium, can be visualized just below the right border of the heart. In the left anterior oblique projection, the spine is to the left of the cardiac silhouette, as is the barium-filled stomach.

LEFT ANTERIOR OBLIQUE (LAO) PROJECTION

When this view is taken, the left anterior chest wall abuts the film cassette and the right chest wall is rotated away from the film holder to a 45° angle (Fig. 3-4). This view places the interventricular septum parallel to the course of the x-ray beam and bisects the cardiac silhouette, so that the sizes of both the right and left ventricles may be appreciated. The left cardiac border is formed mainly by the left ventricle, except for the uppermost portion, which is formed by the left atrium. The arch of the aorta is clearly visualized in this projection and can be seen curving from right to left towards the spine. If a proper 45° obliquity is made, the shadow of the normal left ventricle should not extend to the left of the shadow of the spine. The left-atrial portion of the cardiac contour is usually straight or minimally convex and is defined by the inferior border of the left main bronchus. It can be noted that the best view of the arch is obtained in this obliquity, with dye in the aorta, and therefore on the plain chest film this is the best view for identifying aneurysms of the aortic arch. The right border of the cardiac silhouette is formed by the right ventricle, which merges superiorly with the right atrial border. The ascending aorta can be appreciated to emerge from the right atrial shadow. As mentioned previously the spine is to the left of the cardiac silhouette, as is the gastric shadow. The sternum can be noted to partially overlie the right border of the heart.

CARDIAC FLUOROSCOPY

A discussion of cardiac fluoroscopy is beyond the scope of this chapter. This study is performed by the radiologist as an integral part of the cardiac series and

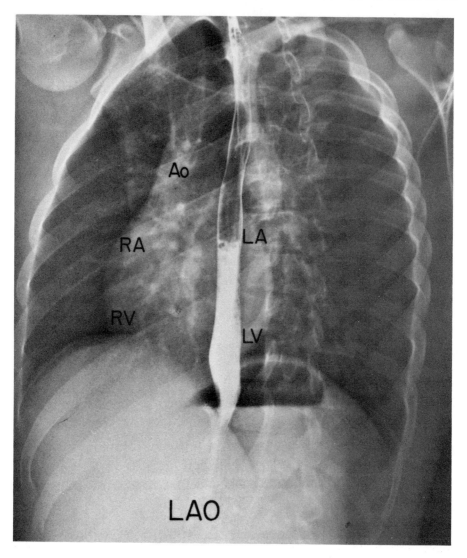

FIG. 3-4.
Chest film showing normal anatomy with left anterior oblique projection. **LAO,** left anterior oblique view; **Ao,** aorta; **RA,** right atrium; **LA,** left atrium; **RV,** right ventricle; **LV,** left ventricle.

may be helpful in allowing him to identify calcium within either the aortic or the mitral valve and also involving the coronary arteries. Fluoroscopy is the least reliable means of identifying a ventricular aneurysm and has become outmoded with the advent of newer techniques, such as the nuclear medicine ventriculogram and cardiac catheterization with angiography, from which more detailed and definitive information concerning the presence of a ventricular aneurysm can be obtained.

THE CHEST ROENTGENOGRAPH IN CONGESTIVE HEART FAILURE

Multiple means of estimating the presence or absence of cardiomegaly on the basis of roentgenographic examination have been developed, some of which entail quite intricate formulas. For the nonradiologically trained observer, the simplest of these would be the cardiothoracic index, which is a ratio relating the diameter of the heart to the diameter of the thorax. It is determined by dividing the maximum transverse cardiac diameter by the maximum transverse diameter of the thorax. The transverse cardiac diameter is the sum of the maximum extension of the heart to the right and to the left of the midline. Pericardial fat pads may be present in the cardiophrenic angles and should not be included in the measurement. The transverse diameter of the thorax is the maximum width of the thorax as measured between the inner margins of the ribs.

The normal cardiothoracic ratio is frequently quoted as being 50%; ratios above this are considered to indicate cardiomegaly. However, several authors have found ratios up to 58% to be normal. The use of this ratio has obvious limitations, when differences in chest contour of individuals are taken into account. Also, whether the cardiac silhouette has a vertical or a transverse lie will greatly influence the cardiothoracic index. If these limitations are appreciated, the cardiothoracic index may be very valuable, especially in the serial evaluation of chest films. It should be stressed that the cardiothoracic index and serial evaluations of cardiac size are valid only in the standard PA film.

Radiologic evidence of elevated left-sided pressures includes the following findings: dilated pulmonary veins, with a discrepancy in the venous ratio between the pulmonary veins of the upper and lower lobe; increased pulmonary interstitial density, presenting as clouding of the lung fields, loss of sharp definition of the vasculature, septal lines, thickened fissures due to subpleural collection of fluid, pleural effusion, peribronchial and perivascular cuffing; and confluent alveolar densities due to plumonary edema.

The first abnormality noted as an indication of elevated left-sided pressures is pulmonary venous congestion, also known as pulmonary venous redistribution or pulmonary venous hypertension. It has become clear from physiologic, radiologic, and pathologic studies that in normal, erect subjects the blood flow is greater at the dependent zones of the lung than at the apices. This pattern may be reversed in the presence of an increase in the left-sided pressures such as occurs in left-ventricular dysfunction or mitral-valve disease.

Before the pathologic state can be identified, the normal anatomy and relationships must be understood. In the PA chest film taken with the patient erect, the inability to visualize upper-lobe veins is normal. This is because the upper-lobe veins, in the normal state, are of a relatively small diameter. When redistribution of blood flow occurs, the upper-lobe veins enlarge and become visible in almost all cases. It is possible to distinguish between the pulmonary arteries and the pulmonary veins. The pulmonary arteries are noted to diverge from the hilus well above the point at which the veins converge on the left atrium, and in most adults this is a distance of 3 or 4 cm. The pulmonary arteries emerge from the mediastinal shadow usually at the level of the seventh to eighth posterior ribs, and the pulmonary veins enter the left atrium at the level of the eighth to tenth posterior ribs. In the upper lobes, the arteries and veins are noted to run parallel to each other in a vertical direction, with each vein lateral to its corresponding artery. In the lower lobes, the pulmonary veins run in a less vertical course than the pulmonary arteries, because of their lower point of convergence in the left atrium, and each vein is noted to be medial to its corresponding artery.

Several studies have now been performed utilizing tomography to establish a venous index. Pulmonary veins in the upper lobes and lower lobes, the same distance from the periphery, were studied in normal individuals and in individuals with left-ventricular dysfunction or with mitral-valve disease. From these studies a venous index has been proposed which is a ratio of the diameter of an upper-lobe pulmonary vein to that of a corresponding lower-lobe pulmonary vein the same distance from the periphery. The venous index in normal individuals was found to be between 0.6 and 0.95, with a mean value of 0.8. In individuals with mitral stenosis and with pulmonary capillary wedge mean pressures greater than 15 torr, this index was > 1.0. In a diverse group of individuals with left-ventricular failure, with symptoms ranging from mild to severe, the index gave results ranging from normal to abnormal. The primary feature to note here is that an increase in the diameter of the upper-lobe vessels was accompanied by a decrease in the diameter of the lower-lobe vessels. In making these measurements on the plain chest film, it is important that the individual be in the upright position and that measurements be made at corresponding distances from the periphery of the lung. The reversed relationship between the upper- and lower-lobe vessels is more striking than the absolute change in the caliber of a single vessel. Radioisotope studies have shown that there is a linear relationship between left-atrial pressure and the blood flow in the upper and lower lobes. Several theories have been formulated to explain the redistribution that occurs with elevated left-atrial pressure, but currently the explanation remains controversial.

Another manifestation of elevated pulmonary capillary pressure is an increase in pulmonary interstitial density. This may manifest itself as Kerley lines, pulmonary clouding, perivascular and peribronchial cuffing, subpleural edema as noted by the thickened fissures, and the presence of pleural effusions. Septal lines were first described by Kerley in 1933, and in the early 1950s, with the advent of right-heart catheterization, the presence of these lines was correlated with the pulmonary capillary wedge pressure in individuals with mitral stenosis and chronic left heart failure. These early studies indicated that Kerley septal lines were not present unless the mean pulmonary capillary wedge pressure was $\geq$ 18 torr. Three types of septal lines have been described, and labelled *A*, *B*, and *C*. Kerley A lines are linear, centrally placed, dense lines up to 4 cm in length. They are most frequently seen in the upper lobes directed towards the hilus. Kerley B lines are fine, dense, parallel lines 1.5 to 2 cm in length, most frequently seen in the lateral portions of the lung bases (Fig. 3-5). Kerley C lines are represented by a diffuse reticular pattern. The existence of Kerley C lines is currently questionable. The Kerley lines, then, are a radiographic manifestation of interstitial edema and are thought to be caused by the thickening of the interlobular fibrous septa of the lungs. Septal lines may result from any process which thickens the fibrous-tissue septa. When secondary to congestive failure, they will resolve when the patient becomes compensated, if the failure is acute. The terms **peribronchial cuffing** and **perivascular cuffing** indicate accumulation of interstitial fluid around these structures. This phenomenon can be appreciated when either a vascular or bronchial structure is seen on end.

Clouding of the lung fields is noted when the central lung zone shows a slight increase in density, as minimal fluid accumulates in the interstitial tissues. Fluid transudes into the interstitial space and is deposited within the perivascular sheath and the interlobular septa, resulting in the previously described radiologic findings. All of the above described manifestations of interstitial edema may be noted on both the standard PA and lateral chest films and also on the portable supine film.

There are two major compartments of the lung in which excess fluid may accumulate, the interstitial space and the air space. Their distinction is important, since the pathophysiologic and clinical manifestations of edema of these compartments differ, and an interstitial phase of edema exists for a variable period before alveolar flooding occurs. Air-space edema is manifested by an acinar shadow. In most cases, these shadows are confluent, creating irregular, rather poorly defined, patchy shadows scattered randomly throughout the lungs. It should be noted that pulmonary alveolar edema may have a number of causes other than elevated left-sided pressures. These include infection, neoplasms, central nervous system disease, pulmonary emboli, the effects of high altitude or toxic gases, aspiration, rapid reexpansion of the lungs, traumatic fat embolism, narcotic abuse, radiation damage, and lung contusion, among others. Note that with these causes associated findings such as interstitial edema and vascular redistribution are absent.

The advent of the Swan-Ganz catheter has allowed for the determination

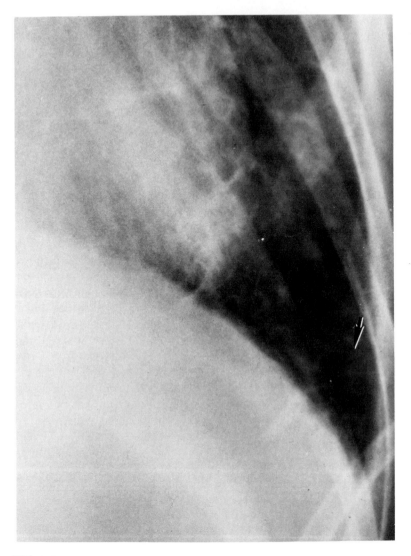

FIG. 3-5.
Kerley B lines. **(arrow)**. Note the dense parallel lines 1.5 to 2 cm in
length in the lateral portion of the base of the lung.

of the left-ventricular end diastolic pressure at which radiographic manifestations occur in individuals with left-ventricular dysfunction. The earliest change
to occur is pulmonary venous redistribution, which corresponds to a pulmonary
capillary wedge mean pressure of between 12 and 18 torr. The development of
interstitial edema occurs as pressures become further elevated, and the presence
of Kerley B lines have been found to correspond to a pulmonary capillary

wedge mean pressure of between 18 and 20 torr. Other signs of interstitial edema, such as perivascular and peribronchial cuffing, have not been correlated with hemodynamic data. Some investigators have suggested a range of 18 to 25 torr for the appearance of these early signs of interstitial pulmonary edema. The critical wedge pressure necessary for the development of alveolar pulmonary edema has been postulated to be between 22 and 25 torr by some investigators and from 25 to 35 torr by others.

A significant problem in evaluating the chest film in persons who are undergoing hemodynamic alterations, either worsening (as in an evolving myocardial infarction) or improving as a result of therapy, is that a lag phase may occur. A "posttherapeutic lag phase" has been demonstrated in the chest film; this refers to the time interval required for the chest film to become normal after an elevated wedge pressure has returned to normal. In certain patients the change in wedge pressure may not be reflected immediately radiographically, and up to 4 days may be required to demonstrate resolution. A second type of lag, a "diagnostic lag," may be responsible for a further lack of correlation between the hemodynamic data and the roentgenographic evidence. In some patients, a clearly documented elevation in wedge pressure may not be reflected immediately on the film; instead there may be a 12-hour delay before it reflects this abnormality. Therefore, although the chest film may be of invaluable help in determining the hemodynamic status of a given individual, the lag phases that occur in an acutely changing hemodynamic situation make this form of evaluation less useful for certain patients.

CHAMBER ENLARGEMENT

With a knowledge of the normal anatomic relationships, specific chamber enlargement can be identified utilizing the cardiac series.

LEFT-VENTRICULAR ENLARGEMENT

The left ventricle may respond to a pathologic state by hypertrophy or by dilatation. Hypertrophy without concomitant dilatation does not result in an increase in the size of the left-ventricular chamber but may be accompanied by increased rounding of the left-ventricular portion of the left heart border in the PA projection. Dilatation of the left ventricle causes both an increase in size and a change in contour of the heart. This results, in the chest film, in an increase in the transverse cardiac diameter and a downward extension of the left-ventricular apex below the diaphragm. In the lateral view, left-ventricular enlargement is present when the posterior border of the left ventricle extends posteriorly to the posterior border of the inferior vena cava more than 1.8 cm, at a level 2 cm cephalad to their crossing. This measurement is made on a plane which parallels the horizontal plane of the vertebral bodies. In the left anterior oblique projection it is generally considered that the left-ventricular shadow should not extend to the left of the vertebral column unless left-ventricular enlargement is present. A note of caution is appropriate in that in the presence of enlargement of multiple chambers, the ability to interpret enlargement of a specific chamber is limited.

RIGHT-VENTRICULAR ENLARGEMENT

Hypertrophy of the right ventricle without concomitant dilatation cannot be identified roentgenographically. In the PA projection, there may be little change in the cardiac silhouette in the presence of right-ventricular enlargement. The most valuable sign of right-ventricular dilatation in this view is therefore an indirect one—an increase in the prominence of the main pulmonary artery. Such evidence is significant, since it is rare to find marked changes in the pulmonary artery without accompanying changes in the right ventricle. An increase in the cardiothoracic index may also occur. In the lateral projection, the enlarged right ventricle encroaches upon the superior retrosternal space, which may be compromised or obliterated by it. Dilatation of the pulmonary artery or ascending aorta may result in the same findings, however. In the LAO projection, there may be an increased convexity of the lower portion of the right heart border. However, right-atrial enlargement may result in this chamber's forming the right contour of the cardiac silhouette. In the RAO projection, marked convexity may be noted in the area of the right-ventricular outflow tract. It is generally accepted that the radiographic evaluation of the size of the right ventricle is of limited value.

LEFT-ATRIAL ENLARGEMENT

In the PA projection, a number of valuable signs indicate enlargement of the left atrium. Because of its thin walls, it may attain giant proportions, especially in mitral regurgitation. With enlargement of the left atrium, a double density which is actually an atrial contour may be identified inside the right heart border, and an increase in the convexity of the left cardiac border beneath the pulmonary artery segment may occur as a result of enlargement of the left-atrial appendage. With barium in the esophagus, displacement of the esophagus to the right may be identified, and more rarely it may be displaced to the left. Occasionally the left atrium may attain gigantic proportions and form the entire right border of the cardiac silhouette. Another valuable sign is widening of the carina, with upward displacement of the main left bronchus. In the lateral projection, with barium in a well-distended esophagus, displacement of the esophagus posteriorly can be identified in the region of the upper cardiac silhouette. Displacement of the esophagus in the lower portion of the cardiac silhouette may indicate left-ventricular enlargement. In the LAO view, the enlarged left atrium can be noted to displace the left main bronchus superiorly. This is associated with an outward bulging of the left-atrial silhouette, which is usually straight or slightly convex in its outline against the left main bronchus.

In the RAO view, displacement of the esophagus can be identified as in the lateral view and is associated with a posterior displacement of the cardiac silhouette in the region of the left atrium. Of the four cardiac chambers, enlargement of the left atrium is the one most reliably demonstrated by radiologic evaluation.

RIGHT-ATRIAL ENLARGEMENT

Of the four chambers, enlargement of the right atrium is the one least reliably demonstrated by the cardiac series. Studies have shown that in the PA view, there are no consistent specific findings for right-atrial enlargement. The diagnosis may be suspected when there is increased convexity, and also increased length, of the right heart border. In the RAO projection, right-atrial enlargement is said to be present if the posterior cardiac border extends behind the esophagus. However, this sign was found to be positive in only one-third of the patients with documented right-atrial enlargement and was falsely positive in 13% of cases. In the LAO view, right-atrial enlargement may present as an increased convexity of the upper right cardiac border. Once again, however, the sensitivity and specificity of this finding is less than ideal.

THE AZYGOS VEIN AND ITS IMPORTANCE

Enlargement of the azygos vein may be considered analogous to dilatation and engorgement of the neck veins on physical examination. On the PA chest film, the azygos arch appears as a spindle-shaped shadow located in the right tracheobronchial angle and can be visualized in up to 56% of normal individuals. The partially straight posterior-anterior course of the azygos vein as it enters the posterior aspect of the superior vena cava makes possible its visualization on the routine chest film. Measurement is made at its widest diameter, as measured perpendicular to the wall of the trachea. Because the shadow of the azygos vein and tracheal wall blend imperceptibly, the measurement includes the tracheal wall. Dilatation of the azygos arch is known to occur in cases of venous congestion, as in congestive heart failure, right-ventricular failure, or organic and functional tricuspid insufficiency. The maximum size of the normal azygos arch in the erect PA projection has been found to vary considerably. Therefore the most reliable use of this structure is made by a change in its diameter as an indication of changing hemodynamic status.

PERICARDIAL EFFUSION

The diagnosis of a pericardial effusion on the basis of a chest film may be made or tentatively formulated because of enlargement of the cardiac shadow, a characteristic "water-bottle" configuration of the cardiac silhouette, and diminished pulsations of the left cardiac border at fluoroscopy. However, none of these signs is completely reliable, and all may be caused by generalized cardiomegaly. The delineation of the epicardial fat-pad line on the lateral chest roentgenograph provides an extra dimension for the diagnosis of either pericardial thickening or pericardial effusion. A knowledge of anatomy and a good-quality lateral chest film are necessary for this. Beneath the visceral pericardium (epicardium) is a variable amount of subepicardial fat which extends from the interventricular groove separating the right and left ventricles to the apex of the left ventricle. The visceral pericardium is in intimate contact with the parietal pericardium, the two layers of pericardium being separated only by a thin film of fluid. Normally there are 25 to 30 ml of this fluid within this space. Adjacent to the parietal pericardium is a layer of anterior-mediastinal fat. It would appear that in a lateral chest film these fat planes would be visible and distinguishable from the soft-tissue density of the heart and the bony structures of the sternum, since the radiodensity of fat is less than that of the other soft tissues, and therefore its roentgen shadow is more lucent (darker) than that of the myocardium or fibrous tissue. The two layers of pericardium will then be depicted as a thin line of soft-tissue density interposed between the anterior-mediastinal fat in front and the subepicardial fat behind. In the presence of pericardial thickening or of pericardial effusion, the two fat layers will become further separated, depending upon the amount of fluid or thickening present. In a series of normal chest films which include lateral chest films, the pericardium, interposed between the two fat lines, could be identified in approximately 40% of cases. In a series of 42 cases of proven pericardial effusion, the fat stripes could be identified in 27 of the 42, or 65%. In these cases the fat stripes were separated by 1.0 to 3.5 cm. Normal separation is accepted as 2 mm. Moderate displacement may be seen with pericardial thickening, but if the fat stripes are displaced much more than 1 cm, a significant amount of pericardial fluid is almost certainly present. In the presence of a normal separation of the fat pads, a pericardial effusion can be excluded.

Concerning the enlargement of the cardiac silhouette and the water-bottle configuration, it has been estimated that at least 250 cc of fluid is necessary to cause a recognizable change in the cardiac silhouette.

In recent years the development and use of the echocardiogram and of nuclear medicine techniques have greatly increased the diagnostic accuracy of predicting a pericardial effusion. The most sensitive means of detecting a pericardial effusion is with the echocardiogram, in which experimentally 50 ml of fluid may be detected.

ELECTROCARDIOGRAPHY

4

C. Thomas Fruehan and Robert H. Eich

DEFINITION

The electrocardiogram is a graphic recording showing voltage variations in relation to time. The voltage is ordinarily recorded from the body surface, and represents different electromotive potentials (voltage) between various sites on the body surface, caused by the flow of tiny currents through the body. These tiny currents are generated by cardiac electrical activity.

In recent years, much of the electrophysiologic mechanisms underlying electrocardiography has been clarified. However, the use of electrocardiography as a clinical tool remains an empiric art. Electrocardiograms are clinically useful because certain electrocardiographic patterns have frequent association with certain specific types of heart disease. Certain electrocardiographic patterns have high specificity for particular diseases; other electrocardiographic patterns have low specificity and serve the primary function of differentiating the tracing as "normal" or "abnormal." Further, it is well known that patients with severe heart disease may have normal electrocardiograms. Thus, it should *not* be inferred that the absence of a particular electrocardiographic finding excludes the disease in question. Within these limitations, however, electrocardiography is a highly useful clinical laboratory test, without exception part of the clinical evaluation of any patient suspected of having heart disease.

ORIGIN OF THE ECG SIGNAL

The ultimate source of the ECG signal is the electrical activity present in heart cells. In all living cells, there is a difference in electrical potential (that is, volt-

43

age) between the interior and exterior of the cell. Because the cell membrane is considered the dividing boundary between the interior and exterior of the living cell, this property is called the **transmembrane potential.** The transmembrane potential exists because of differences in ion concentration between the interior and exterior of the cell. These differences in ion concentration are, in turn, the result of differences in membrane permeability to ionic flow across the cell membrane. The ions responsible for transmembrane potential include potassium, sodium, calcium, and, probably, magnesium.

In its resting state, the living cell maintains a transmembrane potential of approximately 90 millivolts (mv). By convention, this is measured by comparing the voltage of the cell interior to that of the exterior, so that the transmembrane potential of the resting cell is approximately −90 mv. The internal ionic concentration is approximately sodium, 20 mEq/liter, and potassium, 120 mEq/liter. In the resting state, the cell membrane is relatively impermeable to sodium ion flux and relatively more permeable to potassium ion flux. This disequilibrium of ion concentration across the semipermeable cell membrane establishes the transmembrane potential. During activation of the cell, the permeability of the cell membrane is altered. Sodium and calcium flow into the cell and potassium out. This process is called **depolarization.** During recovery, or **repolarization,** the opposite occurs.

The recording of intracellular potential variation with respect to time, for an individual cell, during one cycle of depolarization and repolarization is called the **action potential** of that cell.

DEPOLARIZATION-REPOLARIZATION SEQUENCE

A normal heartbeat is initiated in the sinoatrial node, located in the right atrium, which depolarizes spontaneously and periodically in its function as the heart's normal pacemaker. This sinoatrial-node depolarization has no representation in the body surface ECG.

Depolarization (activation) probably spreads from the sinoatrial to the atria by two routes: 1) by direct spread through atrial muscle, in a concentric fashion through both atria, and 2) along three internodal tracts, groups of fibers which conduct electrical activity faster than direct muscle-to-muscle spread. These three internodal tracts connect the sinoatrial node to the atrioventricular node; they are labelled the anterior, middle, and posterior internodal tracts. A fourth tract, Bachmann's bundle, comes off the posterior internodal tract and spreads into the left atrium.

The normal depolarization process proceeds from the atria to the ventricles only through the atrioventricular node, and then passes through the common bundle of His and finally both bundle branches. These processes, likewise, do not produce sufficient electrical activity to be recorded at the body surface.

The ventricular depolarization process begins via a twig of the left bundle branch at the lower third of the interventricular septum. Thereafter ventricular

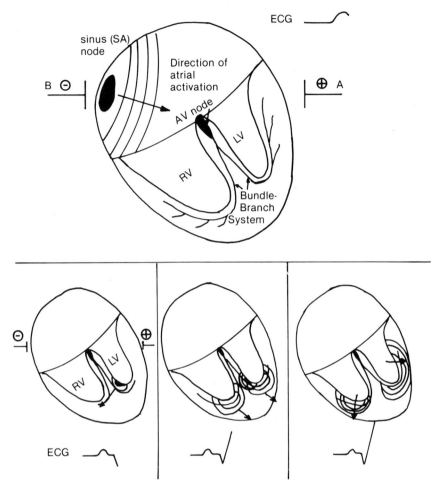

FIG. 4-1.
Sequence of activation of the atria (*top*) and ventricles (*bottom*). At three
instances during ventricular activation, a representative Lead I ECG is shown
which corresponds to that stage of activation. **RV,** right ventricle, **LV,** left
ventricle; **A** and **B,** recording electrodes.

activation spreads rapidly, and nearly simultaneously, through both ventricles,
proceeding more rapidly along the endocardial surfaces and spreading from
endocardium to epicardium. Because of its thinner wall and lesser muscle mass,
the right ventricle completes its depolarization first. The last portion of the heart
to be depolarized is the free wall of the left ventricle and a small portion of the
interventricular septum near the base. The depolarization process is depicted in
Figure 4-1.

Repolarization of the atria proceeds in roughly the same sequence as did
atrial activation. Because atrial repolarization usually takes place at the same

time as ventricular depolarization, the ECG representation of atrial repolarization is usually completely obscured by ventricular depolarization and is little used in clinical electrocardiography.

In contrast, ventricular repolarization occurs in a different sequence than ventricular activation. Actually, the ventricular recovery process begins as soon as each depolarized cell completes depolarization; but the *duration of repolarization* differs for cells in different parts of the myocardium. In general, cells in the center of the myocardium recover the fastest, while those in the endocardial layers have the longest duration of action potential repolarization. This means that, at a given instant in ventricular repolarization, cells in one area of the heart may be at a different stage of repolarization from cells in a different area of the ventricles. This difference between cells in varying phases of recovery results in a potential difference between cells in different areas of the heart at each instant. As can be appreciated, slight localized differences in action potential duration can greatly affect the repolarization signal recorded on the ECG (see Fig. 4-2).

The ECG wave caused by atrial depolarization is called the P wave. Q, R, and S waves are caused by ventricular depolarization (Fig. 4-3). By definition, the first upward deflection due to ventricular activation is the R wave. A downward deflection (below the baseline) preceding an R wave is a Q wave. A

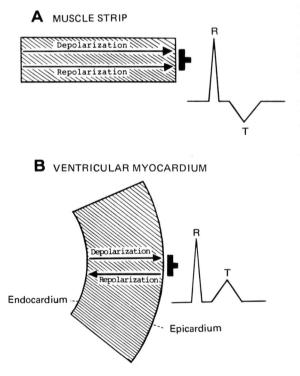

A MUSCLE STRIP

Depolarization

Repolarization

R

T

B VENTRICULAR MYOCARDIUM

Depolarization

Repolarization

Endocardium

R

T

Epicardium

FIG. 4-2.
(A) Depolarization and repolarization of a muscle strip, both proceeding in the same direction. The repolarization wave produces an ECG of opposite polarity to that of the depolarization wave, but of equal area.
(B) For contrast, in the ventricular myocardium it is assumed that the direction of repolarization is *opposite* to that in activation. With these directions of depolarization and repolarization, the repolarization ECG wave would be in the *same* direction as the activation wave (and would have the same area). (Chung EK: Electrocardiography: Practical Applications with Vectorial Principles, ed. 2. Harper & Row, 1980, p 17)

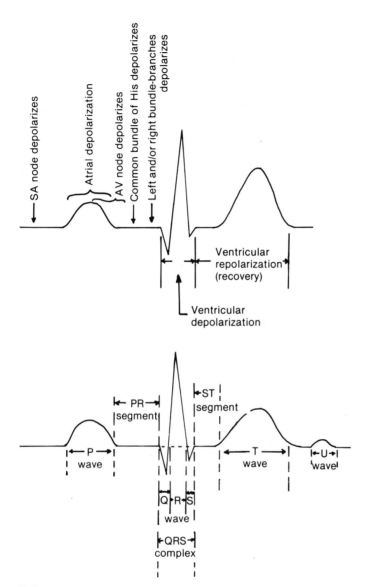

FIG. 4-3.
Names of ECG waves and segments; relationship of
physiologic events to ECG.

downward deflection following an R wave is an S wave. Collectively, the entire ventricular activation process forms what is called a **QRS complex.** A QRS complex may consist solely of a Q wave or an R wave, or it may have both an R wave and an S wave. It may have Q, R, and S waves. Some QRS complexes have a second upward deflection following the S wave, called an R' wave.

Ventricular repolarization produces both the T wave and the entire signal after the QRS complex before the T wave becomes large. This portion of the tracing is called the **ST segment.** In most normal tracings, the ST segment is nearly isoelectric (on the baseline).

Finally, a wave with an upward defection may occur after the T wave; this is called a U wave. The genesis of this wave is still in some doubt.

RECORDING TECHNIQUES AND CONVENTIONS

A **lead** is a combination of two or more electrodes attached to the recording galvanometer. Multiple ECG leads have been developed because each lead is most sensitive to cardiac electrical activity proceeding in a certain direction, and each lead is insensitive to activity perpendicular to that direction. Thus, each ECG lead has a directionality, and use of multiple leads permits recording of activity in all directions.

Twelve leads are used in routine clinical electrocardiography. Six of these leads have directions of maximal sensitivity (their "lead direction") in the frontal plane. These are referred to as the **standard** and **unipolar limb leads.** The three standard leads are I, II, and III. The three unipolar limb leads are AVR, AVL, and AVF. The directions of these leads are depicted in Fig. 4-4. The direction of lead I, horizontal to the left side, is taken as the reference 0°. The other six leads, named the **precordial leads,** named V_1 through V_6, have directionality strongest toward the recording electrode placed on the chest wall (Fig. 4-5). Lead V_1, for instance, is recorded with an electrode placed at the right sternal border at the fourth intercostal space. It is most sensitive to anterior-posterior cardiac electrical activity.

The ECG recording paper is marked as shown in Figure 4-6. The timing intervals shown are for the commonest recorder paper speed of 25 mm/sec. Periodically, the recording technician should put a calibration signal on the recording. The 1.0-mv calibration mark is rectangular and should measure 1 cm in height.

APPROACH TO READING AN ECG

GENERAL OVERALL IMPRESSION

First, the tracing should be examined for proper recording technique and freedom from artifact. Identify the individual P waves, QRS complexes, and ST-T deflections in each lead.

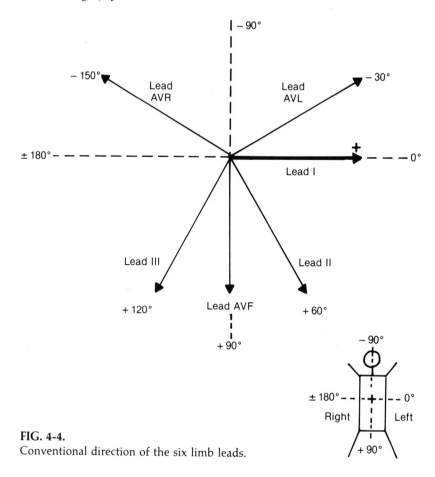

FIG. 4-4.
Conventional direction of the six limb leads.

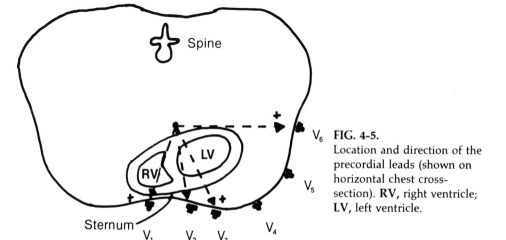

FIG. 4-5.
Location and direction of the precordial leads (shown on horizontal chest cross-section). **RV,** right ventricle; **LV,** left ventricle.

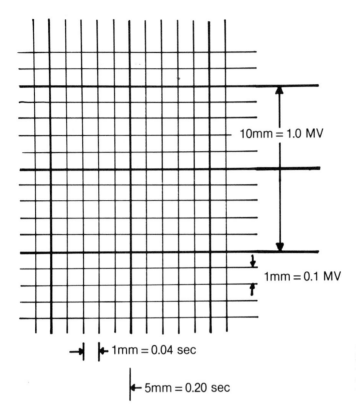

10mm = 1.0 MV

1mm = 0.1 MV

→| |← 1mm = 0.04 sec

|← 5mm = 0.20 sec

FIG. 4-6.
Markings of
conventional
ECG paper.

HEART RATE

Determine atrial rate and ventricular rate independently. Rate can be determined in any of several simple ways:

1. Count beats in 6 sec, multiply by 10.
2. Determine number of "big boxes" on the recording paper between consecutive QRS complexes; 3=rate 100, 4 boxes=rate 75, 5 boxes=rate 60, and so forth.
3. Count the number of "little boxes" between successive QRS complexes; divide 1500 by this number. Example: 21 little boxes between beats; 1500/21 = 72 beats/min.

MEASUREMENT OF STANDARD INTERVALS

Three standard intervals are related to conduction and recovery properties; they are the PR interval, the QRS interval, and the QT or QTc interval. The measurement should be the longest such interval found in a limb lead (I through AVF). Because not all waves are well demarcated in every lead, the determination should be made in a lead where the individual waves have clearly defined starting and stopping points. The intervals are depicted in Figure 4-7.

The PR interval measures the time between the onset of atrial activation and the onset of ventricular activation. Thus, it ends at the first deflection of the QRS complex, whether that is a Q wave or an R wave. The PR interval includes the time it takes for impulses to pass through the atria, the atrioventricular node, the common bundle of His, and at least one of the bundle branches; gross prolongation of any of these transit times may prolong the PR interval. Because a large part of the normal PR interval is transit time through the atrioventricular node (up to two-thirds of the PR interval), it is often forgotten that the interventricular conduction system also contributes to the PR interval.

In the adult, the PR interval is normally 0.12 sec to 0.20 sec, inclusive. At heart rates below 60, PR interval may normally be as long as 0.21 or 0.22 sec. Abnormally short PR intervals may occur with ectopic atrial or atrioventricu-

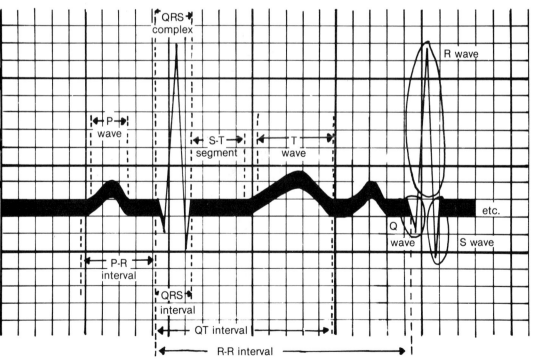

FIG. 4-7.
Determination of standard ECG intervals: PR, QRS, and QT.

lar-node (junctional) P-wave origin, or with a "pre-excitation syndrome" (Wolff-Parkinson-White and Lown-Ganong-Levine syndromes), in which the atrioventricular node is bypassed by a faster accessory conduction tract between atria and ventricles.

A prolonged PR interval is called **first-degree atrioventricular block.** It may indicate a diseased atrioventricular node or His bundle, or slow conduction in the bundle-branch system, or the effect on the atrioventricular node of increased parasympathetic (vagal) tone, or the effects of drugs. Drugs which may prolong atrioventricular conduction include digitalis, procainamide, quinidine and other antiarrhythmics, sympathetic blockers such as guanethidine, and potassium.

The normal adult QRS interval is 0.10 sec or less. The QRS interval may be prolonged by bundle-branch block (left or right); diffuse Purkinje network or ventricular muscle disease (as in cardiomyopathy, for example); ventricular enlargement (left or right); and by drugs which slow ventricular conduction time. These drugs include quinidine, procainamide, disopyramide, and potassium. A standard indicator of possible quinidine or procainamide toxicity is an increase in QRS interval greater than 25% above the pretreatment figure.

The QT interval is measured from the beginning of the QRS complex, whether this begins with an R wave or a Q wave, until the end of the T wave. It measures the entire "electrical systole" of the ventricles, from beginning of depolarization to the end of repolarization. Because the duration of repolarization is affected by heart rate, the normal QT interval range is quite different at different heart rates. To simplify this problem, a **QTc**—computed QT interval—is determined. The QTc is the QT interval which a given heart would have if its rate were 60/min. This can be determined from an empiric formula which is reasonably accurate for most heart rates clinically encountered:

$$QTc = QT \text{ (measured)} \times \frac{1}{\sqrt{R\text{-}R \text{ interval}}}$$

where R-R is the time between the two preceding QRS complexes.

Example: Heart rate, 94 (R-R interval 0.64 sec)
Measured QT, 0.36 sec
$$QTc = 0.36 \times \frac{1}{\sqrt{0.64}} = \frac{0.36}{0.80} = 0.45 \text{ sec.}$$

In our laboratory, the normal QTc range is 0.35 to 0.45 sec.

Unusually short QTc intervals are rare. Digitalis and hypercalcemia may shorten the QTc. Prolongation of the QTc may have a large number of causes. These are summarized in the accompanying list.

Causes of Prolonged QTc

1. Electrolyte disorders
   a. Hypokalemia
   b. Severe hyperkalemia
   c. Hypocalcemia
2. Drugs
   a. Quinidine, procainamide, disopyramide
   b. Guanethedine, reserpine
   c. Phenothiazines (chlorpromazine, thoridazine)
   d. Some antihistamines
3. Central nervous system disorders: trauma, subarachnoid hemorrhage, drug overdoses, and so forth.
4. Myocarditis, myocardiopathy
5. Gross metabolic, acid-base disorders
6. Gross prolongation of QRS interval
7. Hypothyroidism
8. Hypothermia
9. Congenital or hereditary disorder

One of the chief clinical values of the QTc is in suggesting one of these causes to the physician when it might not have been apparent. There is some disagreement among cardiologists as to whether prolonged QTc in the presence of quinidine or procainamide represents *toxicity* of the drug or merely an *effect* of the drug. It is generally accepted that patients who suffer from "quinidine syncope"—ventricular tachycardia or fibrillation caused by quinidine—are patients who have a long QTc *before* quinidine administration. It is not clear whether patients are likewise at risk for ventricular dysrhythmias if the normal QTc before quinidine is prolonged after quinidine administration.

QRS AXIS

QRS axis is primarily a descriptive term which has some clinical utility. It is an attempt to summarize the directionality of the entire QRS complex in one single vectorial direction, as determined by the amplitude of the QRS in ECG leads of several lead directions. For example: if the entire QRS complex is oriented inferiorly, towards the feet, the QRS amplitude will be maximal in lead AVF (which has a similar lead direction), and the QRS will be small or isoelectric in lead I (which has a lead direction perpendicular to the QRS orientation).

There are several ways to determine QRS axis. One simple way is illustrated in Figure 4-8. In this case, in Lead I there is a net 3-mm positive deflection (R wave minus S wave); thus, whatever the QRS direction, its representation in the lead-I direction is + 3mm. In Lead II, there is a net 0-mm deflection (R wave minus S wave), so the QRS complex has zero representation in the lead-II direction. When plotted on a triaxial lead reference map, the intersection of the two dotted lines determines the location of the QRS axis. (It is mandatory to plot the third standard lead similarly, because the three plots do not always meet at a single point.)

A QRS axis to the right of + 90° is called **right-axis deviation.** An axis to the left (counterclockwise), between 0° and − 90°, is called **left-axis deviation.** The normal adult range of the QRS axis is between − 30° and + 90° (notice that left-axis deviation between 0° and − 30° is normal). Some normal adolescents may have deviation of the QRS axis as far right as + 105°; infants and young children normally have deviations of the QRS axis even further to the right. The clinical significance of these deviations will be discussed in a later section.

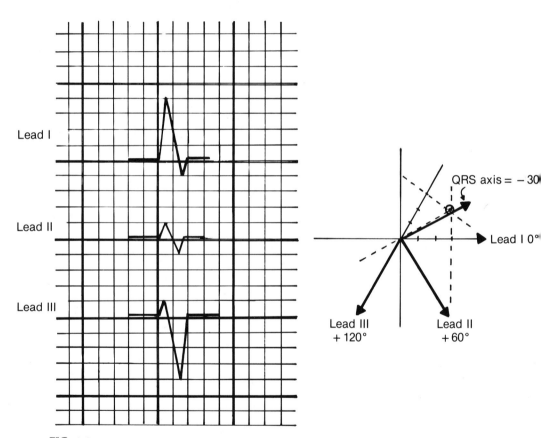

FIG. 4-8.
Determination of QRS axis by plotting QRS amplitudes on triaxial lead reference map (see text for details).

RHYTHM DETERMINATION

After determination of rate, standard intervals, and QRS axis, the next step in ECG-reading is to determine the predominating rhythm and any arrhythmias which might be present. (Arrhythmias are discussed in more detail in Chapters 11 and 12.)

The normal heart rhythm is sinus rhythm. Sinus rhythm has several characteristics:

1. All cycles begin with P waves.
2. All PR intervals are normal and constant (except when there is a conduction defect, which, while not normal, can be present even with sinus rhythm).
3. P waves have the characteristic form indicating sinus-node origin (see the section on P-wave form, below).
4. The rhythm is generally regular.
5. There are no "extra" P waves (P waves which do not conduct to the ventricles).
6. In a resting adult, the sinus rate is rarely over 160/min.

If not all of these characteristics are present, there is a good probability that the rhythm is not a sinus rhythm.

NORMAL ECG WAVE FORM

P Waves

P waves of sinus rhythm normally have a direction ("P-wave axis") between $+25°$ and $+65°$. This is the result of atrial activation, which begins in the right-atrial sinus node and spreads leftward and inferiorly. Consequently, a normal sinus-rhythm P wave will always be upright in leads I and II. If a P wave is inverted in lead I or II, it is likely that the atrial beat is of ectopic atrial origin (or that the ECG leads have been attached incorrectly).

P waves in sinus rhythm may vary in shape and amplitude from beat to beat within the same lead. This may reflect a shifting pacemaker location *within* the sinus node, and is not abnormal so long as the P-wave orientation remains consistent with sinus-node origin.

Left-atrial enlargement may be diagnosed when P-wave duration is longer than 0.12 sec in any lead. Most commonly this can be appreciated in the inferiorly oriented leads (II, III, AVF). Such P waves often are "double-humped" or "notched," but this is not essential for the diagnosis. Such P waves have been called "P-mitrale," because of their *M*-shape and their frequent association with mitral-valve disease. Often, left-atrial enlargement will produce, in lead V_1, a diphasic P wave with a broad and deep negative component. It should be remembered that diphasic P waves in V_1 are normal; it is the large area of negativity, more than 1 mm deep and broad, which suggests left-atrial enlargement.

Right-atrial enlargement may be diagnosed when P-wave amplitude in any sinus beat in any lead exceeds 0.25 mv (2.5 mm). Such P waves may be pointed or peaked. They have been called "P-pulmonale," because of their frequent association with right-sided cardiac disease (cor pulmonale or pulmonic stenosis).

Normal QRS Form

Unfortunately for the beginner, there is a wide range of normal QRS forms. The range of normal amplitudes for adults is summarized in Figure 4-9.

Some generalizations may be drawn about the normal QRS form. The normal QRS axis is between $-30°$ and $+90°$, inclusive. The QRS duration

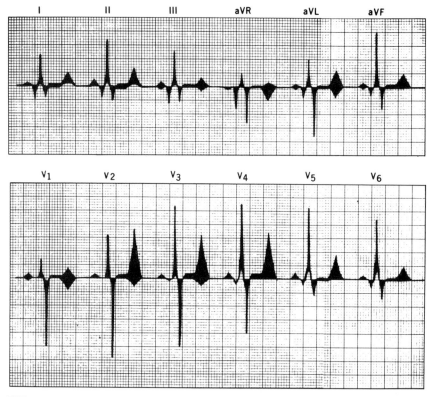

FIG. 4-9.
The composite normal electrocardiogram. The shaded areas for each lead represent the extremes of normal amplitudes for each wave in adults. Properties of time, wave form, and proportional relationships between waves are necessarily not included. (Ezra PS: The normal composite electrocardiogram. Circulation 24:710, 1961. Used by permission of the American Heart Association, Inc.)

does not exceed 0.10 seconds. The QRS complexes have an amplitude sufficient to exceed "low voltage" but not so great as to suggest ventricular enlargement (both of these subjects will be discussed later). The initial portion of the QRS complex does not have Q waves large enough to suggest myocardial infarction (also discussed later). In the precordial leads, V_1 is predominantly a negative deflection; as one proceeds leftward, toward V_4, the R waves gradually increase and S waves gradually decrease in size. By V_4 or V_5, the QRS complex is predominantly a positive deflection. By V_5 or V_6, there is little or no S wave.

QRS Abnormalities

Right-Axis Deviation. Abnormal right-axis deviation usually indicates right-ventricular enlargement, unless it is caused by other recognizable abnormalities, which include lateral-wall myocardial infarction, intraventricular conduction defects (especially right bundle-branch block), an occasional Wolff-Parkinson-White syndrome, and rarities such as dextrocardia.

Left-Axis Deviation. Abnormal left-axis deviation is *not* necessarily associated with left-ventricular enlargement. Most commonly, it is a nonspecific abnormality of the ECG, and there is not universal agreement that it is necessarily associated with heart disease. A slight amount of left-axis deviation, but rarely to an abnormal degree, is often encountered in obesity, pregnancy, ascites, or chronic lung disease.

Marked left-axis deviation, greater than $-50°$, is often indicative of delay or block in the anterior fascicle of the left bundle branch ("left anterior hemiblock"). Such complexes customarily show small R waves and deep S waves in the inferior leads (II, III, AVF) and may have deep S waves in all of the precordial leads.

Other specific causes of abnormal left-axis deviation include inferior-wall myocardial infarction, left-ventricular enlargement (in some patients), and occasionally the Wolff-Parkinson-White syndrome.

Low Voltage. Low voltage is defined as no limb-lead QRS total amplitude (sum of positive and negative) as big as 0.5 mv (5 mm). It does not specifically indicate disease or an abnormal heart; indeed, it is most frequently associated with conditions that affect conduction of cardiac electrical activity to the body surface. Some conditions associated with low voltage are:

1. Massive obesity
2. Emphysema
3. Pericardial effusion
4. Pleural effusion
5. Pneumonia
6. Pneumothorax
7. Cardiomyopathy
8. Hypothyroidism
9. Ascites

There are two circumstances in which low voltage assumes clinical importance. If a patient with previously normal QRS amplitudes has a new finding of low voltage, representing a marked decrease from previous amplitudes, the above clinical associations should be strongly considered.

The second circumstance in which low voltage has great clinical importance is during cancer chemotherapy with doxorubicin hydrochloride (Adriamycin), a drug with severe cardiotoxic potential. Low voltage of the ECG is the most reliable known simple indicator of the onset of such toxicity, and its onset is grounds for stopping the use of the drug.

Intraventricular Conduction Disorders. Intraventricular conduction disorders can be grouped into a few types:

1. Left bundle-branch block
2. Right bundle-branch block
3. Hemiblocks
4. Nonspecific intraventricular conduction defect
5. Wolff-Parkinson-White syndrome

Left Bundle-Branch Block. In this disorder, conduction to the ventricles from the atrioventricular node is through the right bundle branch only, or else conduction through the left bundle branch is so slow that the ECG cannot distinguish the delay from complete left block. In either event, activation of the ventricles is *not* simultaneous; the onset of activation of the right side occurs first, and left-sided activation does not begin until at least 0.04 sec later. The terminal portion of the QRS is entirely from left-ventricular activation. This produces the characteristic ECG picture:

1. QRS duration 0.12 sec or longer
2. Broad positive QRS in the "lateral leads" (I, AVL, V_{5-6}), often slurred or notched
3. Terminal portion of QRS oriented leftward and posteriorly—that is, deep S waves in V_{1-3}
4. No small "septal Q wave" in I or V_{5-6}
5. "Poor R-wave progression" in V_{1-3}—that is, R waves in these leads may be entirely missing, producing complexes of Q waves only, or the R waves will be low, not exceeding 2 mm
6. Associated abnormalities of ST segments and T waves

Left bundle-branch block is nearly always associated with heart disease, most commonly coronary artery disease. Other frequently associated disorders are aortic-valve disease, hypertensive disease, and idiopathic degeneration of the cardiac conduction system (Lenegre's disease). Left bundle-branch block rarely occurs as a congenital defect or in the absence of heart disease. Except in the setting of acute myocardial infarction, it requires no specific therapy. When it occurs in association with acute anterior-wall myocardial infarction, many cardiologists believe that insertion of a temporary artificial pacemaker is indicated (in case the right bundle branch subsequently fails).

The presence of left bundle-branch block renders the ECG valueless for any other diagnosis based on QRS form. This fact cannot be overemphasized. Thus, a patient with left bundle-branch block may have a myocardial infarction, and yet his ECG may give no reliable evidence of infarction. Similarly, the diagnosis of ventricular enlargement cannot be made in the presence of left bundle-branch block.

Right Bundle-Branch Block. In this disorder, conduction is either delayed or blocked in the right bundle branch, so that ventricular activation is through the left bundle. Thus, the onset of right-ventricular activation is delayed, and the terminal portion of the QRS complex is generated by right-ventricular activation. This produces the characteristic ECG:

1. QRS duration 0.12 sec or longer
2. The terminal QRS is oriented anteriorly and towards the right, producing:
   a. Broad S waves in the "lateral leads" (I, AVL, V_{5-6})
   b. Terminal R waves in AVR and V_{1-2}; V_1 often has R-S-R' complexes or may consist entirely of a broad, slurred R wave, or a Q wave followed by an R wave
3. The initial portion of the QRS complexes is relatively unaffected by right bundle-branch block.
4. Associated ST-T abnormalities, most commonly ST depression and inverted T waves in V_{1-3}

Right bundle-branch block is not rare as a congenital defect, occurring in an estimated 1 in 750 to 1 in 1000 apparently normal individuals. When it occurs in middle age, it most commonly is associated with coronary artery disease. It may also occur in Lenegre's disease, aortic-valve disease, and in association with right-ventricular enlargement. It requires no specific therapy except that when it occurs in association with acute anterior-wall myocardial infarction, many cardiologists feel that a temporary pacemaker should be inserted.

In contrast with left bundle-branch block, right bundle-branch block does *not* interfere with the ECG diagnosis of infarction, chamber enlargement, or other diagnoses based on QRS form.

The variant on the theme of right bundle-branch block is called **incomplete right bundle-branch block pattern.** This superficially resembles right bundle-branch block in that the terminal QRS direction is anterior and rightward, producing R' waves in lead AVR, and V_1 and S waves in leads I and V_{5-6}; however, the QRS duration is less than 0.12 sec., so that complete right bundle-branch block cannot be present. In other words, this term describes a wave pattern and not a bundle-branch block. Incomplete right bundle-branch block, pattern with normal QRS duration, is a fairly common finding in normal adolescents and young adults. When associated with heart disease, incomplete right bundle-branch block pattern may be the only ECG finding in patients with right-ventricular enlargement. It may occur transiently in patients with

pulmonary embolus. It is the commonest ECG finding in atrial septal defect.
Hemiblocks. In the middle 1960s, the Argentinian cardiologist Mauricio Ro-
senbaum discovered that the left bundle branch could be *functionally* subdivided
into two groups of fibers, which have been labelled the **left anterior fascicle** and
left posterior fascicle. Block of conduction in either of these fascicles produces
a characteristic ECG picture. These fascicular blocks have colloquially been
called **"hemiblocks,"** because they involve a conduction defect in "half" of the
left bundle. They do *not* ordinarily cause a prolonged QRS duration; rather,
they alter the QRS form characteristically.

Left anterior hemiblock has already been described, in the paragraph on
abnormal left-axis deviation, and includes a marked left-axis deviation over
− 45°. When left anterior hemiblock occurs in association with right bundle-
branch block, there is presumptive evidence of disease in both left and right
bundle branches. Patients with such findings should be followed closely, with
attention to an unusually slow pulse rate, and to any complaint of syncopal
episodes or dizzy spells. The combination of right bundle-branch block and left
anterior hemiblock is fairly common, and most patients with this combination
will *not* progress to complete bilateral bundle-branch block.

Left posterior hemiblock produces a rightward shift of the QRS axis, to
+ 105° or further right, in the absence of other disorders which could cause
right-axis deviation. Typically, lead I has a low R wave and a deeper, broader S
wave. Lead III has a Q wave, often impressively deep, and a tall R wave which
usually has a slurred or notched downstroke. Left posterior hemiblock is more
readily recognized in combination with right bundle-branch block, when the
combination indicates bilateral bundle-branch disease. Except for its relative
rarity, and more frequent progression to bilateral bundle-branch (complete
atrioventricular) block, the clinical implications of right bundle-branch block
and left posterior hemiblock are similar to those for left anterior hemiblock,
described above.

Nonspecific Intraventricular Conduction Defect. In addition to the disorders of
left and right bundle branches described in the preceding paragraphs, a wide
variety of other disorders can produce an abnormally long QRS duration (over
0.10 sec). These include:

1. Left- or right-ventricular enlargement
2. Cardiomyopathy, myocarditis
3. Disease of peripheral Purkinje network, without specific proximal
   bundle-branch block
4. Drug toxicity (quinidine, procainamide, disopyramide)
5. Hyperkalemia
6. "Peri-infarction block"

These conditions have no specific characteristics of QRS form which we
will consider here, except for their wide QRS and association with other evidence of heart disease.

Wolff-Parkinson-White Syndrome. This syndrome, named for those who first described it, is characterized by a short PR interval and a long QRS interval. Both are produced by an atrioventricular-node bypass tract, conducting an impulse from atrium to ventricle while the normally conducted impulse is still traversing the atrioventricular node. The QRS complex is prolonged because this "early" activation produces a small, slurred deflection at the beginning of the QRS, called a **delta wave.** The delta wave may be in any direction, in any lead; its direction depends on the location of the atrioventricular-node bypass tract, which may be at any location between the atria and either ventricle.

The Wolff-Parkinson-White syndrome is of clinical significance for two reasons: patients with it are commonly prone to paroxysmal supraventricular tachyarrhythmias, and the QRS form may be misdiagnosed, in some instances, as myocardial infarction.

MYOCARDIAL INFARCTION

The electrocardiogram is the single most useful tool in the diagnosis of myocardial infarction, in part because of its specificity. When myocardial infarction is properly diagnosed by ECG, one is nearly certain of the diagnosis. (Myocardial infarction, in this discussion, is limited to left-ventricular infarction. Infarctions of the atria and right ventricle occasionally happen, but these are not readily diagnosable by routine electrocardiography.) Unfortunately, the ECG has been estimated to be only 75% to 85% sensitive in diagnosis of infarctions, since a certain percentage of infarctions do not produce a definitively diagnostic ECG. However, even in cases in which the ECG is nondiagnostic, patients with an acute myocardial infarction will virtually never have normal, consecutive ECGs.

There are three general elements to the ECG diagnosis of acute myocardial infarction:

1. Characteristic change in QRS form; most often, this is the new appearance of abnormal Q waves not previously present
2. Characteristic evolutionary changes in ST segments and T waves
3. Localization of the above abnormalities to leads indicating a specific wall location—anterior, inferior, lateral, posterior

When all three of the above elements are present, the diagnosis is nearly 100% certain.

Lateral-Wall Infarction

Infarction in this location produces Q waves in leads I, AVL, and V_{5-6}. The Q waves are usually 0.04 sec, or wider. Their depth should be greater than 25% of the QRS amplitude in the lead in which they are measured. It should be remembered that lead AVL may, in some normal individuals, have large Q waves.

Inferior-Wall Infarction

Infarction in this location produces Q waves in leads II, III, and AVF. Remember that lead III may frequently have large Q waves in normal persons, and that lead AVF may have large Q waves in some normal persons. When all three inferior leads have Q waves 0.04 sec and wider, and greater than 25% of the QRS amplitude, inferior infarction is present. Sometimes the diagnosis can be made when new Q waves appear only in leads III and AVF which are clearly different from previous tracings, and the clinical setting and ST-T evolution are also compatible.

Anterior (anteroseptal) Infarction

Infarction in this location may have several forms in the precordial leads V_{1-3}:

1. Deep Q waves in leads V_{1-3} (some normal persons have Q waves in V_{1-2}.)
2. Decreasing R-wave height from V_1 to V_2, from V_2 to V_3, and V_3 to V_4
3. Marked reduction in V_{1-3} R-wave height from previous tracings
4. Small Q waves followed by R waves in V_{1-3}

If the Q waves of anterior infarction include V_1, some cardiologists believe that the anterior portion of the interventricular septum is also infarcted and label such an anteroseptal infarction. The pathologic confirmation of this differentiation is uncertain.

Posterior Infarction

Infarction of the posterior wall is quite uncommon, except in combination with inferior infarction. Since there is no conventional ECG lead peculiarly sensitive to posteriorly oriented cardiac activity, such infarctions cause "inverse" or "reciprocal" findings in the so-called anterior leads: unusually tall R waves in V_{1-3}.

Once the QRS complex has become deformed by infarction (has formed Q waves) it usually remains diagnostic of infarction for the remainder of the patient's life. On occasion, most often with inferior-wall infarction, the Q waves gradually disappear over a few years, and the QRS forms revert to normal. In such cases, estimated to be 10% to 15% of old inferior-wall myocardial infarctions, the ECG will revert to normal and show no evidence that there has been a previous infarction. The mechanism by which the QRS complex reverts to normal remains obscure.

ST-T Evolution of Infarction

A definite sequence of repolarization abnormalities occurs in acute infarction, in the same leads which show the Q waves of infarction. Although the time course of these repolarization abnormalities is quite variable, the sequence in which they occur is similar for all infarctions. The first finding of acute infarction is increased height of the T wave, perhaps associated with ST-segment elevation. This usually occurs before any change has occurred in QRS form and is not definitive evidence of infarction, but may serve as a strong suggestion of possible infarction in the appropriate clinical setting.

Within the next few minutes or hours after infarction, the ST segments become more elevated. Within one or more days, T-wave height decreases and the T waves become inverted. Usually within 2 to 7 days, the ST segments return to baseline and may become depressed.

The repolarization forms may remain like this, with ST depression and inverted T waves, for years or may gradually return to normal. It is the lack of sequential change on successive serial tracings that permits one to determine that the infarction is "old."

"Subendocardial Infarction"

In a small but definite minority of myocardial infarctions, the physician is reasonably certain that infarction has occurred; the clinical picture is typical, the serum enzymes have risen appropriately, and the ECG shows the typical ST-T evolution of infarction; yet the ECG never shows typical and diagnositic Q waves of infarction. Perhaps the infarction is too small to cause Q waves, or involves an area of left ventricle where the initial part of the QRS is not altered, or involves such a broad area as to lose the localized specificity of Q waves (as in a circumferential or "global" infarction, for example). Over the years, such infarctions have come to be called **subendocardial infarctions,** even though the pathology of such infarctions may be little different from infarctions with which the ECG developed Q waves. It would seem more accurate to call such infarctions **non-Q-wave infarctions,** since they are in every sense myocardial infarctions, act like infarctions, and should be treated as infarctions, regardless of whether or not the ECG develops Q waves.

VENTRICULAR ENLARGEMENT

Left-Ventricular Enlargement

Many sets of criteria are used to diagnose left-ventricular enlargement. In general, all are based on increased amplitude or duration of the QRS complex, especially in the leftward and posterior direction. In our laboratory, we have used the criteria of Sokolow; they combine simplicity, a reasonable sensitivity (admittedly undersensitive), and fairly good specificity (few false positives). The criteria are:

1. R wave in V_5 over 26 mm
2. R wave in V_5 plus S wave in V_1 over 35 mm

3. R wave in AVL over 12 mm
4. R wave in AVF over 19 mm
5. ST-T abnormalities

Any one of the above voltage criteria suffices. If there are no ST-T abnormalities, the diagnosis of left-ventricular enlargement is uncertain. (Some patients with pure aortic regurgitation may have left-ventricular enlargement voltage without the ST-T abnormalities.) These voltage criteria are not appropriate for young adults under age 35, who may normally have larger QRS amplitudes.

Right-Ventricular Enlargement

There are several quite different ways that right-ventricular enlargement may affect the electrocardiogram. Right-ventricular enlargement may manifest itself as a slowing or delay of right-ventricular activation, causing right bundle-branch block or an "incomplete right bundle-branch block pattern." Other possible manifestations of this condition may include the following:

1. **Right-Axis Deviation.** In general, in the absence of an interventricular conduction defect, lateral-wall infarction, Wolff-Parkinson-White syndrome, or other gross alteration of QRS form, right-axis deviation greater than $+105°$ in an adult is evidence of right-ventricular enlargement.

2. **Systolic Overload Pattern.** In lead V_1, R waves are taller than the S waves are deep, and the R waves are greater than 5 mm tall. R waves progressively *decrease* in height as one goes leftward across the precordium. Also, S waves may get progressively deeper as one goes leftward across the precordium. A voltage criterion in this respect is that S-wave depth in lead V_5 plus R-wave height in lead V_1 will be greater than 10.5 mm. The typical clinical picture causing this type of EKG is pulmonic stenosis.

3. **Diastolic Overload Pattern.** This may produce an incomplete or complete right bundle-branch block pattern, perhaps with more pointed R' waves in lead V_1 and S waves in leads V_{5-6} than usual for the typical right bundle-branch block.

4. **QRS Form of Cor Pulmonale or Chronic Lung Disease.** This is characterized by low voltage in the limb leads; the QRS axis may be right-deviated, left-deviated, normal, or indeterminate. There are deep S waves in all standard and precordial leads, often with poor R-wave progression in the precordial leads and a late QRS transition from predominantly negative to predominantly positive in the precordial leads. This transition may occur in leads V_5 or V_6 ("clockwise rotation").

Right-ventricular enlargement is usually accompanied by T-wave abnormalities, most often inverted T waves in leads V_{1-3} ("the leads over the right ventricle").

PULMONARY EMBOLUS

There are many manifestations of pulmonary embolism on the EKG. Nearly all patients with pulmonary embolism will have an EKG abnormality; unfortunately, only rarely will the EKG be sufficiently characteristic to suggest the diagnosis by itself. All or none of the following EKG abnormalities may occur in a patient with documented pulmonary embolism:

1. Atrial tachyarrhythmias, often transient; this may be atrial flutter, atrial fibrillation, or paroxysmal atrial tachycardia. There may be frequent premature atrial contractions.
2. Transient evidence of right-atrial enlargement (tall, peaked P waves)
3. Rightward shift of the QRS axis from its previous value, not necessarily to an abnormal right-axis deviation. (Some patients with pulmonary embolus get a *left*ward QRS axis shift.)
4. Transient new Q waves in lead III and perhaps in lead AVF. Occasionally, inferior-wall infarction may be mimicked.
5. Rightward shift of the terminal QRS direction, causing new appearance or increase in size of S waves in the lateral leads I, AVL, and V_{5-6}
6. Transient right bundle-branch block or incomplete right bundle-branch block pattern
7. ST-segment depression and T-wave inversion in the right precordial leads

None of these findings is specific or diagnostic, and the findings are often transient. It is the transient occurrence of several of the above EKG features which should suggest the possibility of pulmonary embolus.

ABNORMALITIES OF ST-SEGMENT AND T-WAVE FORM (ST-T ABNORMALITIES; REPOLARIZATION ABNORMALITIES)

The commonest abnormalities encountered in the ECG laboratory are those involving the ST segment and T-wave form. As described previously, slight alterations in recovery properties of the myocardium, either localized or widespread, may profoundly affect the repolarization waves of the ECG.

A wide variety of clinical disorders, both cardiac and noncardiac, may affect ST-T forms. Depending on how one counts, upward of 80 separate clinical diagnoses have been associated with repolarization abnormalities. For illustration, these conditions include, but are not limited to:

1. Heart disease: ischemic, valvular, inflammatory, traumatic, hypertensive, fast heart rates
2. Pericardial disease
3. Lung disease
4. Gastrointestinal disease: hiatus hernia, esophagitis, pancreatitis
5. Metabolic disorders: hypothyroidism, hypothermia
6. Electrolyte disorders
7. Drug effects: digitalis, quinidine, procainamide, disopyramide, phenytoin, tranquilizers, antihistamines
8. Central nervous system disorders
9. Normal variants

Unfortunately, the ST-T abnormalities so produced will only rarely be so typical of a single clinical entity as to be diagnostically useful by themselves. Most of the time, ST-T abnormalities are truly nonspecific. Any attempt to attach specific diagnostic content to these nonspecific abnormalities, out of the clinical setting in which they occur, is to be done with restraint. We deplore the practice, prevalent in some institutions, of labelling nonspecific ST-segment depression on routine resting ECGs as "evidence of cardiac ischemia" or "evidence of 'strain' " (whatever that is).

Despite this lack of specificity, findings of ST-T abnormalities serve several useful functions. First, they differentiate between "normal" and "abnormal" tracings. What this means is that 95% of "normal" individuals, with no evidence of heart disease or other illness, will have a normal ECG, including normal ST-T forms. When the ECG is normal (including ST-T forms), it is highly unlikely that there is any major structural abnormality of the ventricular myocardium. Note that one may often have a normal ECG in the presence of severe three-vessel coronary disease, but the ECG is rarely normal if myocardial "damage" (infarction) has occurred, or if there is left-ventricular enlargement or other structural defect.

Second, ST-T abnormalities may alert the clinician to the possibility of cardiac or other illness when it is not suspected.

Third, on occasion there may be an ST-T abnormality so typical of a clinical condition as to suggest it strongly to the clinician.

ST-T abnormalities have been classified by Abildskov as "primary" and "secondary." Primary repolarization abnormalities are those caused by an intrinsic alteration of recovery sequence in the ventricles, whether caused by localized myocardial disease (such as localized ischemia or segmental hypertrophy, for example) or by a more generalized effect on the ventricular myocardium (such as digitalis, hyperkalemia, or hypothyroidism, for example). Secondary ST-T abnormalities are those caused, or contributed to, by disorders of ventricular activation. If the ventricle is depolarized in an abnormal sequence, the onset of repolarization will also be in an abnormal sequence. Some examples of secondary repolarization abnormalities are those associated with left bundle-branch block or Wolff-Parkinson-White syndrome.

Some typical ST-T abnormalities (far from all of them) are described below; for illustrations, the student is referred to any standard ECG text.

Ischemia. Characteristically, ischemia causes ST depression in the leads associated with the ischemic area. For example, inferior-wall ischemia produces ST depression in leads II, III, and AVF. Unfortunately, this is not a unique form; it is indistinguishable from the ST depression of many other disorders.

(In exercise electrocardiography, this ST depression is diagnostically useful because exercise—an ischemia-inducing event—may produce a characteristic *change* from a normal preexercise control.)

Acute Pericarditis. This condition causes "nonlocalized," widespread ST elevation in most leads (AVR excepted)

Cardiac Drugs. Digitalis may cause ST depression and low or inverted T waves in many leads; unfortunately, this is not typical enough to be diagnostically useful. Neither can one estimate the "state of digitalization" from the amount of ST deviation. Quinidine causes prolongation of the QT and T wave, lower T waves, slight ST depression, and larger U waves, in most leads. Procainamide has an effect similar to that of quinidine. Propranolol, in most patients, has little effect on ECG wave forms.

Electrolyte Abnormalities. In general, the ECG is sensitive only to severe electrolyte disorders. Slight electrolyte abnormalities will not affect the ECG enough to be recognized. Hypokalemia causes QTc prolongation, low-amplitude T waves, and large U waves. Hyperkalemia produces very tall, pointed T waves; the QTc may be prolonged, in severe hyperkalemia. Hypocalcemia causes a prolonged QTc, in which a long, straight ST-segment is followed by a relatively normal T wave. Severe hypercalcemia produces a short ST-segment, with the T wave appearing to begin at the end of the QRS complex. The QTc may be abnormally short.

Left-Ventricular Enlargement. Characteristically the ECG has ST depression and inverted or low T waves in the "lateral leads" (I, II, AVL, and V_{5-6}). In former days, this was called "left-ventricular 'strain' pattern."

Right-Ventricular Enlargement. The ECG may have ST depression and deeply inverted T waves in V_{1-3}.

Central Nervous System Disorders. Severe injury or disease may produce the most striking of all repolarization abnormalities. The QTc may be extremely prolonged. T waves may be either upright or inverted, and extremely broad and symmetrical, lacking the normal skewed shape.

SUGGESTED READING

Chung EK: Electrocardiography: Practical Applications with Vectorial Principles, ed. 2. Hagerstown, Harper & Row, 1980

Friedman HH: Diagnostic Electrocardiography and Vectorcardiography, ed. 2. New York, McGraw-Hill, 1977

Marriott HJL: Practical Electrocardiography, ed. 6. Baltimore, Williams & Wilkins, 1977

CLINICAL APPLICATIONS
OF ECHOCARDIOGRAPHY

James L. Potts

5

The application of the reflected ultrasound technique to medical diagnosis was begun in 1954 by Edler and Hertz. Ultrasound examination of various organs of the body had been performed prior to this time, but it was the collaboration of Edler and Hertz that marked the real beginning of echocardiography. In 1961, Edler, Gustafson, Karlefors, and Christenson published a comprehensive review of the entire field of echocardiography in a supplement of *Acta Medica Scandinavia*. A tremendous undertaking, this review described the ultrasound technique for the detection of mitral stenosis, left-atrial tumors, anterior pericardial effusion, and (quite remarkably) motion of the tricuspid valve, which is still difficult to visualize. This work stood as the most comprehensive review of the field of echocardiography for several years.

Dr. Claude Joyner is credited with the initial application of ultrasound for cardiac diagnosis in the United States. In 1963, while at the University of Pennsylvania, he collaborated with John Reid, who had built an ultrasonoscope, and they published the results of their assessment of the mitral valve in patients with normal hearts and in patients with mitral stenosis. In the latter part of 1963, Dr. Harvey Feigenbaum began to examine the posterior left-ventricular wall with ultrasound, and he later described the characteristic echo patterns in patients with pericardial effusions. Interestingly, he spent some time in Dr. Joyner's laboratory refining his own technique for echocardiography. These two men, Joyner and Feigenbaum, are primarily responsible for the growth and development of echocardiography in the United States.

Today echocardiography has attained a high degree of precision as a diagnostic tool. A major recent advance in echocardiography has been the development and clinical application of real-time two-dimensional or cross-sectional echocardiography, which displays cardiac events as they are occurring. This technique also provides specific information on spatial relationships of echo-

69

producing cardiac structures which serves to supplement the information attained from the standard M-mode echocardiogram.

TECHNIQUE AND PRINCIPLES OF
ULTRASOUND IMAGING

Detailed information on the physical properties of ultrasound and ultrasonic
transducers is beyond the scope of this text. Readers are referred to the standard textbooks of echocardiography for detailed information on the physical
properties of ultrasound and the principles of ultrasound imaging.

The apparatus employed for cardiac ultrasound imaging is an ultrasonoscope, which utilizes the same principles as the old sonar equipment which was
used to detect submarines. The sound emitted is called **ultrasound** because it is
above the level of the human hearing range, which is 18,000 Hz or 18,000 cycles
per second. The essential components of any ultrasonoscope are: 1) a transducer for the generation and reception of sound waves; 2) an oscilloscopic
screen for the display of the echo pattern; 3) an electrocardiogram system for
timing of the echocardiographic events; and 4) a recorder, which is used to
make a permanent graphic display of the ultrasound data.

The ultrasound impulses are generated by a piezoelectric crystal, located in
the transducer. This crystal has the unique property of being able to expand and
contract when an electric current is passed through it. The change in shape of
the crystal creates a series of compressions and rarefactions in the air—the ultrasound waves. The waves travel away from the transducer in a straight line,
and a portion of the ultrasound is reflected back to the transducer at each interface which the waves encounter. Sound waves ("echoes") return to strike the
piezoelectric crystal, setting up electrical impulses which are fed into a receiver,
where they are processed, amplified, and displayed as echo signals on an oscilloscopic screen. The crystal is therefore responsible for both the generation and
reception of the ultrasound waves.

The ultrasound waves or signals are usually displayed in "A-mode" or
"M-mode" for cardiac imaging. *A* stands for amplitude; the display for the
standard A-mode presents the ultrasound waves or echoes as a series of spikes.
M stands for motion; in the M-mode, the ultrasound waves are displayed as
constantly moving objects. The B-mode (brightness mode) is used primarily for
nonmoving structures. It utilizes intensity modulation to convert the amplitude
of the ultrasound wave (spike) to intensity, represented by a dot.

The sound emitted by the crystal located in the transducer has a frequency
of 1 to 5 million Hz, which is well above the human hearing range. Basically the
crystal emits ultrasound in 1-μsec bursts at a repetition rate of 1000 times per
sec. This means, then, that the crystal emits ultrasound only 0.1% of the time
and receives or "listens" 99.9% of the time. The velocity with which the ultrasound wave travels through a medium is related to the density of the medium.

The physical properties of the ultrasound wave are similar to those of light in that the wave travels in a straight line and is reflected back by an interface of adjacent structures of varying densities. For example, air and skin act as a reflecting interface; so do blood and heart valves, and also the walls of the lung and heart. The velocity at which ultrasound travels through specific tissues is constant; in human tissues this velocity is 1540 m per sec. If one knows the velocity at which sound is traveling through a medium and the time that it takes for the ultrasound to leave the transducer, strike the interface, and return to the transducer, then it is possible to calculate the distance between the reflecting surface and the transducer. By calibrating the ultrasonoscope for the velocity of sound traveling through tissue, then conversion of time to distance is automatically done, and the distance between each reflecting surface can be measured, so that the dimensions of various cardiac structures can be calculated. These principles represent the basis for ultrasound imaging.

The ultrasound examination is performed with the patient in a reclining position. The transducer is applied to the anterior chest wall in the third or fourth intercostal space. An airless contact is facilitated by the use of a coupling gel. The transducer is held perpendicular to the heart, and various technical adjustments are made until the cardiac structures are identified.

APPLICATIONS OF ECHOCARDIOGRAPHY

By definition, the echocardiogram is a graphic representation of the motion and characteristics of heart valves and heart walls that is obtained with the use of the ultrasound. In addition, precise measurements of cardiac dimensions and motion velocities of various cardiac structures are obtainable from the echocardiogram.

Echocardiography is an important diagnostic technique because it provides precise information about cardiac structure and cardiac function with a noninvasive procedure. For orientation, a diagrammatic representation of the heart is made with the echo patterns produced by the various cardiac structures as the transducer angle is changed. By making a continuous sweep along a straight line from the base of the heart and aorta to the cardiac apex with the hand-held transducer and simultaneously recording the echo patterns, a one-dimensional echo scan is produced. As the transducer is angled from a superior medial position to an inferior lateral position, the ultrasound beam successively encounters the aortic root and walls, aortic cusps, posterior left-atrial wall, right-ventricular chamber, interventricular septum, anterior mitral leaflets, posterior mitral leaflets, left-ventricular chamber, and posterior left-ventricular wall. A schematic representation of a one-dimensional sector scan is shown in Figure 5-1. This one-dimensional scan is essential for the accurate interpretation of the echocardiogram and for definition of anatomical relationships among the various cardiac structures.

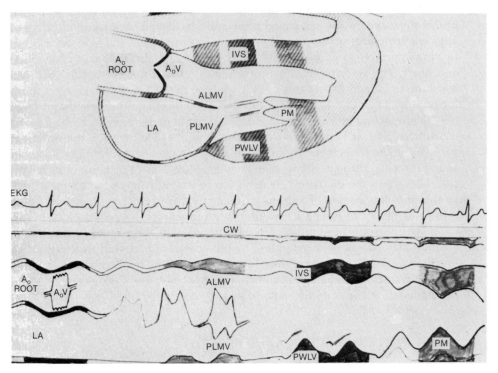

FIG. 5-1.
Schematic of a one-dimensional sector scan. **CW,** chest wall; **Ao Root,** aortic root; **AoV,** aortic valve; **LA,** left atrium; **ALMV,** anterior mitral leaflet; **PLMV,** posterior mitral leaflet; **IVS,** interventricular septum; **PWLV,** posterior left-ventricular wall.

ASSESSMENT OF VALVULAR FUNCTION AND CHARACTERISTICS

Mitral-Valve Assessment

The mitral valve is an important structure to identify on the echocardiogram. It is easy to record but, more important, the distinctive *M*-shaped pattern of the mitral valve also makes it easy to recognize, so that it serves as a point of reference, and the motion of the mitral leaflets and leaflet characteristics are important in many pathological conditions. Figure 5-2 shows an example of a normal mitral-valve echogram. The letter designations represent specific physiologic cardiac events. The A wave is the mechanical component of the P wave on the electrocardiogram and represents atrial systole; the B-point represents the beginning of left-ventricular systole; the C-point represents mitral closure; the D-point represents the beginning of diastole and the onset of mitral-valve opening; the E-point represents the peak opening of the mitral valve, and the F-point represents the end of the rapid filling wave of the left ventricle which results in

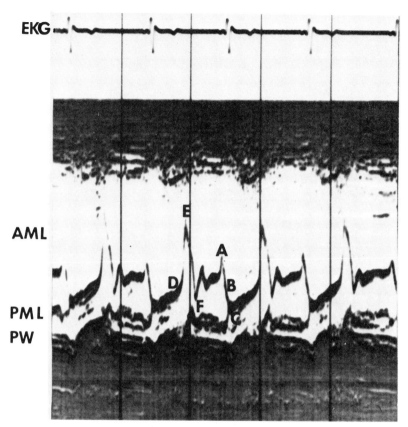

FIG. 5-2.
Normal mitral-valve echogram. **AML,** anterior mitral leaflet; **PML,**
posterior mitral leaflet; **PW,** posterior ventricular wall; **Sep,**
interventricular septum.

partial closure of the mitral valve. The following examples are some of the specific echocardiographic manifestations of pathological conditions affecting the
mitral valve.

Pathological Conditions of the Mitral Valve

Mitral Stenosis. It was the assessment of mitral stenosis that launched echocardiography as a diagnostic tool. There are several important points concerning
the echocardiographic features of mitral stenosis that deserve to be emphasized.
Edler and Hertz first observed in 1954 that the echo pattern of the mitral valve
in patients with mitral stenosis showed a distinctive distortion when compared
to the pattern of normal persons. They found that the typical double-peaked,
M-shaped pattern found in normal individuals was replaced by a plateaulike

distortion of the pattern in patients with mitral stenosis, which results in a reduction in the mitral valve E-F slope, which is the maximal slope obtained by drawing a line from the E-point to the F-point on the anterior mitral-leaflet echogram (Fig. 5-3). In addition, the echoes from the mitral leaflet in patients with mitral stenosis appeared to be more dense than in those patients with normal mitral valves. It then became apparent that there was a correlation between the E-F slope of the mitral valve and the severity of mitral stenosis. Joyner believed that this correlation was precise; however, more recent data indicate that there is only a rough correlation between the E-F slope and the mitral-valve area. It is not surprising that the correlation is less than perfect, since the E-F slope of the mitral valve is related to several different factors: 1) flow across the mitral valve; 2) heart rate; 3) pressure changes between the left atrium and left ventricle; 4) movement of the atrioventricular ring; 5) left-ventricular compliance. Cope studied the correlation between the E-F slope and the mitral-valve area in 61 patients in 1975 and found that the correlation is only fair. Analysis of data from this study showed that 75% of the patients with E-F slopes < 15 mm/sec had mitral-valve areas < 1.1 cm^2.

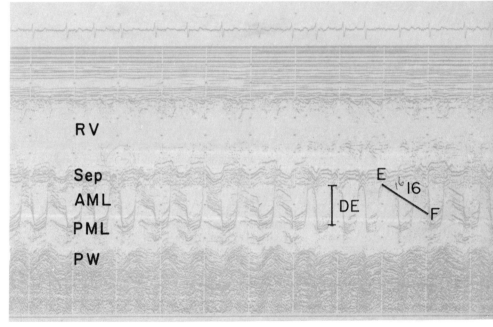

FIG. 5-3.
Mitral stenosis demonstrating a reduced EF slope. **RV,** right ventricle; **Sep,** interventricular septum; **AML,** anterior mitral leaflet; **PML,** posterior mitral leaflet; **PW,** posterior wall; **DE,** opening excursion of the anterior mitral leaflet; **E—F,** E-F slope.

The characteristic echocardiographic features of mitral stenosis are:

1. Reduction of the E-F slope
2. Thickened mitral leaflets
3. Poor mitral-valve excursions
4. Anterior movement of the posterior mitral leaflet

In summary then, the E-F slope may be an unreliable basis for quantitating the severity of mitral stenosis in the individual patient, but it is extremely useful for determining whether mitral stenosis is present. Formerly, the anterior movement of the posterior leaflet was considered an essential finding for the correct diagnosis of mitral stenosis. However, Levisman found that the posterior leaflet of the mitral valve exhibited normal motion in 10% of the patients in his study with proven mitral stenosis.

Mitral-Valve Prolapse. **Mitral-valve prolapse** and **Barlow's syndrome** are the terms most widely used to describe the disorder which produces distinctive auscultatory findings and a myriad of associated signs and symptoms. The prevalence rate of the syndrome in the general population, according to echocardio-

Mitral Valve Prolapse

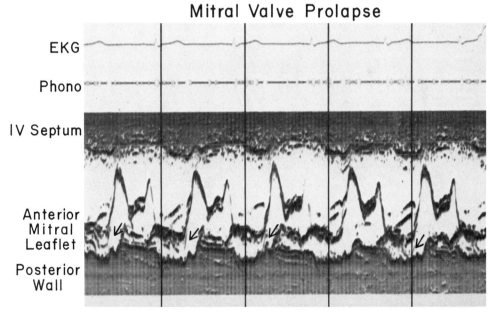

FIG. 5-4.
Mitral valve prolapse. **Arrows** indicate prolapsing mitral leaflets (**IV,** interventricular).

graphic studies, ranged between 8 and 17%. The echocardiographic features include posterior buckling of one or both leaflets in systole, absence of the normal
anterior rise of the anterior mitral leaflet, pansystolic or "hammocklike" bowing
of the mitral leaflets, and a profile of the prolapsing leaflets against the left-atrial
wall (Fig. 5-4). The echocardiogram is diagnostic for this condition, and angiographic studies are no longer necessary to confirm the diagnosis of mitral-valve
prolapse.

The echocardiogram is not a reliable tool for diagnosing mitral regurgitation produced by other varieties of cardiac disorder such as rheumatic mitral
regurgitation, cardiomyopathy, and mitral regurgitation secondary to papillary-
muscle dysfunction.

Aortic-Valve Assessment

The normal characteristics of the aortic valve, as well as abnormalities of the
aortic valve, can be accurately assessed by echocardiography. Figure 5-5 shows
an echogram of a normal aortic valve and demonstrates that the dimension of
the left atrium can be accurately measured in this view. Thickening of the aortic
cusp and decreased aortic-cusp separation can be accurately determined by

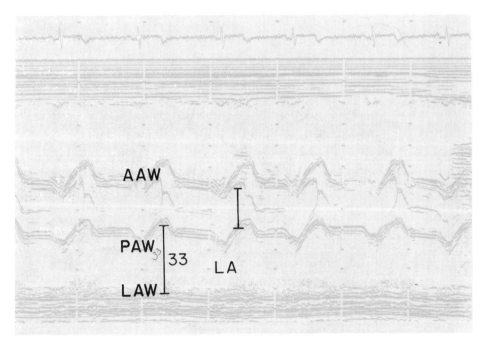

FIG. 5-5.
Normal aortic-valve echogram with left atrial dimension. **AAW,** anterior aortic wall;
PAW, posterior aortic wall; **LAW,** left atrial wall; **LA,** left atrium.

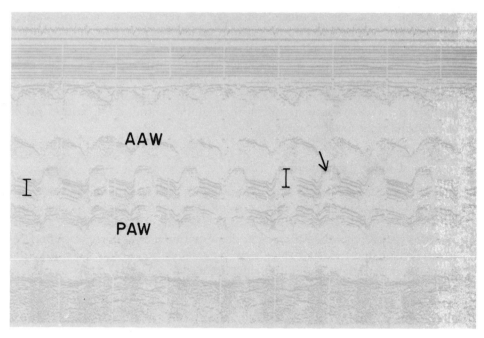

FIG. 5-6.
Abnormal aortic-valve echogram. **Arrow** indicates thickened aortic leaflets with thickened echoes in diastole (**I**) and a reduced cusp separation in systole (**I**). (**AAW,** anterior aortic wall; **PAW,** posterior aortic wall.)

echocardiography (Fig. 5-6). It has been disappointing that there is a poor correlation between the separation of the aortic cusp and hemodynamically derived calculations of aortic-valve areas. Chang and her coworkers recently studied echocardiographic determination of cusp separation in patients with aortic stenosis and concluded that cusp deformity invalidated the measurement of midsystolic cusp separation as an index of the severity of aortic stenosis.

The dimension of the aortic root can be determined by echocardiography, and it is also possible to detect bicuspid aortic valves. The technique cannot be heavily relied on for the diagnosis of aortic dissection, however, since it has yielded a large number of both false negative and false positive diagnoses of aortic dissection.

Aortic regurgitation produces a characteristic echocardiographic pattern, but it is the mitral leaflet that reflects evidence for aortic regurgitation. In chronic aortic regurgitation, the anterior leaflet of the mitral valve demonstrates high-frequency oscillations in diastole. These oscillations are produced when the regurgitant jet of blood from the aorta strikes the anterior mitral leaflet and causes it to vibrate. In acute aortic regurgitation, the mitral leaflets demonstrate premature closure before the end of the diastolic filling period. The premature closure of the leaflets is caused by a rapid reversal of the normal diastolic pressure gradient between the left atrium and left ventricle, as a consequence of the acute volume load imposed on the left ventricle.

Figures 5-7 and 5-8 are examples of the mitral-valve echo pattern in chronic, and acute, aortic regurgitation. It is important to list other conditions in which fluttering of the anterior leaflet of the mitral valve has been seen: these include mitral stenosis with calcification of the mitral valve, mitral insufficiency, and right-to-left shunts.

Tricuspid-Valve Assessment

The tricuspid valve will show the same abnormalities as the mitral valve. The tricuspid valve is technically more difficult to record because of its anatomical position. A reduction of the E-F slope of the tricuspid valve has the same significance as reduction of the E-F slope of the mitral valve. The correlation between the E-F slope and tricuspid-valve stenosis is much poorer, however, than that between the E-F slope and mitral-valve stenosis.

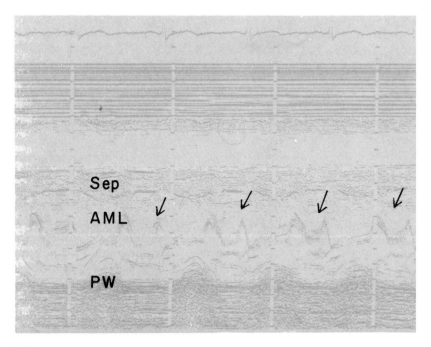

FIG. 5-7.
Mitral-valve oscillations in chronic aortic regurgitation. **Arrows** indicate high-frequency oscillations of the anterior mitral leaflet seen in chronic aortic regurgitation. **Sep,** interventricular septum; **AML,** anterior mitral leaflet; **PW,** posterior wall.

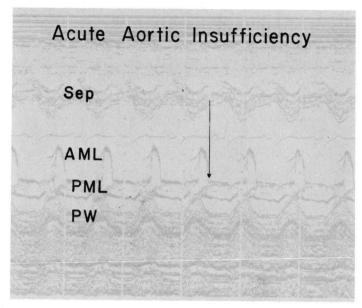

FIG. 5-8.
Mitral-valve echogram in acute aortic regurgitation. **Arrow** indicates premature closure of the anterior and posterior mitral leaflets in acute aortic regurgitation. **Sep,** interventricular septum; **AML,** anterior mitral leaflet; **PML,** posterior mitral leaflet; **PW,** posterior wall.

When echocardiograms of the mitral and tricuspid valves are recorded simultaneously, the results can be diagnostic for Ebstein's anomaly of the tricuspid valve. Figure 5-9 is an example, showing exaggerated motion of the tricuspid leaflet and tricuspid closure occurring 0.08 seconds after mitral closure.

Pulmonic-Valve Assessment

The pulmonic valve is recordable in 40 to 60% of normal persons and the percentage of diagnostic pulmonic-valve echograms increases with patients who have pulmonary hypertension. Figure 5-10 shows a normal pulmonic-valve echogram. The A wave of the pulmonic valve is usually > 4 mm, the opening slope is usually < 300 mm, the pulmonic-valve excursions are usually > 9 mm, and the diastolic E-F slope on the pulmonic valve is steep. The pattern of motion characteristics of the pulmonic valve is altered by pulmonary hypertension in a predictable manner. There is loss of the A wave with an increased velocity of the opening slope, and decreased excursions of the pulmonic valve with a flat pulmonic-valve E-F slope.

FIG. 5-9.

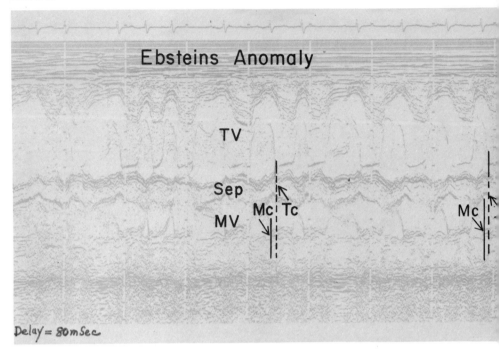

Ebsteins Anomaly

TV

Sep

MV   Mc Tc   Mc

Delay = 80 mSec

FIG. 5-10.

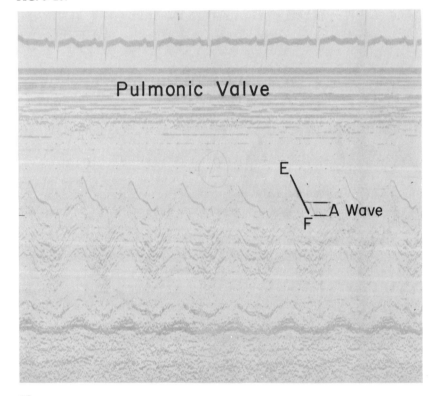

Pulmonic Valve

E

F ⎽ A Wave

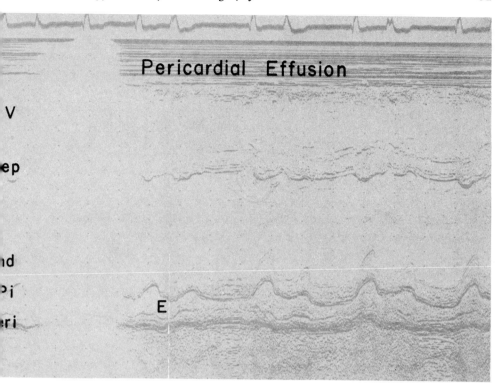

V

ep

ıd

ɔi

ɛri

FIG. 5-11.
Pericardial effusion. **RV,** right ventricle; **Sep,** interventricular septum; **End,** endocardium; **Epi,** epicardium; **Peri,** pericardium; **E,** effusion.

PERICARDIAL EFFUSION

One of the most frequent uses of echocardiography is for the detection of pericardial effusion. Normally the posterior left-ventricular wall and the pericardium are not separated and can be expected to produce a single echo. With accumulation of fluid in the pericardium, the left-ventricular epicardium and pericardium each produce separate, distinctive echo patterns. This is because both the pericardium and epicardium individually act as strong reflecting surfaces when they are separated by an accumulation of pericardial fluid (Fig. 5-

◀**FIG. 5-9.**
Ebstein's anomaly of the tricuspid valve. Tricuspid-valve closure is delayed by 80 msec or 0.08 sec. (**TV,** tricuspid valve; **Sep,** interventricular septum; **MV,** mitral valve; **Mc,** mitral closure; **Tc,** tricuspid closure.)

◀**FIG. 5-10.**
Normal pulmonic-valve echogram. **A,** pulmonic valve A wave; **E—F** indicates the diastolic slope of the pulmonic valve.

11). The echocardiogram is probably the most accurate and the most sensitive tool for the detection of pericardial effusions. As little as 20 cc of pericardial fluid can be detected by this method.

CARDIAC TUMORS

Effert is credited with the original echocardiographic diagnosis of an atrial tumor or clot in 1959. The echocardiographic features of an atrial myxoma are particularly distinctive. The mitral valve is used as a landmark, and a mass or cloud of echoes beneath the mitral valve is the distinctive finding most commonly present in patients having an atrial myxoma. Prior to 1972, only nine reported cases of atrial myxoma had been diagnosed previous to operation by echocardiogram. We studied patients with atrial myxoma in our laboratory. One important finding was that the size of the myxoma affected certain key features of the echocardiogram. More specifically, the length of the echo-free interval and the change in the mitral valve E-F slope appeared to be related to the size of the atrial myxoma. Figures 5-12A and B are pre- and post-operative examples of a patient with an atrial myxoma which was surgically removed. The diagnosis of atrial myxoma is now made much more frequently and with greater accuracy with echocardiography.

LEFT-VENTRICULAR FUNCTION

One of the most promising areas for application of echocardiography has been in the noninvasive assessment of left-ventricular function. A word of caution is warranted, however, because the derived echocardiographic parameters for de-

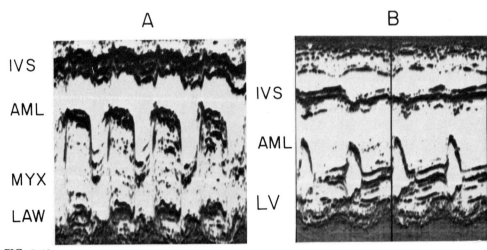

FIG. 5-12.
(A) Atrial myxoma before surgery. (B) Atrial myxoma after surgery. **IVS,** interventricular septum; **AML,** anterior mitral leaflet; **MYX,** myxoma; **LAW,** left-atrial wall; **LV,** left ventricle.

termining left-ventricular function are based on the assumption that the left ventricle—obviously untrue—is a symmetrically contracting chamber which has the configuration of a prolate ellipse.

The left-ventricular dimensions are obtained by measuring the distances between the endocardial surfaces of the septum and the free wall of the left ventricle at end diastole and peak systole (Fig. 5-13). The other parameters of left-ventricular function are derived from these two basic measurements: these include the ejection fraction, the percentage of cord-shortening, the rate of circumferential fiber-shortening, and posterior-wall velocities.

Echocardiographically Derived Left-Ventricular Function Parameters

Ventricular volumes

$$\text{End diastolic volume} = \text{EDD}^3$$

$$\text{End systolic volume} = \text{ESD}^3$$

$$\textit{Percentage (\%) of cord-shortening} = \frac{\text{EDD} - \text{ESD}}{\text{EDD}} \times 100$$

$$\textit{Ejection fraction} = \frac{\text{EDD}^3 - \text{ESD}^3}{\text{EDD}^3} \times 100$$

$$\textit{Posterior-wall velocity} = \text{slope mm/sec}$$

$$\textit{Circumferential fiber-shortening} = \frac{\text{EDD} - \text{ESD}}{\text{EDD} \times \text{ET}}$$

Key: EDD = end diastolic dimension
　ESD = end systolic dimension
　ET　= ejection time

The rate of circumferential fiber-shortening is accepted as one of the most accurate measurements of the level of left-ventricular function. Quinones and his coworkers found that the rates of circumferential fiber shortening derived echocardiographically correlated well with those derived angiographically. In addition, the mean rate derived from the echocardiogram separated normal from abnormal cases in eleven of twelve patients with coronary artery disease.

In cases where there is segmental disease of the left ventricle, the volumes and ejection fractions derived from the echocardiogram may be unreliable. Fortunately, the rate of circumferential fiber-shortening still appears to be reliable, even in patients with this condition.

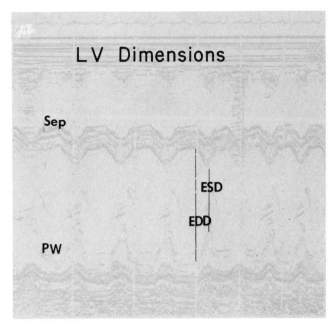

FIG. 5-13.
Left-ventricular dimensions. **Sep,** interventricular septum;
PW, posterior wall; **ESD,** end systolic dimension; **EDD,**
end diastolic dimension.

CONGENITAL HEART DISEASE

Echocardiography is particularly useful in helping to determine cardiac anatomy in patients with congenital heart disease. Pediatric cardiologists rely heavily on the echocardiogram for the detection of such complicated congenital
anomalies as transposition of the great vessels, Ebstein's anomaly, atrio-ventric-
ular cushion defects, atrial septal defect, hypoplastic left heart syndromes, and
for detection of left-ventricular outflow obstruction.

In adult cardiology, two of the most common congenital cardiac defects are
accurately diagnosed by echocardiography. These are the atrial septal defect
and asymmetric septal hypertrophy, with or without outflow obstruction.

Atrial septal defect is the third most common congenital cardiac disorder
found in the adult population. In patients with atrial septal defect, one looks for
evidence of right-ventricular volume overload, which includes an increased
right-ventricular dimension, paradoxical motion of the interventricular septum,
and a normal pulmonic-valve a-wave amplitude when there is no pulmonary
hypertension. Figure 5-14 shows an example of these features.

Asymmetrical septal hypertrophy is the congenital abnormality characterized by an increased thickness of the interventricular septum, out of proportion

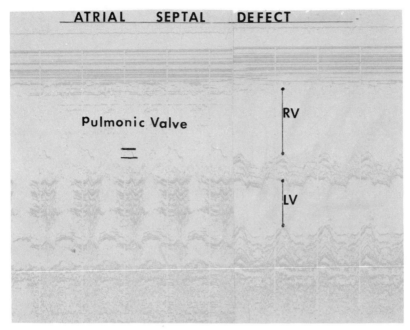

FIG. 5-14.
Echogram features of atrial septal defect. = indicates height of
pulmonic-valve A wave; **RV**, right ventricle; **LV**, left ventricle. (Note:
interventricular septal motion is paradoxical.)

to the thickness of the left-ventricular free wall. The echocardiographic features
of asymmetric septal hypertrophy are:

1. A markedly thickened interventricular septum, with a septal to
   free-wall thickness ratio > 1.5
2. Systolic anterior motion of the mitral valve, if there is outflow
   obstruction
3. Fusion of the anterior mitral leaflet with the septum, indicating a
   small left-ventricular cavity dimension.

It is now possible to quantitate the degree of outflow obstruction and to assess
the effect of various interventions on the amount of outflow obstruction caused
by motion of the mitral valve. Figure 5-15 is an example of this abnormality.

VALVULAR VEGETATIONS

One of the newer applications of echocardiography has been the detection of
vegetations on cardiac valves caused by endocarditis. The echo patterns are var-
ied, but the most commonly found features are:

IHSS

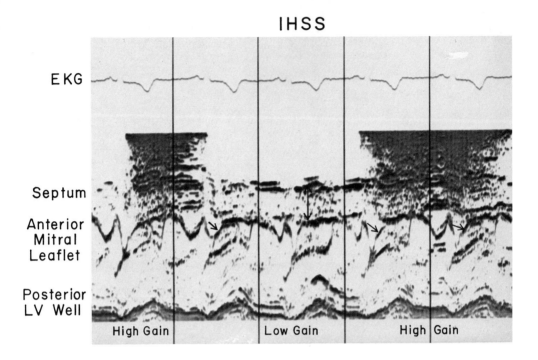

EKG

Septum

Anterior
Mitral
Leaflet

Posterior
LV Well

High Gain   Low Gain   High Gain

FIG. 5-15.
Echogram features of idiopathic hypertrophic subaortic stenosis. **Arrows** indicate left-ventricular septal thickness and systolic anterior motion (SAM) of mitral valve.

1. Thickened, shaggy echoes from the valve leaflets
2. Flail leaflets with evidence of fluttering of the involved leaflets
3. Increased excursions of the septum and free wall, indicative of volume overload

In cases of acute aortic regurgitation caused by valvular vegetations, there is premature closure of the mitral valve. Figures 5-16 and 5-17 are examples of vegetations on the mitral and aortic valves, respectively.

All of these findings are extremely helpful in evaluating patients with fever and new heart murmurs, since one is somewhat hesitant to catheterize these extremely ill patients because of the high risk of causing systemic embolization of the bacterial vegetations and because more profound congestive heart failure may be produced during the catheterization procedure itself. A word of caution is warranted: normal echocardiograms have been found in cases of proven endocarditis in studies performed in our laboratory and in other laboratories.

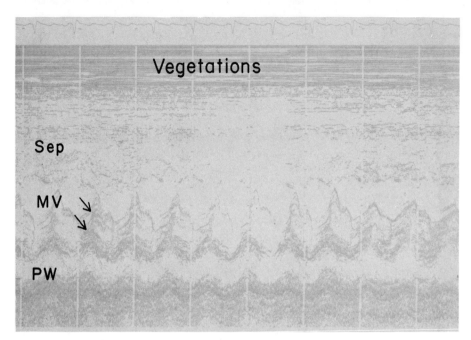

FIG. 5-16.
Mitral-valve vegetations. **Arrows** indicate vegetations in diastole. (**Sep,** interventricular septum; **MV,** mitral valve; **PW,** posterior left-ventricular wall.

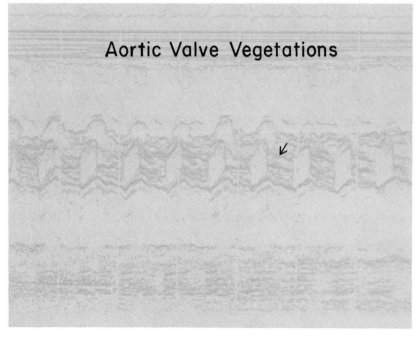

FIG. 5-17.
Aortic-valve vegetations. **Arrow** indicates vegetations in diastole.

SECTOR SCANS

The newest development in echocardiography is marked by the use of two-dimensional real-time sector scans of the heart. This allows for cross-sectional visualization of the heart by use of a single crystal or multiple crystals. It is a complex arrangement but provides highly resolved two-dimensional scans of the heart in real time.

There are three basic systems for obtaining real-time cross-sectional scans of the heart. They are:

1. The multi-element transducer array system
2. The mechanical driven transducer system
3. The phrased array transducer system

Sector scans, or cross-sectional echocardiography, have been used clinically for about 3 years. The method has served to clarify some anatomical relationships which conventional echocardiograms had been unable to show.

The basic principle for obtaining two-dimensional cross-sectional images by ultrasound is the same, regardless of the system which is used. Whereas the M-mode echocardiograms visualize the bodily structures in a single straight line, the two-dimensional systems visualize the structures along many straight lines in a plane. Multiple B-scan (brightness-mode) recordings of a section of the heart build up a composite image in which each bright dot represents a structural interface encountered by the echo beam.

A somewhat oversimplified view of this process is that a single bright dot represents each structural interface encountered by the ultrasound beam. For example, the right-ventricular endocardium would produce a dot, the right-ventricular septum a dot, and so on, until a brightness scan of the heart is produced through that plane. If one multiplies these lines and obtains B-mode images, then a sector scan of the heart is produced. Figure 5-18A and B represents a schematic drawing and an actual example of a two-dimensional sector of the long axis of the left ventricle.

Popp and his coworkers reported on the diagnostic accuracy of the multi-element transducer system and were able to obtain studies of diagnostic quality in 62% of the patients studied. The correct diagnosis was obtained in 45 of 47 patients with structural cardiac disease.

There are several reports of the measurement of mitral-valve orifice areas in patients with mitral-valve disease by real-time, two-dimensional echocardiography. Henry and his coworkers found that the mitral-valve area measured by two-dimensional echocardiography was within 0.3 cm^2 of the orifice area measured at operation in 86% of their patients who came to surgery for mitral-valve disease.

Measurement of aortic orifice areas by two-dimensional echocardiography has been less precise. The aortic valve is more difficult to localize and record because the valve orifice passes rapidly through the echo beam in a superior-inferior direction during left-ventricular systole. Weyman and his coworkers re-

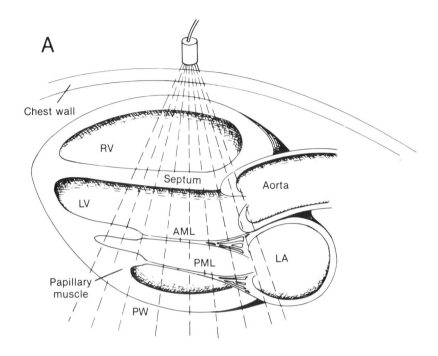

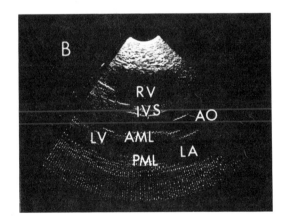

FIG. 5-18.
(A) Schematic of sector scan. **RV**, right ventricle; **LV**, left ventricle;
AML, anterior mitral leaflet; **PML**, posterior mitral leaflet; **LA**, left
atrium; **PW**, posterior left-ventricular wall. **(B)** Example of long-axis
sector scan. **RV**, right ventricle; **IVS**, interventricular septum; **AO**, aorta;
LV, left ventricle; **AML**, anterior mitral leaflet; **LA**, left atrium.

ported that there is a good correlation between the measured aortic-valve diameter obtained from two-dimensional echocardiography and the severity of aortic stenosis found at cardiac catheterization.

SUGGESTED READING

Chang S, Clements S, Chang J: Aortic stenosis: echocardiographic cusp separation and surgical description of the aortic valve in 22 patients. Am J Cardiol 39:499–504, 1977

Edler I: The diagnostic use of ultrasound in heart disease. Acta Med Scand [Suppl] 308:32, 1955

Edler I, Hertz CH: Use of ultrasonic reflectoscope for continuous recordings of movements of heart walls. Kungl Lysiogr Sallsk Lund Fiorhandl 24:5, 1954

Edler I, Gustafson A, Karlefors T, Christensson B (eds): Ultrasound cardiography. Acta Med Scand [Suppl] 370:5–123, 1961

Fortuin VJ, Hood WP, Sherman ME: Determination of left ventricular volumes by ultrasound. Circulation 44:575–584, 1971

Henry WL, Griffith JM, Michaelis LL, McIntosh CL, Morrow AG, Epstein SE: Measurement of mitral orifice area in patients with mitral valve disease by real-time two dimensional echocardiography. Circulation 51:827–831, 1975

Joyner CR, Hey EB, Johnson J, Reid JM: Reflected ultrasound in the diagnosis of tricuspid stenosis. Am J Cardiol 19:66–73, 1967

Linhart JW, Mintz GS, Segal BL, Kawai N, Kottler MN: Left ventricular volume measurement by echocardiography. Am J Cardiol 36:114–118, 1975

Quinones MA, Gaasch WH, Alexander JK: Echocardiographic assessment of left ventricular function with special reference to normalized velocities. Circulation 50:42–51, 1974

Weyman AE, Feigenbaum H, Dillon JC, Chang S: Cross sectional echocardiography in assessing the severity of aortic stenosis. Circulation 52:828–834, 1975

CARDIAC CATHETERIZATION

6

Robert H. Eich

This chapter is intended to be a basic introduction to the subject of cardiac catheterization, appropriate for students. In order to keep the presentation simple, I have deliberately left out many details which might have been included in a discussion intended for specialists.

The development of cardiac catheterization has been a milestone in the understanding of heart disease. The ability to precisely measure pressure and flow and to determine anatomy by angiography has represented a "quantum leap forward." Since Forssmann first demonstrated that a catheter could be safely passed from the arm vein to the right atrium in himself in 1929, and Cournand showed that the catheter could then be safely passed from the right atrium to the pulmonary artery in 1941, the advances have been enormous. Beginning in the fifties, pressures were measured directly in the left side of the heart, in addition to the rightsided pressures, and finally, in 1962, Sones first reported selective catheterization of the coronary arteries. All of these techniques are, of course, invasive. Cardiologists are now trying to develop noninvasive techniques to obtain the same information. However, the "gold standard" to which all noninvasive techniques must be compared is the valuable data obtained from cardiac catheterization.

The information obtained varies, depending on what kind of catheterization is done. The first studies were right heart catheterizations; the catheter was introduced through a cutdown on the antecubital vein. This technique yielded information about rightsided pressures, cardiac output, and oxygen saturation. In occasional patients, radiopaque dye was injected and angiography carried out to evaluate the pulmonary circuit, or, by delaying the films, to visualize the left heart and aorta.

PRESSURES

Pressures are measured in mmHg and compared to a zero hydrostatic pressure set at the mid-anterior–posterior line of the chest with the patient supine. The normal pressures are given in Table 6-1. The rightsided pressures are low, since the pulmonary circuit is highly distensible.

Flow in the normal subject must at least triple before pulmonary-artery pressure increases. A rise of 10 mmHg above normal is significant. The upper normal pulmonary-artery systolic pressure is 30 to 35; mmHg; therefore, 40 to 45 mmHg is clearly an elevated value. Likewise, the diastolic pressure is low in the right ventricle and right atrium, and a 5 to 10 mmHg increase would be clearly abnormal. Note the absence of valve gradients. Right-atrial equals right-ventricular diastolic pressure, and right-ventricular systolic pressure equals pulmonary-artery systolic pressure. We will discuss gradients in more detail in the section on valvular stenosis.

Using the right heart catheter, if the catheter is advanced in the pulmonary artery, the tip will wedge in a small branch of the artery. The catheter shaft effectively occludes the artery and the pressure measured at the catheter tip is called the **pulmonary capillary pressure,** or **pulmonary wedge pressure.** This equals the left-atrial pressure, as long as there is no pulmonary venous disease. Further, if there is no mitral-valve disease, the left-atrial pressure equals the left-ventricular diastolic pressure. Thus, the pulmonary capillary pressure, or pulmonary wedge pressure, is normally the same as the left-ventricular diastolic pressure. Also, if there is no pulmonary vascular disease, the pulmonary-artery end diastolic pressure equals the left-atrial pressure, which, in turn, equals the left-ventricular diastolic pressure, since there is no flow, in diastole, throughout the system. Thus, in a sick patient with a myocardial infarction, a catheter can be left in the pulmonary artery and the pulmonary artery diastolic pressure can be used to monitor left-ventricular diastolic pressure. This is of great value in assessing fluid intake and the ability of the left ventricle to accept it.

Table 6-1.   Normal Pressures and Resistances

SITE	PRESSURE (mmHg)
Right atrium	Mean: 7
Right ventricle	Systolic: 30
	Diastolic: 7
Pulmonary artery	Systolic: 30
	Diastolic: 10
	Mean: 9–16
Left atrium or wedge	Mean—under 10
Left ventricle	Systolic—120
	Diastolic—10
Cardiac index	2.5 to 4.5 liters/min/M2
Resistances (units)	Total systemic resistance 20 < units
	Total pulmonary resistance 3.5 < units
	Pulmonary vascular resistance 1.5 < units

As cardiac surgeons developed techniques for operating on the mitral valve, it became apparent that knowledge of the pulmonary capillary pressure was not adequate to permit the physician to judge the condition of the mitral valve or the left ventricle. It was necessary, therefore, to devise a way to measure left-ventricular systolic and diastolic pressure directly. The new technique developed involves passing a catheter through a systemic artery retrograde across the aortic valve. If the brachial artery is used, it is usually necessary to cut down and expose the artery. However, if the femoral artery is used, it is possible to employ the percutaneous technique developed by Seldinger. Here no cutdown is necessary, but a needle is placed in the femoral artery, a guide wire is then threaded through the needle, the needle is withdrawn, and the catheter is advanced into the artery following the guide wire. Both techniques have advantages; obviously, a retrograde femoral-artery catheterization cannot be done in patients with extensive peripheral vascular disease. In terms of speed and simplicity, we prefer the femoral artery route, if it can be used. In the early sixties, Braunwald developed the transseptal technique, in which a catheter is passed from the right atrium to the left atrium through the fossa ovalis. This is an extremely useful technique in patients with an artificial valve in the aortic position or with very tight aortic stenosis, both of which preclude retrograde catheterization.

The left-ventricular diastolic pressure, measured after atrial systole, most accurately reflects left-ventricular diastolic properties. The normal end diastolic pressure is 10 mmHg, and elevations due to changes in the left-ventricular compliance are associated with dilatation, fibrosis, or hypertrophy.

It is important to understand the concept of valvular pressure gradients. Normally, there is no pressure differential across the cardiac valves. Thus, in diastole there is no difference between the left-atrial and the left-ventricular diastolic pressure or the right-atrial and right-ventricular diastolic pressure. Similarly in systole, pulmonary-artery systolic pressure is equal to right-ventricular systolic pressure, and aortic systolic pressure equals left-ventricular systolic pressure. As the valves narrow with disease, a gradient or difference develops, and the left-ventricular systolic pressure becomes greater than the aortic, or the left atrial diastolic pressure becomes greater than the left ventricular diastolic pressure. The same process holds for the right side. An example of a diastolic gradient across the mitral valve, associated with mitral-valve stenosis, is shown in Figure 6-1. Figure 6-2 shows an example of an aortic systolic gradient. I will deal further with gradients in the discussion of valve areas.

FLOW

In addition to pressure, we measure flow, or actually cardiac output. This can be measured by using either the Fick principle or the dye dilution technique. Each has its particular advantages and disadvantages.

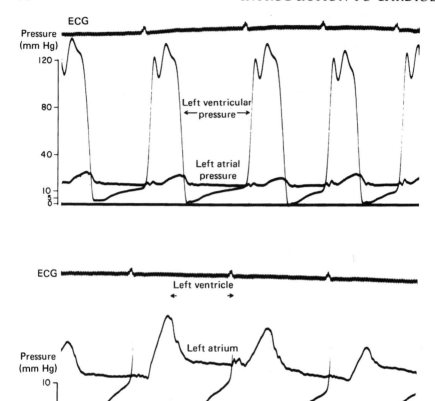

FIG. 6-1.
Simultaneous left atrial and left ventricular pressure recordings in a patient
with mitral stenosis and atrial fibrillation. Normal left ventricular systolic and
end-diastolic pressures are found in the absence of other disease **(top)**. As
shown at **bottom** there is a pressure difference across the mitral valve
throughout diastole. The mean left atrial pressure is elevated. Large A waves
characteristic of mitral stenosis are absent in the presence of atrial
fibrillation. (Fowler, NO: Cardiac Diagnosis and Treatment, ed. 2.
Hagerstown: Harper & Row, 1976, p. 125)

THE FICK TECHNIQUE

Dr. Adolph Fick first suggested the technique named for him in 1870. He was
never able to actually validate his theory because it was not possible at that time
to catheterize the pulmonary artery, but the concept was valid. Fick reasoned
that when the oxygen consumption and the blood arteriovenous difference for

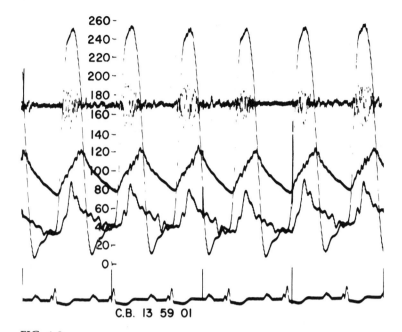

C.B. 13 59 01

FIG. 6-2.
Hemodynamic data in aortic stenosis. The left ventricular systolic
pressure is 250 mm Hg and the end-diastolic pressure 40 mm Hg.
The peak systolic pressure gradient across the aortic valve is 130
mm Hg. The aortic pressure shows a slow upstroke which does not
peak until it intersects the downslope of left ventricular pressure.
The upstroke shows coarse vibrations which represent the aortic
systolic thrill. Above the aortic pressure tracing an external
phonocardiogram records an ejection systolic murmur. Pulmonary
aterial pressure is recorded below the aortic pressure. Note
considerable pulmonary hypertension (80/40). Also note that the
pulmonary artery diastolic pressure is equal to the left ventricular
end-diastolic pressure. (Fowler NO: Cardiac Diagnosis and
Treatment, ed. 2. Hagerstown: Harper & Row, 1976, p. 130)

oxygen across the lungs can be measured, flow can be determined. He reasoned
that if the amount of oxygen taken up by the lungs is measured and also the
concentration of oxygen in the pulmonary artery and any systemic artery, one
has a measure of the cardiac output. Thus, if the oxygen consumption is 200
cc/min of oxygen taken up by the pulmonary circuit, the pulmonary artery oxygen content 160 cc/liter, and the brachial artery content 200 cc/liter, then the
200 cc/min oxygen consumption divided by 40 cc/liter, the arteriovenous difference, yields a cardiac output of 5 liter/min. Five liters of blood have to flow
through the pulmonary circuit, 40 cc of oxygen being added to each liter, in
order to account for a 200 cc total oxygen consumption.

Oxygen consumption is measured by a timed collection and analysis of expired air. The expired air is compared with inspired room air the oxygen concentration of which is known. Collecting expired air requires the use of a mouthpiece and a nose clip, and the gas is collected over a period of 2 to 3 min. This can be quite bothersome for patients, especially if they are dyspneic.

Blood oxygen is often reported in terms of percentage of saturation but can easily be converted to cc/liter if the oxygen-carrying capacity, that is, the oxygen content of the blood when fully saturated, is known. This, in turn, depends on the hemoglobin concentration, since each gram of hemoglobin holds 1.34 cc of oxygen. Therefore, to find the oxygen capacity, one multiplies the hemoglobin concentration in the blood by 1.34. Then the oxygen content of any blood sample is figured by multiplying the percentage of saturation by the oxygen-carrying capacity. For example, if the oxygen capacity is 210 cc of oxygen/liter of blood and the pulmonary artery blood is 70% saturated, the oxygen content of pulmonary artery blood is 147 cc of oxygen/liter of blood.

The Fick principle is especially accurate in low-cardiac-output states in which the arteriovenous difference is wide. Actually, the arteriovenous difference alone is a reflection of cardiac output, since as output falls, the arteriovenous difference increases. We often will follow cardiac output just by observing repeated arteriovenous differences in patients where we have reason to believe the oxygen consumption does not change. If an intervention widens the arteriovenous difference, the cardiac output has fallen.

THE DYE DILUTION TECHNIQUE

The second technique used to measure flow is the dye dilution technique. This was developed by Hamilton and Stewart in the 1920s and 30s. If an indicator is added to the bloodstream, dilution of the indicator is a function of volume flow; the higher the flow, the more diluted the indicator. The indicator must stay in the bloodstream for at least one circulation, must—obviously—be nontoxic, and its concentration must be measureable. Currently, indocyanine green dye is used, since it binds promptly to plasma albumin and remains in the bloodstream for at least one passage through the lungs. A major problem is that because of recirculation, the area under a time-concentration curve of a single circulation is obscured as shown in Figure 6-3. Hamilton showed that the obscured portion of the downslope is predictable and is an exponential function. Therefore, if some points on the initial portion of the downslope are known, the rest of the downslope can be extrapolated (Fig. 6-4), and the area of a single circulation can be determined.

The dye dilution technique is somewhat more convenient than the Fick technique, since it can be done without the need for an oxygen-consumption determination. However, the downslope becomes nonexponential both in low flow states and with valvular regurgitation, and the technique thus is less accurate than Fick's in evaluating sick people with low cardiac outputs.

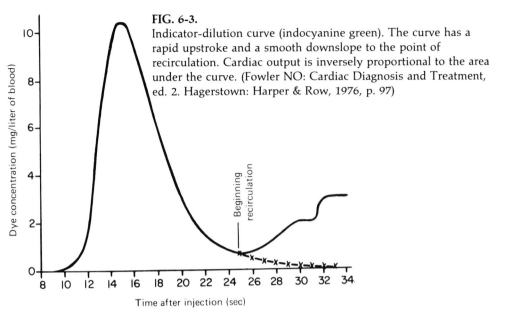

FIG. 6-3.
Indicator-dilution curve (indocyanine green). The curve has a rapid upstroke and a smooth downslope to the point of recirculation. Cardiac output is inversely proportional to the area under the curve. (Fowler NO: Cardiac Diagnosis and Treatment, ed. 2. Hagerstown: Harper & Row, 1976, p. 97)

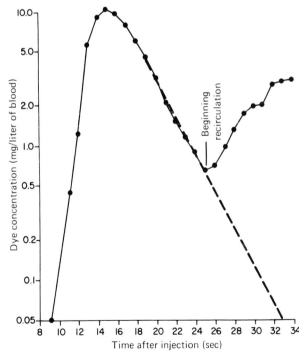

FIG. 6-4.
Indicator-dilution curve depicted in Fig. 6–3 replotted on a semilogarithmic ordinate. The point at which recirculation begins is much more distinct, and the curve may be extrapolated toward zero. The extrapolated curve represents a single circulation of the indocyanine green. The points along the dotted portion of the curve, which assume an exponential disappearance of the indicator, are used in most methods of calculating cardiac output from indicator-dilution curves. (Fowler NO: Cardiac Diagnosis and Treatment, ed. 2. Hagerstown: Harper & Row, 1976, p. 97)

Recently, iced saline injected into the right atrium has been used as the indicator instead of dye, with a thermistor catheter in the pulmonary artery to detect temperature change. Since the iced saline is warmed in the capillary bed, there is no recirculation. However, the method is still not accurate in low flow states, because the downslope is irregular. In our experience, methodology alone can produce a 10% variation in the figures for cardiac output; therefore, only changes of 20% or more should be considered significant.

A normal cardiac output is usually corrected for body-surface area, thus accounting for variations in cardiac output due to body size. The formula used is: "cardiac output divided by body surface area equals cardiac index." The normal range for this index is 2.5 to 4.5 liters/min/m^2. There is an extraordinarily wide range for this cardiac index, and most people with heart disease will fall within the normal range. In our experience, an isolated cardiac output measurement has not been particularly useful in determining the presence of heart disease.

CALCULATIONS DERIVED FROM PRESSURE, FLOW, AND HEART RATE

If pressure, flow, and heart rate are known, several other calculations can be made which have proved useful and are often part of a standard catheterization report.

1. *Stroke volume:* stroke volume $= \dfrac{\text{cardiac output cc/min}}{\text{heart rate}}$

2. *Stroke work:* stroke work = blood pressure (mean) × stroke volume

3. *Resistance:* if you can measure the pressure drop across a vascular bed, and the flow, resistance can be calculated, using the Poiseuille equation.

   a) $P1 - P2 = \dfrac{8\ L\ V\ F}{r\ 4}$

where L = length
       V = viscosity
       r = radius
       F = flow

   b) These are combined into a *term resistance:*

   term resistance $= \dfrac{P1 - P2}{\text{flow}}$

For the *systemic vascular resistance,* the arterial pressure is high enough so that P2, the venous pressure, does not have to be subtracted. Resistance is given in resistance units.

   c) resistance $= \dfrac{\text{mean arterial pressure}}{\text{cardiac output (liters/min)}}$

The normal systemic resistance is less than 20 units. Resistance may also be expressed in dynes:

$$\text{d) resistance (dynes/cm } -5/\text{sec)} = \frac{\text{mean arterial pressure} \times 1332}{\text{cardiac output (cc/sec)}}$$

The 1332 is a conversion factor. The range for systemic vascular resistance in dynes is 1200 ± 200 dynes/cm 5/sec.

Another important resistance unit is the *pulmonary vascular resistance.* Pulmonary resistance may be calculated in units:

$$\text{e) total pulmonary resistance} = \frac{\text{PA systolic} - \text{left-atrial pressure}}{\text{cardiac output (liters/min)}}$$

The normal range is under 3.5 units.

$$\text{f) pulmonary vascular resistance} = \frac{\text{PA mean} - \text{left-atrial pressure}}{\text{cardiac output (liters/min)}}$$

The normal range is less than 1.5. Again, the resistance can be given in dynes/cm 5/sec, and the normal range is 150 to 250.

4. *Valve area:* The open areas of the cardiac valves can be calculated, using the hydraulic formula developed by Gorlin. While the hydraulic formula assumes laminar nonpulsatile flow, the calculated valve areas do compare very well with areas measured at surgery.

$$\text{a) mitral-valve area} = \frac{\dfrac{\text{cardiac output (cc/min)}}{\text{diastolic time (sec/min)}}}{\div 31\sqrt{\text{LA} - \text{LV diastolic pressure}}}$$

where LA = left atrial
LV = left ventricular

$$\text{b) aortic-valve area} = \frac{\dfrac{\text{cardiac output (cc/min)}}{\text{systolic time (sec/min)}}}{\div 44.5\sqrt{\text{LV systolic} - \text{aortic systolic}}}$$

The normal mitral-valve area is 5 cm^2; under 1.5 cm^2 is significantly stenotic. A normal aortic-valve area is 3 cm^2; 0.75 cm^2 or less is significantly stenotic. Valve-area calculation is not accurate when significant regurgitation is present, since the cardiac output measures only effective forward flow and does not include regurgitant volume. Cardiac output therefore underestimates valve flow and then underestimates the calculated valve area.

Still other calculations can be made using derivatives of pressure and flow. The rate of pressure rise in the left ventricle, dP/dT, has been used as an estimate of left-ventricular contractility but is not particularly useful. Efforts to study the heart-muscle performance have been extremely important in our understanding of myocardial performance but have not been particularly useful in solving clinical problems.

In patients who are suspected to have a left to right shunt of oxygenated blood into the right heart, multiple blood samples are taken from the pulmonary artery for oxygen saturation, and then sequentially from the right ventricle, the right atrium, and the superior vena cava. A 10% increase in oxygen saturation in the sequential blood samples indicates a significant left to right shunt. For example, if the pulmonary artery saturation is 80%, right-ventricular saturation is 80%, and the right atrium is 60%, then there is a ventricular septal defect with left to right shunt at the ventricular level. By applying the Fick principle, the shunt flow can actually be calculated.

ANGIOGRAPHY

The final procedure that can be carried out at cardiac catheterization is angiography. This involves the injection of contrast agents, containing organic iodides, which are radiopaque and can thus be visualized on x-ray film. The film may be taken either as a movie (*cineangiography*) or using cut films and a rapid film changer. Both techniques have advantages. In general, cineangiography is preferred for rheumatic and coronary artery disease, where evaluating flow and matter is most important, but for congenital heart disease, where anatomic detail is more crucial, cut films are more widely used.

CORONARY ARTERY ANATOMY

Angiography can be carried out to evaluate both anatomy and function. Although it has been in use for 25 years to evaluate valve function and congenital heart disease, the major advance in the application of this technique was the development of selective coronary angiography by Sones in 1962. With this technique, the coronary arteries above 200 μ diameter in size can be safely and accurately visualized. This has led to an explosion of knowledge about coronary artery disease and has provided a solid data base for the understanding of this disease. The relationship between anatomy, function, symptoms, and prognosis are now being clearly defined. Today, as mentioned earlier, we are working to develop noninvasive techniques for obtaining the same information, but cardiac catheterization and coronary angiography remain the standard investigative tools.

In the Sones technique, a cutdown is made on the brachial artery and a flexible catheter tip is manipulated directly into the orifices, successively, of the left and right coronary arteries. About 8 cc of contrast agent are injected by hand and the cineangiography films are exposed. Films are taken in multiple projections in order to obtain complete evaluation of the coronary circulation.

Subsequent to the Sones's innovation, Judkins developed a technique using preshaped catheters introduced percutaneously into the femoral artery. One shape permits easy cannulation of the left coronary artery, and then the catheters are changed to a different shape which is better suited for the right coronary artery. Again, hand injections of dye are carried out in multiple projections. This technique is often faster than the Sones method and is less difficult to learn. If meticulous attention is given to technique, including heparinization during the procedure, it is as safe as the Sones method.

For both techniques, mortality should be under 0.1% and lesions can be determined with observer variability for the degree of stenosis no more than 20%. Anatomy is well standardized although there are, of course, individual variations. The main left coronary artery branches immediately into the circumflex artery and the left anterior descending artery, which supply the anterior and lateral walls of the left ventricle. If the right coronary artery is dominant, it supplies the inferior wall of the left ventricle. Otherwise, this is supplied by the circumflex artery.

Artherosclerotic lesions involve the major epicardial coronary arteries. The plaques are often eccentric, requiring multiple views in different obliques to assess the degree of obstruction. We grade lesions by quantitative quadrant: 0 to 25%, 25 to 50%, 50 to 75%, 75 to 99%, and 100% occlusion. In general, a degree of obstruction 75% or greater is considered to be significant. Both the degree of obstruction and the presence of collaterals from normal to diseased vessels are usually evaluated after nitroglycerin has been given.

LEFT-VENTRICULAR FUNCTION

In addition to its usefulness in defining coronary artery anatomy, angiography is used to determine left-ventricular function. The contrast agent is power-injected into the left ventricle and films are taken in the right anterior oblique projection; then a second injection is made while films are taken in the left anterior oblique projection. By placing the x-ray tube at a predetermined distance from the patient, ventricular volume in systole and diastole can be measured, using formulas developed by Sandler and Dodge. It is possible then to calculate the ejection fraction. Normally the heart empties two-thirds of its end diastolic volume; thus the ejection fraction = stroke volume divided by end diastolic volume = 66% ± 0.08 (S.D.). Two standard deviations below 66% is 50%, and an ejection fraction below 50% is abnormal. The ejection fraction is usually obtained both before and after nitroglycerin has been given, and more recently its response to exercise has been extensively evaluated.

The calculation of ventricular volume involves some major assumptions. First, the heart is considered to be a prolate ellipsoid, which, of course, it is not. Second, the two minor diameters of the ellipsoid are assumed to be equal. In a single projection, one can be measured but the other cannot. Coronary artery disease, especially with the development of abnormal left-ventricular shape, may invalidate both assumptions. Third, the landmarks used to measure left-ventricular volume have never been completely standardized from one laboratory to another. However, even with these limitations, measurement of the ejection fraction is a remarkably useful measure of ventricular function and is universally used.

The ventriculogram also gives information about segmental wall motion and viability. In the right anterior oblique projection, the ventricle is divided into six segments. In the left anterior oblique projection, the septum and the posterior basilar segment are visible. Wall motion is evaluated as normal, hypokinetic, akinetic, or dyskinetic (aneurysmal). If defective wall motion improves after nitroglycerin is given, some viable muscle is presumed to be present.

OTHER USES OF ANGIOGRAPHY

Angiography is also used to evaluate valvular insufficiency. For mitral insufficiency, dye is injected into the left ventricle, and regurgitation is observed into the left atrium in both the right and left anterior oblique projections. The amount of regurgitation is graded from 1 to 4+. Four+ is complete opacification of the left atrium, with reflux into the pulmonary veins, while 1+ is just a trace of regurgitation. Obviously this system is somewhat subjective, but it is quite useful. Likewise, for the study of aortic regurgitation, dye is injected into the aorta, usually in the left anterior oblique position, and films are taken to detect regurgitation of dye from the aorta to the left ventricle. This is graded, again, on a scale ranging from 1 to 4+, with 4+ describing complete left-ventricular opacification. Similar techniques can be used to measure tricuspid insufficiency or pulmonic insufficiency, but in these cases the catheter traverses the tricuspid or pulmonic valve and could affect its closure function.

The value of cardiac catheterization for congenital heart disease and rheumatic heart disease is well established. Patients with these two conditions are catheterized prior to surgery. With many of the congenital heart diseases, the presence of the lesion alone is an indication for surgery. With rheumatic heart disease, it is customary to wait for symptoms before considering surgery.

There is some controversy over the indications for coronary angiography. These indications were reviewed in *Circulation* (June, 1977). We are in complete agreement that not everyone with angina or chest pain needs to be catheterized. With coronary artery disease, catheterizations are sometimes done for anatomy and prognosis, even if no surgery is indicated. In general, the indications for catheterization are severe angina for which surgery is being considered; chest pain, when the diagnosis is uncertain; myocardial infarction in selected patients, including young patients, those who have complicated infarcts, and some patients with infarcts who have developed angina.

The physician should remember, before sending a patient to catheterization, that it is a frightening and expensive procedure, which does carry some morbidity and mortality. No patient should be asked to undergo an invasive procedure unless there is reasonable certainty that the procedure will yield information which will help in the patient's management.

CONGESTIVE FAILURE: PATHOPHYSIOLOGY

7

Robert H. Eich and Robert Warner

Congestive heart failure is the syndrome that results when the cardiac output is inadequate to supply the metabolic needs of the body at rest or during ordinary activity. The manifestations of the syndrome are the result of the inadequacy of the cardiac output in combination with elevation of the left-ventricular diastolic pressure. The diagnosis of congestive heart failure is made by clinical evaluation of the patient, utilizing the history, physical examination, and, at times, the chest film. Invasive studies are generally not needed to make the diagnosis.

PATHOPHYSIOLOGY

In order to understand the pathophysiology of congestive failure, it is necessary to examine the factors that regulate cardiac output. In addition to heart rate, which has complex effects on cardiac output, the output is determined by three factors that affect stroke volume: contractility, preload, and afterload. *Contractility* refers to the speed and forcefulness of cardiac contraction, independent of myocardial diastolic fiber length. *Contractility* is increased by enhanced activity of the sympathetic nervous system. Preload has to do with the Starling mechanism, that is, with the relationships between pressure and volume in the ventricle, which determine the force of concentration. Specifically, up to a point an increase in the ventricular volume in diastole and thus in myocardial fiber length is associated with an increase in the force of systolic contraction. This differs from contractility in that the changes in force of contraction with variations in preload are related to changes in myocardial fiber length, whereas in contractility they are not. *Afterload* is directly related to resistance to emptying of the ventricle and is directly related to wall tension. Since we cannot measure tension, we relate afterload to blood pressure. Since a reduction in afterload will result in an increase of stroke volume independent of changes in contractility and preload, there has been much recent interest in lowering the resistance to ventricular emptying with vasodilators in the acute and chronic treatment of congestive failure.

In normal subjects, cardiac output is regulated primarily by the sympathetic nervous system; changes in preload and afterload play secondary roles. The preload, or Starling mechanism, becomes important if the ventricle cannot empty completely, as a result of loss of muscle or increased mechanical burden on the heart. The resultant increase in diastolic volume and diastolic fiber length causes an increased force of contraction. The price for the increased diastolic volume is, eventually, an elevation of the ventricular filling pressure. The preload mechanism is an extraordinarily effective compensatory mechanism for maintaining cardiac output. However, its capacity can be exceeded, and at some point further elevation of ventricular volume results in a decrease in stroke volume. The reasons for the fall in stroke volume have not been completely elucidated but are partly related to an increase in tension in the ventricular wall, resulting from the increase in radius of the ventricle. In addition, excessive stretching of myocardial fibers results in diminished contact between the actin and myosin filaments. The net result is a combination of inadequate cardiac output and elevated filling pressures, a combination which leads to the changes responsible for the signs and symptoms of congestive heart failure.

The elevation of left-ventricular diastolic pressure resulting from excessive preload is responsible for the dyspnea experienced by patients with congestive failure. Since the mitral valve is open during diastole, the elevated diastolic pressure is transmitted directly to the left atrium, pulmonary veins, and pulmonary capillaries. When the left-atrial pressure exceeds 18 mmHg, fluid leaves the pulmonary capillaries and enters the interstitial space at a rate that exceeds the capacity of the lymphatics to remove it. The accumulation of this interstitial edema reduces pulmonary compliance and increases airway resistance, producing the sensation of dyspnea. Shortness of breath is considered to be true dyspnea if the patient's sensation of difficulty in breathing is inappropriately great for his level of activity at the time. When the left-atrial pressure exceeds 25 mmHg, fluid enters the alveolar space and eventually results in clinical pulmonary edema. A sustained increase in pulmonary capillary pressures increases the pulmonary artery pressure and may lead to failure of the right ventricle. Failure of the right ventricle is manifested by a rise in right-ventricular diastolic pressure and, therefore of right-atrial pressure. The latter is responsible for the neck-vein distension often seen in heart failure. It is important to emphasize, however, that left-ventricular failure may be present without right-ventricular decompensation, and that right-atrial pressure can be normal in patients in overt pulmonary edema. This is commonly seen in acute myocardial infarction.

Whereas the rise in left-ventricular diastolic pressure in heart failure is responsible for the symptom of dyspnea, the fall in cardiac output results in the symptom of fatigue. Fatigue is due to inadequate tissue flow, and it most often manifests itself as a feeling of tiredness in the legs while walking. In addition, the decreased cardiac output results in decreased renal bloodflow, and consequently in sodium and water retention. The increase in intravascular volume results in a greater overload of the ventricle and the accumulation of edema.

DIAGNOSIS OF CONGESTIVE FAILURE

The diagnosis of congestive failure depends upon clinical evaluation and can usually be made with a high degree of certainty using the history, physical examination, and a chest film.

HISTORY

The primary symptom of congestive heart failure is dyspnea. In the earliest stages of congestive failure, dyspnea is produced only by effort and the patient is comfortable at rest. As the congestive failure increases in severity, the patient experiences dyspnea with progressively less strenuous types of exertion and may eventually have symptoms at rest. Thus the extent of the patient's disability can be determined by correlating the sensation of dyspnea with the amount of physical activity with which it is associated. It should be emphasized that acute and chronic pulmonary disease often results in impressive dyspnea, which is difficult to distinguish from that of congestive failure on the basis of the history alone.

An important feature of the dyspnea of congestive failure is its increase with recumbency. The mechanism of this seems to involve fluid shifting into the lungs when the patient is lying down. A related manifestation of congestive failure is paroxysmal nocturnal dyspnea, which again results from the redistribution of fluid into the lungs when the patient is recumbent. Paroxysmal nocturnal dyspnea typically occurs 1 to 2 hours after lying down, wakes the patient with severe shortness of breath, and requires him to assume an upright posture in order to obtain relief. The most advanced stage of dyspnea resulting from heart disease is acute pulmonary edema. At this stage, not only are lung mechanics abnormal, but blood-gas exchange is impaired, so that arterial hypoxemia and even CO_2 retention may occur.

Besides dyspnea, a common symptom of congestive failure is cough. This may occur with exertion or with rest at night, is generally productive, and may seriously interfere with sleep.   *pink, frothy*

The symptoms associated with a decrease in cardiac output are more difficult to quantitate. Although not a specific symptom, fatigue generally occurs with exercise and tends to worsen later in the day. The symptom is caused by decreased bloodflow to skeletal muscle and may actually limit the patient's tolerance for exercise more than dyspnea.

Another symptom commonly associated with congestive failure is swelling of the peripheral tissues, owing to the formation of edema. One of the mechanisms responsible for this development of edema is the retention of sodium and water as a result of the diminished renal bloodflow associated with the low cardiac output. The decreased renal bloodflow results in increased secretion of aldosterone by activation of the renin-angiotensin system. In addition, the formation of edema is favored by elevation of right-atrial pressure, with retrograde transmission of the increased pressure to the peripheral capillaries. Because the intravascular hydrostatic pressure is augmented by gravity, transudation of fluid into the interstitial space tends to occur in the dependent portions of the body. Therefore the edema associated with heart failure is found predominantly in the feet and ankles in upright individuals and over the sacrum in patients who are supine. Occasionally, abdominal swelling from the development of ascites may occur in patients with congestive failure.

The symptoms of congestive failure in the elderly may differ significantly from those in younger patients. The onset of heart failure may be more subtle, manifested by restlessness and irritability at night. In older patients, chronic cough is often a more prominent complaint than dyspnea. Because of the variability of the many symptoms of heart failure in the elderly, the physician must keep this possibility well in mind, in order to make the diagnosis.

PHYSICAL EXAMINATION

The physical examination is a valuable tool for evaluating congestive heart failure, but many of the classical physical findings are seen only in advanced stages. The patient with congestive heart failure generally appears chronically ill, often with rather marked muscle wasting and cachexia, owing to both an associated anorexia and reduced perfusion of the peripheral tissues, resulting from the low cardiac output. With acute pulmonary edema, the patient is in obvious, marked distress, sitting up, gasping for air, and coughing up pink sputum. In congestive failure, there is reflex augmentation of sympathetic tone in order to attempt to compensate for the reduced cardiac output. As a result of the enhanced sympathetic activity, a rapid pulse rate often coexists with cold, pale, sweaty skin and an elevated blood pressure. Pulsus alternans, a relatively strong systolic impulse alternating with a relatively weak one, may be detected by simply palpating the peripheral pulse. However, the use of a blood-pressure cuff increases the ease with which beat-to-beat variation in the amplitude of the systolic impulse can be demonstrated. Increased right-atrial pressure may be identified by noting the presence of distended neck veins, and an accurate estimate of the right-atrial pressure may be made (see Chap. 2). In most individuals in sinus rhythm, the "a" wave is the most prominent component of the jugular venous pulse. However, in patients with right-ventricular failure, tricuspid insufficiency may occur owing to dilatation of the right ventricle, and "cv" waves become the dominant component of the jugular venous pulse. Another feature of right-ventricular failure is dependent edema, which "pits" on pressure.

Examination of the lungs helps to substantiate the diagnosis of congestive failure. Rales may be heard; however, left-atrial pressure may be significantly elevated and yet not high enough to produce alveolar flooding and rales. Furthermore, the presence of rales is not specific evidence of congestive failure, since these sounds may also be produced by pulmonary atelectasis. Before rales may be attributed to heart failure, they must persist after coughing and must be associated with other signs and symptoms of failure. The rales from pulmonary edema tend to be basilar at first. As the pulmonary edema worsens, the rales become audible at progressively higher levels of the chest and eventually may be present over the entire lung fields. Wheezing (cardiac asthma) may be produced by left-ventricular failure, owing to reduction of the size of the bronchiolar lumina from submucosal edema. Pleural effusion due to venous hypertension may be associated with congestive failure, and manifests itself by dullness to percussion and decreased breath sounds at the lung bases. Pleural effusions caused by heart failure may be bilateral or right-sided, but are seldom left-sided alone.

There is no one finding from examination of the heart that is specific for congestive failure. Since most patients will have cardiomegaly, as a result of the increase in preload, the point of maximal impulse can usually be palpated outside the midclavicular line. However, in right heart failure and in patients with acute left-ventricular failure in whom chamber enlargement has not yet occurred, there may be no discernible left-ventricular enlargement. In the absence of left bundle-branch block, paradoxical splitting of the second heart sound is indicative of impairment of left-ventricular function. When left-ventricular failure results in pulmonary hypertension, accentuation of the pulmonic component of the second heart sound may occur.

The presence of a third heart sound is suggestive of heart failure. However, this sound can be heard in healthy young individuals and in patients with mitral insufficiency without heart failure. A fourth heart sound tends to be associated with any process that reduces ventricular compliance and not with congestive failure per se. As a result of ventricular dilatation, some patients will have the murmurs of mitral or tricuspid incompetence.

CHEST FILM

The chest roentgenographic examination may contribute to the diagnosis of congestive failure by showing pathological changes (interstitial edema, for example) before the classical physical findings of failure have developed. (For full discussion of cardiac roentgenology see Chap. 3.) It is important to note, however, that the appearance of abnormalities on the chest film may lag several hours behind the elevation of filling pressure. Conversely, it may take as long as 24 hours for the radiological abnormalities to resolve, following reduction of an elevated filling pressure to normal levels. To ensure a reliable radiological diagnosis, the chest film should be taken with the patient in the upright position, with the machine six feet away from the patient. The abnormalities of the chest film associated with left-ventricular failure are: pulmonary venous engorgement, interstitial edema, and alveolar edema. Engorgement of the pulmonary veins initially is greater in the upper than in the lower lobes, the reverse of the normal relationship. As pulmonary venous pressure continues to increase, interstitial edema develops. This will be shown on the film as septal edema (Kerley B lines), perihilar haze, and blurring of the margins between the pulmonary vessels and the air-filled alveoli. The appearance of alveolar edema is characterized by nodular or diffuse infiltration in the lung fields. While generally bilateral, alveolar pulmonary edema may be asymmetrical or even unilateral.

ELECTROCARDIOGRAM AND ECHOCARDIOGRAM

The electrocardiogram shows no changes specific for congestive failure but can provide evidence for chamber enlargement, arrhythmias, or other heart disease that commonly accompanies the syndrome. In addition, while not specific, the ECG is seldom normal in congestive failure.

The echocardiogram will often show chamber enlargement and valvular abnormalities that may be associated with heart failure, even though there is no specific echocardiographic pattern for congestive failure.

ETIOLOGY

Once the diagnosis of congestive heart failure is made, the causes of the heart disease should be sought. The causes of left-ventricular failure include hypertension, coronary artery disease, valvular heart disease, and a heterogeneous group of primary myocardial diseases (cardiomyopathy). Two or more pathological processes, such as mitral insufficiency complicating myocardial infarction, may combine to produce heart failure. A variety of diseases may cause the right ventricle to fail independently of the left. These disorders include mitral stenosis, left-atrial myxoma, pulmonic stenosis, multiple pulmonary emboli, and primary pulmonary hypertension. The term **cor pulmonale** has been applied to heart disease secondary to lung disease. It is a relatively nonspecific term, since many pulmonary disorders can result in pulmonary hypertension and thus impose significant afterload stress on the right ventricle.

In addition to the primary etiological diagnosis, precipitating factors must be identified. For example, excessive salt ingestion, omission of medication, arrhythmias, myocardial infarction, increased physical activity, infection, and fever may all be responsible for the onset or aggravation of congestive heart failure.

High cardiac output failure refers to a condition in which there is no depression of cardiac function in absolute terms, but in which cardiac output is inadequate to meet excessive demands. Examples of disorders that may result in high output failure are anemia, thyrotoxicosis, arterial venous fistula, beriberi heart disease, and Paget's disease of the bone. It is crucial to make the diagnosis, since the circulatory disturbance can only be reversed by correcting the etiological factor. As is true in the study of any disorder, the methods used to determine the etiology and precipitating factors of congestive heart failure should be selected in the light of their relative risk to the patient, as well as the value of the information to be obtained. For this reason, noninvasive studies are preferable to invasive diagnostic procedures.

CONGESTIVE FAILURE: TREATMENT

Robert H. Eich and Robert Warner

8

The management of congestive failure is basic to cardiology, and therefore we will devote a separate chapter to the principles and specifics of treatment. Treatment of congestive failure should be based upon a careful clinical evaluation of the patient, with consideration of the severity as well as the etiology and precipitating factors of the heart failure. For example, mild chronic heart failure can be treated on an outpatient basis, while acute pulmonary edema is a medical emergency requiring hospitalization.

BASIC PRINCIPLES OF TREATMENT

We will start with a brief outline of treatment before going into the details of certain aspects of therapy, especially the use of digitalis preparation.

1. **Diagnosis.** As we have said, the diagnosis of congestive failure is a clinical matter and can be made on the basis of the history, physical examination, and chest film. In the course of establishing the diagnosis, the physician also determines underlying causes (type of heart disease), possible precipitating events, and, finally, assesses severity. The usual causes include:

1. Coronary artery disease
2. Hypertensive cardiovascular disease
3. Valvular heart disease
4. Cardiomyopathy
5. (Rarely in adults) congenital heart disease.

However, one should also remember these rare, but curable, forms of heart diseases:

1. Thyrotoxicosis
2. Anemia
3. Atrioventricular fistula

A valuable rule to bear in mind is that something has to precipitate congestive failure, and the precipitating event must be searched for. The following may all be precipitating factors: especially a recent myocardial infarction; tachyarrhythmias or bradyarrhythmias; pulmonary emboli; an abnormal increase in cardiac work due to infection, excitement, or a sodium load; or the patient's failure to follow a therapeutic program prescribed for him. Finally, one needs to assess the severity of the congestive failure and make a decision about whether the patient is to be treated as an outpatient or hospitalized and, if he does require hospitalization, whether he should be assigned to the intensive care unit or to a general clinical floor.

2. **Workup.** In addition to the history, physical examination, and chest film, a standard workup should include complete blood count, urinalysis, and tests to evaluate levels of electrolytes (sodium and potassium), fasting blood sugar, blood urea nitrogen, and uric acid. It is often valuable to know the levels of arterial blood gases in assessing the severity of congestive failure. If the PO_2 is below 50 on room air or if there is CO_2 retention, the patient should be hospitalized in an intensive care unit. Thyroid function should also be determined if there is any question about the thyroid status. Finally, if the patient is febrile, tests (including blood cultures) should be made to determine if infectious diseases are present, especially endocarditis. Eventually an echocardiogram, a radioactive ventriculogram, and even cardiac catheterization may be indicated to establish the type and the severity of heart disease, but these are hardly ever necessary in the treatment of the acute illness.

3. **Treatment.** Once the diagnosis is established and basic laboratory data has been obtained, treatment should be started. We feel that the treatment of congestive failure should start with the administration of digitalis. Other important components of treatment include the giving of diuretics, the restriction of sodium intake and of physical activity, and (obviously) treatment of other factors which have contributed to the congestive failure, such as arrhythmias or anemia.

Digitalis will be discussed at considerable length in the next section. Digoxin, given either orally or intravenously, is the drug of choice because of its short half-life. As with antiarrhythmic agents, all digitalis preparations require a loading dose to reach a therapeutic level. If the patient is ill, we recommend using digoxin intravenously, giving about 1.0 to 1.2 mg over the first 24 hours. If oral digitalization is adequate, we would give about one-third more, orally, over 24 hours, about 1.5 mg. The proper maintenance dose can then be decided upon, depending on renal function.

Diuretics are also one of the mainstays of therapy. By increasing sodium and water excretion, the left-atrial pressure can be lowered and pulmonary edema reversed. The most widely used diuretic now is furosemide. Again, this may be given orally or intravenously, depending on the severity. In long-term management, restricting the sodium intake to under 2 g per day is extremely valuable. Frequently, worsening congestive failure can be traced to dietary indiscretion, with an increased intake of sodium.

Likewise, by systematically decreasing physical activity, many patients can be kept compensated for long periods. Most patients can be compensated in the hospital by bed rest. If the patient is to be kept on bed rest for any length of time, the use of anticoagulants should always be considered.

For intractable failure, the use of afterload reduction to improve cardiac output has been extremely valuable. By adding this program, patients can be kept much more comfortable for many months. We reserve the use of afterload reduction for patients who cannot be compensated by the standard methods. Afterload reduction can be achieved by prescribing hydralazine hydrochloride or can be combined with preload reduction by the use of nitrates or prazosin.

Acute pulmonary edema and severe congestive failure require hospitalization. In addition to receiving the standard digitalis and diuretics, the patient's head should be elevated, and he should be given nasal oxygen at about 4 liters per minute and morphine sulfate, 4 to 6 mg given intravenously; this last is a superb tool to improve shortness of breath. It allays apprehension, decreases the work of breathing, and is in general extremely effective. However, one should monitor blood gas levels, since occasionally morphine sulfate causes increased CO_2 retention; if so, naloxone (Narcan) should be given to reverse the effect of the morphine.

Patients who do not respond to these measures will often respond to tourniquets rotated on the extremities, which decrease preload by pooling blood in the extremities. In an acute situation, the use of a nitroprusside drip to decrease preload and afterload is valuable. For the use of the nitroprusside, the patient should be in an intensive-care setting, almost surely with a pulmonary artery pressure monitor. Finally, the blood gases should be closely observed; a rise in PCO_2 and a fall in PO_2 may be an indication for intubation. Intubation in this situation can be life-saving. The work of breathing is dramatically decreased, atelectasis is overcome, ventilation is improved and patients are truly more comfortable intubated. The tube can be removed in a few days.

DIGITALIS

As we have stated, we feel that the single most effective drug in the treatment of congestive failure is digitalis and its derivatives. While some cardiologists argue that diuretics are more valuable, we do not agree. Digitalis improves myocardial contractility and increases cardiac output. Because the drug thus enables the ventricle to empty more completely, ventricular volume and filling pressure are decreased, and myocardial oxygen needs actually decrease. In addition, the increase in stroke volume caused by the drug makes the patient less dependent upon enhanced activity of the sympathetic nervous system to maintain cardiac output. As a consequence, there is a decrease in the heart rate and in vasomotor tone. The reduction in vasomotor tone results in a decreased afterload, which further increases cardiac output.

There are many excellent articles on digitalis, most of which are included in the list of references published in Circulation 59:837–840, 1979. Since digoxin is the form of digitalis most commonly used in the hospital setting, the present discussion will concentrate on this preparation. Digoxin is the most widely used because of its short half-life. Ninety percent of it is excreted through the kidneys, and in a patient with normal renal function the half-life of digoxin is 36 to 46 hours. Digoxin, like all the digitalis preparations and the antiarrhythmics, follows first-order kinetics, so that 4 half-lives are required for digitalization and a therapeutic level to be achieved. If a patient is treated with a daily maintenance dose, he would require approximately 6 to 8 days to achieve a therapeutic level. The term **digitalizing dose** refers to the amount needed to attain a therapeutic level during the first 24 hours. As previously stated, if the patient is ill, we recommend giving the digoxin intravenously; that way, one is sure that the proper dose is absorbed and that a predictable level can be reached. However, the maintenance dose (the daily dose necessary to maintain the therapeutic level) is almost always given orally. Assuming that the patient has not been on any digitalis preparation prior to the time of therapy, the basic goal is to administer 1 to 1.2 mg of digoxin intravenously over 24 hours for the digitalizing dose. There is no therapeutic threshold below which digitalis is not active, and it has been shown that ½ mg of digoxin given intravenously will raise cardiac output and lower pulmonary-artery pressure in patients in congestive failure. For this reason, a good rule is to give 0.25 to 0.5 mg intravenously during the first two hours and base the subsequent dose necessary for the 24-hour digitalization upon the following considerations:

1. **Serum Potassium Level.** The presence of hypokalemia greatly increases the incidence of serious rhythm disturbances associated with the use of digitalis. Therefore, the serum potassium levels should be maintained within the normal range.

2. **Renal Function.** Since digoxin is excreted largely by the kidneys, patients with significant impairment of renal function should be given a lower digitalizing dose of the drug.

3. **Body Size.** Digoxin is taken up by skeletal as well as cardiac muscle. Consequently, in patients with a decreased skeletal muscle mass, a greater proportion of the administered dose of digoxin will be taken up by the heart, and a lower dose should therefore be used.

4. **Severity of Heart Disease.** It is unfortunate that the more severe the impairment of cardiac function, the more likely the patient is

to suffer digitalis intoxication. The reasons for this are complex but involve diminished renal blood flow, which impairs excretion, and an increased intrinsic sensitivity of the cardiac tissue to the arrhythmogenic effects of digitalis.

5. **Chronic Lung Disease.** Patients with this condition frequently become toxic from digitalis, partly because of the chronic hypoxia, and partly because the dyspnea from pulmonary disease may be attributed to congestive failure and treated with more digitalis.

6. **Age.** Elderly patients are much more susceptible to digitalis toxicity than younger individuals because of their decreased muscle mass, impaired renal function, and greater likelihood of advanced heart disease. In addition, patients on chronic digoxin maintenance who suffer from mental confusion may take more than the prescribed dose.

7. **Myxedema.** These patients metabolize digitalis at a slower rate.

Taking all of the above factors into consideration, the general rule, as we have said, is to give, initially, 0.25 to 0.5 mg of digoxin intravenously and then give supplements of 0.25 mg every 4 to 6 hours until the desired digitalizing dose has been achieved. In seriously ill patients, we again emphasize that it is important to digitalize by using the intravenous route. If the drug is given orally, ⅓ more must be given and, in addition, gastrointestinal absorption is erratic. If acute digitalization is not necessary, then administration of the daily maintenance dose of digoxin for four half-lifes (6–8 days) will result in a steady state in patients with normal renal function.

The maintenance dose of digoxin is widely variable and may be as little as 0.125 mg on alternate days or as much as 0.5 mg daily. Since digoxin is excreted almost exclusively by the kidneys, patients with decreased renal function require a lower maintenance dose. A number of formulas for determining the proper dose of digoxin have been derived, based on renal function. We have not found these formulas particularly helpful, and there seems to be no substitute for clinical judgement. In patients with rapidly changing renal function, digitoxin may be used in place of digoxin, since the former is metabolized primarily by the liver; however, the half-life is 6 days for this preparation. The final determination of the proper maintenance dose is largely an empirical process, and the drug is given customarily until a satisfactory therapeutic response is seen or until toxic manifestations appear.

The toxic manifestations of digoxin are rhythm disturbances in about 70% of patients and extracardiac symptoms in the remaining 30%. Although any arrhythmia may be produced by digitalis, the most common arrhythmias are premature ventricular contractions, paroxysmal atrial tachycardia with block, and accelerated junctional rhythm. One should remember that paroxysmal atrial tachycardia with block may be caused by intrinsic heart disease and not digitalis excess. Digitalis may also produce varying degrees of heart block. The major extracardiac manifestations of toxicity include anorexia, nausea, weakness, and visual disturbances. Because of the potentially lethal outcome of digitalis intoxication, patients with suspected intoxication should be observed in a monitored setting until the toxicity has subsided. The treatment of digitalis toxicity consists of withholding the drug, correcting the potassium imbalance, and, if the arrhythmias are life-threatening ventricular arrhythmias, lidocaine or phenytoin may be given. However, these medications should be given with some caution, and obviously in an intensive-care unit setting.

In recent years, it has become possible to measure the levels of digoxin and digitoxin in the blood. Although the therapeutic range, as measured by the immunoassay technique, is wide, measurement of digoxin blood levels had been an enormous help in the proper dose regulation for this drug.

DIURETICS

Diuretics are also useful in the management of congestive failure. By reducing intravascular volume, diuretics decrease ventricular size and filling pressure, with consequent improvement in the signs and symptoms of circulatory congestion. However, if the administration of the diuretic results in a reduction of ventricular preload below an optimal level, there may actually be a decrease in cardiac output. For example, in most patients with an acute myocardial infarction, the left-ventricular filling pressure should be kept at 15 to 18 mmHg in order to maintain an adequate output. Lowering of the filling pressure below this may decrease cardiac output. Despite these considerations, diuretics are effective agents for reducing the manifestations of pulmonary congestion and for eliminating peripheral edema. There are four types of diuretics:

1. The thiazide and related compounds, including chlorthalidone. These inhibit sodium reabsorption in the ascending distal tubule. Since only 10% of sodium is reabsorbed from this area, these diuretics are in general less potent than the so-called loop diuretics.
2. The loop diuretics, furosemide and ethacrynic acid, act on the ascending limb of the Henle loop, where 20% of sodium is reabsorbed, and are thus more effective. In addition, they are more effective with an increasing dose and also in the presence of electrolyte abnormalities. Most physicians now use furosemide or ethacrynic acid, and as time has gone by, we have used larger and larger doses for patients in refractory failure. Treatment with furosemide starts with 40 mg orally or 20 mg intravenously and the dose is increased as the need arises.
3. The distal-tubular diuretics, triamterene and spironolactone, are less potent than the other diuretics but have a potassium-sparing effect.
4. Finally, there is a new group of compound derivatives of dichlorophenoxyacetic acid. These have natriuretic and uricosuric activ-

ity. They therefore obviate a concern over a rising uric acid level and can be used in patients who have elevated levels of uric acid to start with. In terms of effectiveness, they probably are similar to the thiazide group of diuretics. These drugs may have serious side-effects, however.

When diuretics are used with a digitalis preparation, the potassium level must be carefully monitored and kept in a normal range. Usually this cannot be done by diet alone and will require either a potassium supplement or the use of spironolactone or triamterene, which, as we have said, have a potassium-sparing effect. The choice of a potassium supplement will be influenced by patient tolerance and the cost of the preparation. Although effective, 10% potassium chloride elixir may be rejected by patients because of its unpleasant taste and impressive gastric irritation, which may necessitate the use of preparations such as potassium chloride slow-release tablets (Slow K) or effervescent potassium tablets such as K-Lyte. Patients with chronic failure also may develop significant hyponatremia. The correct treatment for this is fluid restriction rather than the administration of sodium, since total body sodium stores are already increased and the low sodium is dilutional.

MEANS OF TREATMENT

Standard in treatment for congestive failure is sodium restriction to 2 g per day and a reduction in physical activity. Much can be done to keep patients compensated by truly vigorous attention to sodium restriction with the help of a dietician to instruct the patient. Common problems are that the patient confuses sodium and salt, or has in his home a water softener that uses an exchange with sodium, or that he tries to eat in restaurants. It is impossible to follow a low-sodium diet in any kind of a restaurant setting. Reduction in activity may simply consist in cutting out strenuous activities, but certain patients may have to spend long periods of the weekend in bed. In any case, judicious use of rest will certainly enable many people to keep going.

A relatively new addition to the therapy of congestive failure, particularly for those cases refractory to conventional treatment, has been the use of vasodilators. By dilating the systemic arterioles, vasodilators reduce left-ventricular afterload and thereby increase cardiac output and stroke volume. In addition, many vasodilators increase the capacitance of the veins by relaxing the smooth muscle in the venous wall. This venodilatation results in peripheral venous pooling and therefore in diminished return of blood to the heart—that is, decreased preload. Because of the combination of decreased preload and the more complete emptying of the ventricle resulting from the decreased afterload, ventricular volume and filling pressure are reduced. The net result is an improvement in both cardiac output and the manifestations of circulatory congestion.

A variety of vasodilators are available for clinical use. Nitroglycerin (tablets and paste), isosorbide dinitrate (oral and sublingual), and hydralazine are suitable for both acute and chronic use. Prazosin at first appeared to be extremely promising, since it affected both preload and afterload. However, it is now apparent that tolerance develops to the drug fairly quickly, and it may not, after all, prove to be useful for long-term therapy. For patients with severe congestive failure, intravenous sodium nitroprusside is the agent of choice. In severely ill patients, pulmonary as well as systemic arterial pressure should be monitored during the administration of vasodilators. In addition, the effect of the agents on the cardiac output should be assessed, since excessive reduction of the left-ventricular filling pressure may result in a decrease in cardiac output. Besides observing the patient for changes in such clinical features as mental status, skin texture, pulse rate, and urinary output, the cardiac output may be measured directly either by the Fick or dye dilution techniques.

The use of vasodilators is particularly appropriate when congestive heart failure is associated with mitral or aortic valvular insufficiency. In mitral insufficiency, regurgitation of blood into the left atrium not only exacerbates pulmonary congestion by increasing the atrial pressure but results in a decrease in forward cardiac output because a proportion of the left-ventricular stroke volume goes backward into the atrium. Vasodilators, by reducing resistance in the systemic arterial system, increase the relative ease with which blood leaves the ventricle by the normal antegrade route, and therefore decreases the severity of the mitral regurgitation.

In aortic insufficiency, blood in the aorta during diastole goes both antegrade and retrograde. Since vasodilators reduce resistance to flow in the systemic arterial system, the administration of these agents in aortic insufficiency tends to increase the proportion of normal antegrade flow and therefore reduces the relative amount of regurgitation.

As was stated, the most dramatic and immediately life-threatening manifestation of congestive heart failure, acute pulmonary edema, is managed according to the principles already outlined for the administration of digitalis and diuretics and measures designed to achieve afterload reduction. In addition to the administration of the drugs, other methods designed to rapidly correct the hemodynamic abnormalities should be employed. The patient should be allowed to sit up, so that gravitational effects will favor pooling the blood in the legs rather than in the lungs. Oxygen should be administered by nasal cannula to correct the arterial hypoxemia associated with pulmonary edema. Rotating venous tourniquets on the extremities are employed to reduce return of blood by trapping blood in the veins and keeping it out of the central circulation, thus decreasing left-ventricular preload. Morphine is given, not only because of its analgesic and sedative effects, but because it also dilates venous and arteriolar smooth muscle and thus reduces both preload and afterload. In some patients, phlebotomy may be indicated to reduce circulatory congestion. Tachyarrhythmias, such as rapid atrial fibrillation, may result in acute congestive failure because of the shortening of the ventricular diastolic filling period and loss of the atrial contribution to ventricular filling. Such arrhythmias, therefore, should be treated either with drugs or electrical cardioversion. Conversely, extremely slow rates may result in congestive failure, and such patients should be appropriately treated with an artificial pacer. Arterial blood gases should be closely monitored. A rise in PCO_2 or a fall in PO_2 is an indication for endotracheal intubation. This procedure can, indeed, be livesaving because it reduces the work of breathing, allowing the patient to rest by increasing positive pressure to expand atelectatic alveoli, and thus improving oxygenation.

CORONARY ARTERY DISEASE: MYOCARDIAL INFARCTION

Robert H. Eich and Robert Warner

9

Coronary artery disease is the major medical problem in the United States today; it is responsible for 800,000 deaths per year. Several other terms are used for this disease, including **arteriosclerotic heart disease, atherosclerotic heart disease, coronary heart disease,** and **ischemic heart disease.** All are acceptable, and we use the term coronary artery disease only because of our custom. Coronary artery disease may manifest itself in a myocardial infarction, angina pectoris, congestive failure, or sudden death. The latter is almost always the result of an arrhythmia, ventricular tachycardia and ventricular fibrillation or bradyarrhythmia and asystole.

ETIOLOGY

The underlying pathological process responsible for the clinical entities seen in coronary artery disease is atherosclerosis of the large coronary arteries. The initial process appears to involve injury to the vessel wall and the development of an atheroslerotic plaque in response to this injury. Atherosclerosis has been extensively investigated to determine how and why it starts, what factors are involved in accelerating the process, and, more important, whether it can be slowed or reversed. Certain factors greatly influence the rate of development of the disease. Major factors include age, male sex, smoking, hyperlipidemia, hypertension, diabetes mellitus, and a family history of vascular disease. In addition, there are less important risk factors such as obesity, sedentary life, emotional stress, and the Type A personality (characterized by a marked concern over meeting deadlines).

Age is certainly a well-recognized risk factor, since coronary artery disease usually does not manifest itself until the 50s or 60s. However, it is important to point out that the disease is not an inevitable consequence of aging. Many individuals live into the 80s or beyond with no coronary artery disease. The presumption is that other risk factors are necessary, and age is only one.

With respect to hyperlipidemia, several excellent reviews have been published recently.[1, 2] The lipid most clearly associated with coronary artery disease is cholesterol, specifically cholesterol carried in the blood by low-density lipoprotein. Interestingly, an elevated level of high-density lipoprotein cholesterol may actually be protective. It is well-recognized that in America, most patients with coronary artery disease have a "normal" level of cholesterol. This is in part because the normal range established in the United States is probably too high. However, a normal cholesterol concentration tells nothing of the ratio of low- to high-density lipoprotein. When abnormal, this ratio may be an important risk factor in addition to the total cholesterol. A high level of triglycerides is also a risk factor, and Frederickson has developed a system for typing hyperlipidemias using cholesterol and triglycerides.[3]

There is currently great interest in the question of whether modification of risk factors can either slow or actually reverse the disease. This has been most extensively studied in terms of cholesterol. Cholesterol levels can be lowered by both drug and dietary therapy. However, the importance of this effort to prevent and reverse coronary artery disease remains controversial. A well done study in the United States, the coronary drug study, showed that lowering cholesterol with a drug program had no effect on coronary artery disease.[4] However, the results were different in the European studies.[1]

Cigarette smoking (one package per day for at least 10 years) is without doubt a major risk factor and is the one factor that can be eliminated, if the patient stops smoking. However, even without smoking, the patient does not return to a normal level of risk for 10 years. Smoking appears to be even more dangerous when combined with other risk factors. Pipe and cigar smoking, unless the subject inhales, are not significant risk factors.

Diabetes mellitus is a major risk factor, and in our experience a parent or sibling with diabetes mellitus is a risk factor even if the patient has not yet developed full-blown diabetes mellitus. Hypertension is also a risk factor, and both diabetes mellitus and hypertension clearly accelerate vascular disease.

While atherosclerosis and myocardial infarction almost always occur together, it has been argued that the two are not causally related, and that possibly the myocardial infarction occurs for some other reason. Certainly there are patients who develop a myocardial infarction without coronary artery disease. However, this is uncommon, and the presumption at present is that atherosclerosis is necessary for the development of a myocardial infarction. But even once it is agreed that atherosclerosis is necessary, there is no agreement among pathologists as to what actually precipitates the myocardial infarction. The precise role of thrombus in the pathogenesis of myocardial infarction is uncertain. While many believe that thrombosis on the surface of the antherosclerotic plaque is the primary event in precipitating the infarct, several pathologists believe that the thrombus is secondary to stasis from some other process (Roberts, Baroldi).[5,6] Recently, coronary artery spasm has been demonstrated angiographically in patients during the first few hours of the myocardial infarction.

The question of precise etiology is obviously important in developing any kind of program to prevent myocardial infarction. If thrombus were the major factor, anticoagulants should prevent myocardial infarction, but this has never been statistically demonstrated. On the other hand, if thrombus on an atherosclerotic plaque is not the precipitating factor, possibly some process in the arterioles or capillaries starts the event. If indeed the process occurs distal to the atherosclerotic plaque, then coronary-artery bypass surgery might not prevent a myocardial infarction, and it has not been shown to statistically. Obviously, this area is an exciting one for further study.

HISTORY

The history given by the patient with a myocardial infarction is typical and reproducible. Because early in the time course the ECG and laboratory studies are often normal, the patient may have to be admitted to the cardiac care unit on the basis of his history alone. About 50% of patients with myocardial infarction give a history of premonitory symptoms in the preceding 2 to 3 weeks. Such symptoms may be as nonspecific as generalized fatigue or may consist of the onset of new angina pectoris. In patients who already have angina, there is commonly an increase in the severity, frequency, duration, or ease of production of the angina. Because the new onset of angina or a change in the pattern of angina often does lead to a myocardial infarction, it is recommended that patients with unstable angina or new angina be hospitalized in a coronary care unit. Bed rest and vigorous medical therapy will often stabilize the patient and may prevent a myocardial infarction.

Although a relationship between stress, emotional or physical, in the onset of the myocardial infarction has been avidly sought, normally no such relationship can be found. About one-third of myocardial infarctions occur during sleep, one-third when the patient is at work, and one-third when the patient is not at work. Sudden, severe exertion can rarely precipitate a myocardial infarction; more often, such sudden stress appears to precipitate ventricular arrhythmias and sudden death, without an actual myocardial infarction. In our experience, during major snow storms there are always sudden deaths attributable to heart disease, but there are no more admissions to the coronary care unit at that time than at any other.

The most prominent symptom of myocardial infarction is chest pain. As compared to angina, typically this is real pain. While it may come and go at first, the pain will eventually become severe, steady, and oppressive, and will often be associated with diaphoresis and nausea. Classically, the pain is substernal but it may radiate to the arms, shoulder, jaw, or back. The pain is not related to respiration or position, and the patient tends to stay quiet and avoid moving around. Although the classic presentation of myocardial infarction is associated with severe chest pain, there is a wide variation in the intensity of the symptoms. It has been found that about 20% of myocardial infarctions, as diagnosed by routine ECG, were clinically silent, with the patient unaware of any symptoms at the time of the infarction.

FINDINGS AND EVALUATIVE TESTS

A number of techniques beside the history are available to aid in the diagnosis of myocardial infarction; these will be discussed subsequently. However, it must be emphasized again that patients should be admitted to the coronary care unit on the basis of the history alone. First, only the history may be positive early; second, patients in the earliest phase of a myocardial infarction are at an extremely high risk for potentially lethal ventricular arrhythmias. Therefore, it is mandatory to move these patients into a monitored setting as quickly as possible. This permits the identification of such arrhythmias and simplifies their proper management. As many as 50% of the deaths from myocardial infarction occur before the patient can be gotten into the hospital. Many of these deaths are preventable.

A number of studies of the prehospital phase have shown that it takes the average patient 2 to 3 hours from the onset of the pain to take action. Once he decides to do something about the pain, however, he rather quickly arrives in a monitored setting. Efforts to shorten the time of the prehospital phase have included public education about the significance of chest pain, the use of monitored coronary-care ambulances, and the use of portable monitors and defibrillators at places such as sports arenas where large crowds gather. It is still true, however, that a large number of patients with infarctions die of treatable arrhythmias before they get to the hospital.

Physical Findings

The physical findings associated with an acute myocardial infarction are nonspecific and may include an S_4 gallop (almost universal in patients with a myocardial infarction when sinus rhythm is present), decreased intensity of S_1, and S_2, an S_3 gallop, a systolic murmur of papillary dysfunction, and, later in the course, a pericardial friction rub.

ECG

Eventually the ECG of a patient with a myocardial infarction should become abnormal but the initial tracing may be normal. Most myocardial infarctions ultimately produce Q waves of the ECG. However, when subendocardial myocardial infarction occurs, no diagnostic Q waves are seen. ST- and T-wave abnormalities are usually most marked early in the course of the infarction and tend to resolve with time. In addition to its usefulness in establishing the diagnosis, the ECG is obviously of value in identifying arrhythmias and disturbances of conduction. The ECG is further discussed in Chapter 4.

Enzyme Levels

Myocardial infarction is characteristically associated with a release of certain myocardial enzymes into the blood. The enzymes measured in evaluating a patient with suspected infarction are serum glutamic-oxaloacetic transaminase, lactic dehydrogenase, and creatine phosphokinase. The last, creatine phosphokinase, is especially useful, since it is the first of the enzymes whose level rises in the course of a myocardial infarction. Creatine phosphokinase is contained in brain (BB) and skeletal muscle (MM) as well as cardiac muscle. A specific isoenzyme can be identified for myocardial creatine phosphokinase, the MB band. Intramuscular injection, trauma, and even cardiac resuscitation can increase the skeletal muscle creatine phosphokinase, so that ability to identify the cardiac-specific MB isoenzyme is most useful. Elevation of the total creatine phosphokinase to at least 2½ times the normal value, accompanied by a positive MB band, and subsequent elevation of the serum glutamic-oxaloacetic transaminase and lactate dehydrogenase levels, is virtually diagnostic of an acute myocardial infarction. Considerable effort has gone into using the magnitude of the creatine phosphokinase rise as an indication of the size of the myocardial infarction. However, because of the need for a quantitative MB analysis, which is difficult, and variations in release and excretion of creatine phosphokinase, there is not a direct linear relationship between creatine phosphokinase and the size of the myocardial infarction.

CPK (MB)
↓
LDH
↓
SGOT

Radionuclear Studies

Radioisotopes are additional tools for diagnosing myocardial infarction. Radioactive technetium pyrophosphate is taken up by the infarcted tissue, since the pyrophosphate binds to the calcium released by the necrotic muscle. In our experience, however, this has not been a particularly specific or sensitive test, and a negative technetium pyrophosphate scan should not be viewed as excluding the diagnosis of myocardial infarction. Thallium 201, a potassium tracer, does not label ischemic muscle and therefore an area where an infarction has occurred shows up as a "cold area." This test is still being evaluated but appears to be quite promising. In addition, a blood-pool scan, using the patient's red cells tagged with a radioisotope to obtain the radionuclear ventriculogram, can be performed to demonstrate abnormalities of ventricular-wall motion. The use of radionuclear studies is discussed further in Chapter 20.

Other Tests and Findings

Some other nonspecific laboratory tests and physical findings should be mentioned. The patient may have either sinus bradycardia or sinus tachycardia. He will usually have some elevation of temperature. The degree of elevation bears a vague relation to the size of the infarct. The white-blood-cell count is elevated, as are levels of glucose and serum lipids. While still experimental, the echocardiogram appears to offer promise of giving useful information about wall motion. In an acute anterior infarct, poor septal motion suggests a large infarct and a poor prognosis.

TREATMENT

The patient suspected of having a myocardial infarction is admitted to a coronary care unit. The major role of the coronary care unit early in the course of infarction is the management of arrhythmias, primarily ventricular. There is some controversy over the efficacy of the coronary care unit, but in most hospitals which have developed them, the mortality from myocardial infarction has been reduced by about 15% to 20%. This would appear to us to represent sufficient justification for the use of the coronary care unit.

Patients admitted to the unit with an acute infarction are often extremely apprehensive. This, combined with the physical discomfort associated with the infarction, results in increase of sympathetic tone that may worsen the ischemic process. Therefore, the patient should be treated with narcotics and sedatives and given positive emotional support by the nurses and physicians. Above all, he should be reassured that most patients recover from a myocardial infarction and that he can be expected to get out of the hospital and go home and return to work.

Most patients with an acute infarction benefit from oxygen administered by nasal cannulae, 2 to 4 liters/min. There is some experimental evidence that this helps to minimize the size of the infarct, since patients at bed rest commonly experience some fall in Pa_{O2} because of pulmonary atelectasis. Finally, we believe that our patients just feel better and more secure with oxygen running at 2 liters/min. This need not be continued for a long period, but for the first 2 or 3 days it is most helpful. Patients should be started on a clear liquid diet that is advanced to a low-cholesterol, and often a low-sodium, diet during their hospitalization. The low-cholesterol diet is obviously not used for its immediate effect but rather to get the patient familiar with such a diet for long-term use. Physical activity should be begun as soon as the patient is free of pain and consists initially of sitting on the edge of the bed. If this is well tolerated, he may then be allowed to sit in a chair, and finally to ambulate. Bathroom privileges are permitted as early as possible in order to avoid the discomfort associated with the use of the bedpan. Most coronary care units strictly limit visiting hours. However, it has been found that the presence of a relative or friend will sometimes help to allay the patient's apprehension, and in that case the visiting hours should be liberalized.

COMPLICATIONS

The five major complications of myocardial infarction are tachyarrhythmias, congestive heart failure, conduction defects, myocardial rupture, and shock.

Arrhythmias

It is generally recognized that premature ventricular contractions are the necessary precursors of ventricular tachycardia and fibrillation and that effective suppression of the premature ventricular contractions can prevent the latter complications. In some coronary care units, all patients with known or suspected myocardial infarction are given prophylactic antiarrhythmic agents. In other hospitals, these agents are given only to patients who develop premature ventricular contractions, that is, over 5 per min, 2 or more in a row, multifocal, or premature ventricular contraction on the t wave (the "r or t" phenomenon).

Those who favor the more selective, rather than the routine, use of antiarrhythmic agents point out that the drugs are associated with significant side effects. The drug most commonly used for the suppression of premature ventricular contractions is lidocaine, given as an intravenous bolus of 50 to 75 mg, followed by a repeat bolus in 10 to 15 min. As soon as the first bolus is given, the patient is started on a drip of 4 mg/min. The rate of this infusion is reduced as quickly as possible to the minimum required to control the premature ventricular contractions (preferably 2 mg/min). The major side effects of lidocaine consist of central nervous system manifestations. These range in severity from mild paresthesias to grand mal seizures. Elderly patients and patients with liver disease are most susceptible to these adverse reactions.

In addition to ventricular arrhythmias occurring in the acute phase of the myocardial infarction, late arrhythmias (that is, those occurring after the third day) may also develop. These are generally seen in patients with large infarcts, triple-vessel disease, and impaired left-ventricular function, and thus carry an ominous prognosis. If the condition is acute, these would be treated with lidocaine, but in addition they usually require long-term oral therapy. These patients are monitored by telemetry during their entire stay in the hospital, if possible. Their management is always difficult and will usually require more than one antiarrhythmic agent and a good deal of trial and error before the arrhythmias can be satisfactorily suppressed. The further management of premature ventricular contraction is discussed in the section on tachyarrhythmias (Chap. 11). Ventricular tachycardia is an emergency and should be treated with a chest thump followed by electroshock. The ventricular fibrillator should be defibrillated as soon as it is recognized.

Patients with a myocardial infarction may also have supraventricular tachyarrhythmias, most commonly atrial fibrillation and flutter. The recognition and management of these arrhythmias is important because they may result in significant hemodynamic impairment and worsening of the myocardial ischemia. Depending upon the circumstances under which these arrhythmias occur, they may be treated with digitalis or electrical cardioversion. Cardioversion for supraventricular tachyarrhythmias is reserved for those patients who are in difficulty hemodynamically from the fast rate; it is commonly used for atrial flutter and is much less commonly necessary for atrial fibrillation.

Congestive Failure

Congestive failure occurs in 10% to 15% of myocardial infarctions and carries a poor prognosis. The diagnosis is made as described in Chapter 8. The patient develops increasing shortness of breath, often first noticed by the nurses. An S_3 is often present. Basilar rales are heard and the chest film shows interstitial or pulmonary edema. In general, congestive failure represents a large infarct with a loss of 20% to 30% of the myocardium. However, specific conditions such as mitral regurgitation from papillary muscle dysfunction or rupture, a ruptured intraventricular septum, or tachybradyarrhythmias, may cause congestive failure in a patient with a myocardial infarction. The management of tachyarrhythmias has already been discussed. Bradyarrhythmias may be managed by atropine or an artificial pacemaker (to be discussed subsequently). Mitral regurgitation and ventricular septal defects are recognized by their characteristic murmurs. Although medical management can often stabilize such patients, they may, in many cases, require surgical therapy.

Once specific causes have been excluded for the congestive failure, the treatment is well standardized. Although many physicians are reluctant to give digitalis to patients with a recent infarction, the use of digitalis in failure results actually in a net decrease in myocardial oxygen needs by decreasing the size of the heart, and thus is beneficial. The best method of administering the drug (assuming the patient has not previously taken digitalis) is to give 1 mg of digoxin intravenously over 24 hrs, beginning with a bolus of 0.5 mg. Diuretics are used to reduce left atrial pressure and pulmonary congestion. Vasodilators, such as nitroglycerin, isosorbide dinitrate, and nitroprusside are extremely effective in managing refractory congestive failure. They act by reducing preload or afterload and possibly by improving myocardial perfusion. If hypotension is associated with failure, then hemodynamic monitoring with a pulmonary-artery catheter is mandatory. Excessive reduction of left-ventricular filling pressure below 15 to 18 mmHg would further threaten cardiac output and blood pressure. However, the ordinary patient in failure who has a normal blood pressure does not require a pulmonary-artery catheter, and the failure can be treated on a clinical basis. If acute mitral insufficiency or ruptured ventricular septum are suspected, then the pulmonary-artery catheter can be used to diagnose the left-to-right shunt or the large v wave in the pulmonary capillary wedge tracing for mitral regurgitation.

Conduction Defect

Heart block of varying degrees can occur in patients with an acute myocardial infarction, and for these conduction defects the management is well standardized. Sinus bradycardia, defined as a heart rate under 60, is usually benign. We do not treat this unless the heart rate is below 50 or the patient manifests hypotension or failure. The treatment is atropine given intravenously, usually 0.5 mg, repeated in 3 min if there has been no response. Rarely, sinus bradycardia will require a temporary transvenous pacer to control the rate until the sinus node recovers. For atrioventricular block, the treatment depends on the location of the infarction. In general, atrioventricular block in an inferior myocardial infarction is more benign. The block is temporary, and the His bundle will provide a dependable backup pacemaker. Therefore, first degree and second degree (Mobitz I or Wenckebach) block does not require a temporary transvenous pacer. Third degree block generally does, depending on the patient's hemodynamic status. With an anterior or true posterior myocardial infarction, the His bundle is not dependable, and with complete block there is no backup pacer. First degree block is worrisome and the staff of the cardiac care unit should be alerted to the problem. Treatment requires some judgment. If it is 8:00 A.M. Monday, with all of the cardiology staff available, one might not use a pacer; however, if the patient seems in any way unstable, then a temporary transvenous pacer should be inserted. Second degree block (Mobitz II) is an indication for immediate pacing, and third degree is an emergency. However, while waiting for transvenous pacer placement, a rhythm can be maintained using a drip of Isoproterenol at approximately 2 to 6 µg/min.

Controversy remains about the indications for pacing with new bundle-branch block or hemiblock. In general, it is our feeling that a new bundle-branch or hemi-block requires a temporary pacer. However, one may find some disagreement about this among cardiologists. Some patients who require temporary pacing will also require a permanent pacer. These are usually the patients who have anterior or posterior infarcts with high degrees of block.

Myocardial Rupture

Myocardial rupture occurs in only about 3% of myocardial infarctions, but it accounts for about 10% of the deaths from infarction. It generally occurs during the first 5 days, and in older patients and patients who are hypertensive, with a first infarction. Because of the last, hypertension (greater than 150/90) should be treated promptly in the cardiac care unit. Nitroprusside has been proved to be an effective agent in this setting. While there have been a few reports of successful surgery for myocardial rupture, the mortality rate remains virtually 100%.

Shock

Cardiogenic shock occurs in about 9% of all myocardial infarctions but carries with it an 80% mortality, depending on how it is defined. The shock can occur initially, but often the patient's blood pressure will decline gradually during several days before the typical syndrome develops, full-blown shock. The definition of shock includes arterial systolic blood pressure below 100 mmHg and evidence that the patient has reduced systemic flow, such as cold, moist skin, oliguria, and an impaired sensorium. In about 20% of these patients, the left-ventricular filling pressure is low, because the patient is volume-depleted. By using intervenous fluids and raising the left-ventricular diastolic pressure as measured by the pulmonary artery catheter to end diastolic pressure of 16 to 18 mmHg output will improve, and the patient may very well survive. However, in the remaining 80% of the patients with the clinical findings of cardiogenic shock, the filling pressure is elevated, and the mortality is close to 100%. The use of vasoactive drugs such as Dopamine or possibly Dobutamine (more promising recently) and the intraaortic balloon assist have not significantly improved the survival rate. Even if the patient survives to leave the hospital, he has a 50 to 60% mortality in the next year.

A less important but bothersome complication of myocardial infarction which may occur early in the course is pericarditis. This will be associated with new pain, which, however, is different from the pain of the myocardial infarction. it is positional, related to respiration, and associated with a friction rub. While pericarditis usually occurs with a large myocardial infarction, it does not have a significant effect on prognosis. It is almost always a self-limiting complication. Patients with pericarditis should not be given anticoagulants, because of the dangers of hemorrhagic pericarditis and tamponade. Pericarditis responds well to Indocin.

LIMITING THE SIZE OF THE MYOCARDIAL INFARCT

For years the actual pathogenesis of cardiogenic shock was unclear, until it was beautifully demonstrated by Roberts that shock occurs when 40% of the left-ventricular mass is lost. With experience it has become obvious that congestive failure and lethal late arrhythmias are also associated with large infarcts, although a little less myocardium is lost than in cardiogenic shock. Just after Roberts made his discovery, Braunwald began the necessary studies to determine if the loss of myocardium could be limited, thus preventing shock, congestive failure, and the late arrhythmias. It had been shown at autopsy that the entire infarct is not formed at the same time. At first the affected area of the myocardium contains ischemic tissue which is not irreversibly lost and which could potentially be salvaged, thus limiting the size of the infarct. It was reasoned by Braunwald that if coronary flow could be improved to the ischemic area or the oxygen needs decreased, then the ischemic myocardium might be salvaged. In animals, this can clearly be shown for several drugs, including nitroglycerin, beta blockade, and hyaluronidase. In man, before methods of limiting the size of the infarction can be satisfactorily evaluated, reliable methods for measuring the size of the infarct and the amount of dead and salvagable ischemic myocardium must be found. Current techniques that have been employed for this purpose involve ECG ST-segment mapping, serial measurements of creatine phosphokinase released from the infarcted myocardium, and, more recently, radionuclear studies. All have limitations, and at the moment the most promising appears to be the radionuclear studies. However, no complete agreement exists as to whether infarct size can be quantitated. Nevertheless, because of the impressive animal data and some preliminary patient data, several drugs are being used. Nitrates have been most extensively used in attempts to limit the size of the infarct. The mechanism of their action consists of reducing ventricular preload and afterload, thus decreasing myocardial oxygen needs and increasing myocardial perfusion by vasodilatation either of the coronary arterioles or of the coronary collaterals. Recent studies showing coronary artery spasm in acute myocardial infarction make nitrates a really promising mode of therapy. The development of significant hypotension limits the use of nitrates, and they should always be given with caution in an acute myocardial infarction. If hypotension occurs, fluids should be used to raise the blood pressure, and the patient should be flat in bed with the legs raised.

Propranolol has also been utilized to limit the size of the infarction, because of its negative inotropic and chronotropic properties. These serve effectively to decrease myocardial oxygen needs. Propranolol must, however, be used with extreme caution, since it can exacerbate congestive failure and produce conduction defects and hypotension.

Hyaluronidase has been shown to decrease the size of the infarct in some patients, but its use has not been well established on a clinical basis. Solutions of glucose, insulin, and potassium have been used to minimize the size of the infarct by improving anaerobic metabolism; again, their use is controversial. Various mechanical means of supporting the circulation and thus decreasing the burden on the ventricle have been employed successfully in selected patients. The most widely used is intraaortic balloon counterpulsation. This is an invasive technique and should be reserved for very complicated infarcts. It cannot be used routinely. While conclusive evidence that myocardial infarct size can be limited is lacking, in the patient who continues to have pain over 24 hours, aggressive therapy appears to be indicated. Because of the evidence for spasm, we start with nitrates in such patients. The blood pressure should be carefully watched. If the pain persists, we would then add propranolol, starting in low doses and carefully monitoring blood pressure and atrioventricular and interventricular conduction.

Other Aspects of Treatment

The use of anticoagulants in myocardial infarction remains somewhat controversial. Careful reviews of the available data by Feinstein have pointed out that no definitive studies have been done to evaluate the role of anticoagulants. In general, we do not use them routinely; however, they certainly may be used if there are no contraindications. Relative contraindications to the use of anticoagulants, besides pericarditis, include a prior history of gastrointestinal bleeding and significant liver disease. For long-term anticoagulation, one must have both a reliable patient and a reliable laboratory.

After 3 stable days in the cardiac care unit, the patient may be transferred out. We prefer keeping every patient on ECG monitoring by telemetry for the next 2 or 3 days or in a progressive care unit. Actually, all patients should be monitored throughout their entire stay in the hospital. However, as this is not yet possible for all patients, those who have had large myocardial infarctions, as judged by the clinical criteria of failure, hypotension, or complicated arrhythmias, should be monitored for longer. Obviously, if the patient develops a new pain or new arrhythmia, he should be returned to the coronary care unit.

The progress of ambulation once the patient leaves the coronary care unit is somewhat variable. We prefer keeping the patient in his room for 3 or 4 days after he has left the coronary care unit, although he should have bathroom privileges as soon as possible. Then, over the next week to 10 days, he is gradually encouraged to walk, so that by the time is almost ready to go home he is able to walk unassisted in the hall as he likes. Prior to discharge from the hospital, which could be before the full 3 weeks for many patients, the patient should have a 24-hour ECG monitor or be returned to telemetry for 24 hours. We prefer the ambulatory Holter monitor, since this device makes it easier to quantitate the number of premature ventricular contractions. If significant ventricular arrhythmias are shown, patients should be kept in the hospital and started on an antiarrhythmic agent, as discussed in the section on tachyarrhythmias. The principles of therapy are to give a loading dose and judge the response to therapy by telemetry and blood levels. The exact number of premature ventricular contractions requiring treatment have not been determined, but it is believed that more than 30 per hour, multifocal ones, or two in a row, should be treated. The antiarrhythmic therapy should be continued for at least 6 months, and it is important to emphasize that patients will often require multiple drug therapy before the premature ventricular contractions can be successfully suppressed. Whether or not this will have any real effect on mortality is unknown, but our current thinking is that it should be done.

Secondly, we believe that a low-level stress test should be carried out in some patients. This is useful primarily for the uncomplicated myocardial infarction. We use about a 9-min treadmill test with continual ECG monitoring. The workload should not exceed stage I of the Bruce protocol, 1.7 mph at a 10% grade. In addition, the heart rate should probably not be allowed to exceed 110 to 120 beats per min. Patients who cannot walk the necessary 9 min because of angina, ST-segment or t-wave changes, hypotension, or fatigue, require further treatment in the hospital. They should not be discharged until they have been put on antianginal therapy, if they have angina, or on antiarrhythmic therapy if they develop arrhythmias.

After discharge, the average patient should be kept at home for 3 weeks and then allowed to increase his activity for 3 more weeks; at the end of 6 weeks at home he should have a repeat treadmill test. Obviously, in considering the plans for discharge, the home situation is all-important. For example, if the patient lives alone and must climb two flights of stairs to get to the bathroom, hospitalization should be prolonged.

Certain patients, but not all, should undergo cardiac catheterization after myocardial infarction. Generally, we reserve catheterization for patients who have the following features: *1*) Age under 30: often, in this age group, patients have single-vessel disease, the prognosis is good, and they will be helped a great deal by knowing it. *2*) Angina with postmyocardial infarction: it is said that 50% of patients will have angina after myocardial infarction and that not all of these need to be catheterized. However, if the angina is clearly related to minimal exertion, the patient should be studied. Post myocardial-infarction angina may mean that the ischemic process is continuing outside the area of the infarction and that another wall is threatened. *3*) Patients with a positive stress test should, in general, have catheterization. *4*) Some patients with a subendocardial infarction should have a catheterization.

Much has been written about exercise training in patients with a myocardial infarction. Certainly if there is no angina, hypotension, or failure, patients can be trained in the normal way. As with all exercise training programs, patients feel better, but there is no evidence that they live any longer. We do not systematically put all our patients into a jogging or bicycle program. However, exercise has a role in improving patients' morale.

If they do get into a training program, they must have a stress test first and then should be trained at a load below that which leads to abnormalities on the stress test. We recommend exercise training, for both angina and infarctions, only in a hospital setting. The training can be done on an outpatient basis, but exercise should start in the hospital rather than in an office setting. Although, as we have said, systematic exercise training is not routine for all patients, most should be encouraged to do some walking. While this may not in any way enhance survival, it makes patients feel better. Older patients may have to walk in enclosed shopping centers in the winter, but the advantages seem worth the effort.

Finally, certain drugs apparently prolong survival in patients with myocardial infarction; they are the salicylates, sulfinpyrazone, and beta blockers. Practolol, while no longer available, appeared to be clearly effective in improving survival in anterior infarcts. Both aspirin and propronolol are now being carefully studied in a National Institutes of Health program, and the results should be available in the next two years, though incorrect dose selection may render the aspirin study inconclusive. We do not routinely put our patients on beta blockers, aspirin, or sulfinpyrazone. However, many cardiologists are using one of these modes of therapy.

The physician has a good chance to modify risk factors while patients are still under treatment. The patients are frightened and tractable. They have often stopped smoking because of hospital regulations, have been eating a sensible diet, and have had their blood pressure controlled. This is the time to consolidate these gains into permanent behavior changes.

REFERENCES

1. Oliver MF: Cholesterol, coronaries, clofibrate and death (editorial). N Eng J Med 299:1360–1361, 1978
2. Mann GV: Diet-heart: end of an era. N Eng J Med 297:644–650, 1977
3. Fredrickson DS: A physician's guide to hyperlipidemia. Modern Concepts of Cardiovascular Disease 41:31–36, 1972
4. Coronary drug project research group: Clofibrate and niacin in coronary heart disease. J Amer Med Assoc 231:360–381, 1975
5. Roberts WC, Buja LM: The frequency and significance of coronary arterial thrombi and other observations in fatal acute myocardial infarction. Amer J Med 52:425–443, 1972
6. Silver MD, Baroldi G, Mariani F: The relationship between acute occlusive coronary thrombi and myocardial infarction studied in one hundred consecutive patients. Circulation 61:219–227, 1980

CORONARY ARTERY DISEASE: ANGINA PECTORIS

10

Robert H. Eich and Robert Warner

  The term **angina pectoris** means literally a choking or suffocative pain in the chest. Diagnosis is based primarily on the history. Implicit in the diagnosis is ischemia of the myocardium as a cause of the pain. This ischemia is usually the result of coronary atherosclerosis, although it may be present in aortic valve disease with normal coronary arteries and in other diseases of the coronary arteries. For example, luetic involvement of the ostia of the coronary arteries can produce classical angina pectoris. Likewise, spasm of the coronary arteries can produce ischemia in some patients with normal coronary arteries. This chapter, however, will be devoted to angina pectoris as it occurs with coronary artery disease in the form of coronary atheroslerosis.

  Angina pectoris may be the first manifestation of coronary artery disease in a given patient. Although angina has been reported in nearly every age group of patients over 30, it is most commonly seen in patients in their 50s and 60s. While the exact incidence of angina pectoris is hard to determine and depends on the population studied, in one series the incidence of the development of new angina was 4.2:100 in the age group 50 to 54. The diagnosis of angina pectoris carries with it an increased risk of myocardial infarction or sudden death from arrhythmia. The prognosis in patients with angina is clearly related to the number of vessels with significant disease (three-vessel disease is more serious than one-vessel disease) and the quality of left-ventricular function. Mortality is clearly incresed with decreased left-ventricular function.

PATHOPHYSIOLOGY

The symptoms of angina pectoris occur when the demands for oxygen by the myocardium exceed the capacity of the coronary circulation to increase flow

134

and meet the demands. The coronary circulation is such that if oxygen needs are increased, flow must increase. The heart has only a limited tolerance for anaerobic metabolism, and it cannot compensate for increased oxygen needs by increasing oxygen extraction.

Oxygen demand by the myocardium is determined by heart rate, myocardial contractility, and left-ventricular wall tension. Wall tension is difficult to estimate. It is directly related to the impedance to ventricular emptying (afterload, or, more simply, blood pressure) and to ventricular volume, and inversely related to wall thickness. Simplistically, we equate wall tension with blood pressure, since tension, wall thickness, and ventricular volume are difficult to determine. Therefore, myocardial oxygen needs depend on heart rate, contractility, and blood pressure. The oxygen needs can then be roughly estimated by the so-called double product (heart rate × systolic blood pressure), or triple product (heart rate × systolic blood pressure × systolic ejection time). The systolic ejection time is used as an indication of the duration of oxygen needs, since these are greater in systole. Diastolic fiber length plays some role in oxygen needs as well.

Oxygen delivery to the myocardium depends on the oxygen content of the blood, oxygen extraction, and myocardial blood flow. As already mentioned, since extraction cannot be significantly increased, oxygen delivery depends essentially on flow. Consideration of flow involves both total flow and distribution of flow with the myocardium. Blood flow to the endocardium is the most precarious and can easily be jeopardized, not only by coronary artery disease but by shortening diastole or incresing systolic pressure. Coronary flow itself is directly regulated by blood pressure (most importantly, the diastolic blood pressure, since most of the flow occurs in diastole) and by resistance.

Resistance is determined in some part by a systolic throttling of flow. Until recently, however, the major resistance to flow in the coronary circulation was felt to be in the precapillary arterioles. These are under some neurogenic control by the sympathetic nervous system but primarily controlled by local metabolic factors. When myocardial oxygen demand increases, there is a reduction in tissue oxygen tension or pH, and this results in the release of a chemical mediator, probably adenosine, which produces vasodilatation. This vasodilatation in turn, leads to increased flow and thus the increased demands for oxygen are met. With the development of coronary artery disease in the large epicardial arteries, flow becomes limited by the stenosis. Thus when needs are increased, although there is dilatation at the arteriolar level, the fixed narrowing in the lumen of the epicardial arteries prevents flow from increasing. A 50% reduction in the lumen diameter may be sufficient to limit flow with exercise while a 75% reduction would limit flow at rest. When flow is limited and oxygen needs are increased, ischemia develops. The ischemia is more dangerous than hypoxia since because of the reduced blood flow there is an accumulation of metabolic products. These include lactate and hydrogen ions, and potassium which leaks out of the cell. Because of the reduced flow these accumulate in high concentrations and threaten cell viability. With continued ischemia arrhythmias, hemodynamic abnormalities, and myocardial infarction may occur.

The large epicardial arteries were always felt to be passive conduits narrowed only by anatomical obstruction due to coronary atherosclerosis. However, it has now been clearly demonstrated that the large epicardial arteries have autonomic nervous system innervation and that the alpha sympathetic nervous system produces vasoconstriction and the beta system vasodilatation. Spasm or increased neurogenic tone can reduce coronary flow and produce ischemia without any increase in needs. The spasm may occur on a fixed obstruction or, more rarely, it may occur in normal epicardial arteries. Thus the clinical entity of Prinzmetal's angina which occurs at rest has now been shown to be due to spasm and not increased needs. The large epicardial arteries are not under metabolic control and thus the increased vasomotor tone is unopposed and vasoconstriction occurs. Increased vasomotor tone in the epicardial arteries or spasm may also play a role in unstable angina or possibly even in some patients with stable angina.

DIAGNOSIS

HISTORY

The diagnosis of angina pectoris is made chiefly on the basis of the history. While we habitually ask patients about chest "pain," most patients with angina do not refer to the sensation as pain. The majority describe it either as a pressure or a burning sensation in the chest. The closest approximation to this sensation of "burning" is the feeling in the chest that most adults can recall getting as children when they had run hard for a long period of time. Occasionally patients point out that it is not always an unpleasant sensation. The discomfort is usually retrosternal, but it may start in the arms, shoulders, neck, jaw, or back, and if it starts in the substernal region, it may well radiate into the above areas. It is usually not at the cardiac apex. The discomfort may be associated with diaphoresis or shortness of breath, but these are not necessary for the diagnosis. However, it is important to point out that at times patients may confuse shortness of breath with chest discomfort and describe angina as shortness of breath.

Symptoms characteristically occur at times of physical or emotional stress, circumstances which increase myocardial oxygen demands by increasing blood pressure, heart rate, or contractility. In most cases the discomfort will tend to increase if the patient continues the activity, forcing him to stop or slow down. This is an important differential, since patients with chest pain and normal coronary arteries can often keep on exerting, despite the pain. However, in an occasional patient with true angina, the pain will subside despite continued effort. This phenomenon is called *walk through angina*, and subsidence of the pain presumably results from the opening of coronary collaterals as the result of the release of adenosine.

Most patients report that their angina is worse, and comes on more easily, in the cold. This is explained by an increase in left-ventricular afterload as a result of an increase in blood pressure produced by the cold. Similarly, the discomfort may be worse after eating, presumably because eating itself increases myocardial oxygen needs. Additionally, patients often find their angina worse upon first arising in the morning. They will stop, take a nitroglycerin, the pain will subside, and they will have no further episodes for the rest of the day. Many patients will have pain on walking to work in the morning and never have it again throughout the day.

At a given stage in the course of the disease, the amount of exertion required to produce angina remains relatively constant, as measured by treadmill testing. However, patients will often report day-to-day variations in the location, quality, radiation, and duration of the discomfort, as well as in the amount of effort needed to produce it. In addition, 30% of patients will have a spontaneous remission. The production of the angina is often a function of the quality, as well as the type of physical activity. In many cases angina is provoked more readily by activities requiring the use of the arms than those which require the use of the legs, the explanation being that the arms are less well trained and have a lesser muscle mass, so that more activity is necessary. Another important point in the history is that the pain or discomfort subsides fairly quickly after the patient stops the exertion, usually within 2 to 3 min after stopping the activity or taking nitroglycerin. Prompt clearing of the discomfort is an important differential, since in patients with chest pain and normal coronary arteries, activity and nitroglycerin seem to have very little effect on the pain.

Again, for the sake of emphasis, let us repeat that several special features of angina are crucial in the history.

1. There should be some exertional component to the pain. The patient may get it at rest but he also clearly should get it on exertion. Only the variant angina (**Prinzmetal's angina**) or unstable angina occurs at rest without an exercise component.
2. Second, while it may not be described as pain, angina is the kind of sensation that makes the patient stop whatever he is doing. He recognizes that with continued exertion the discomfort would worsen in severity, and therefore he stops.
3. Once he stops, with or without taking nitroglycerin, the discomfort should subside in 1 to 3 min.

These three features—an exertional component, the increase in severity as the patient continues to exercise, and prompt relief with rest and nitroglycerin, are the most useful features which distinguish true angina pectoris.

In our catheterization laboratory, as in most laboratories, about 10% to 15%

of the patients admitted for catheterization with chest pain are found to have normal coronary arteries. The syndrome of chest pain with normal coronary arteries is benign and may have many causes; occasionally it is difficult to separate from coronary artery disease by the history. However, the histories of most patients with this syndrome have unusual features: the discomfort is not burning; it is often sharp; it is not exertional; they can exercise with it; it does not subside with rest; and it is not promptly relieved by nitroglycerin. We must add, however, that occasionally angina itself may become atypical, and failure of nitroglycerin to give relief implies either no disease or severe triple-vessel disease.

The pain pattern of angina can vary. It is well recognized that in about 30% of patients with angina, the pain will subside for long periods and the patients will become asymptomatic. The mechanism for this is either the development of collaterals or the occurrence of a myocardial infarction. Similarly, of course, the angina can increase, and we call angina which develops in this way **unstable angina** or **crescendo angina,** we prefer not to use the term **preinfarction angina** since patients who become unstable do not always go on to develop myocardial infarction. Important signs that the angina is becoming unstable are that less and less exertion is required to produce the pain; the pain may develop at night, or at rest; more nitroglycerin, and more time, are required for relief of the pain. The pain of angina can blend into the pain of myocardial infarction, and the development of myocardial infarction becomes a major concern when patients with angina become unstable. The term **intermediate coronary syndrome** is useful to describe the patient whose angina has become unstable and continues to have pain in spite of maximum medical therapy, including hospitalization. The patient is probably threatened with a myocardial infarction. In our own experience, failure of angina to stabilize with hospital treatment is uncommon but it does occur.

The presence of risk factors for conorary artery disease is helpful in evaluating the history of chest pain. If the patient is under 35, has no family history of coronary artery disease, none of the usual risk factors, and has atypical chest pain, then it is highly likely that he does not have angina pectoris. The risk factors (described earlier in Chapter 1) include:

1. Age: coronary artery disease and angina pectoris increase with age into the 50s
2. Sex: coronary artery disease is more common in men than in women until age 50 to 60 when the incidence becomes equal
3. Hypertension
4. Diabetes mellitus
5. Smoking (*esp* <50 *yrs*)
6. Hyperlipidemia
7. A positive family history

In the age group under 50, smoking (more than a pack daily for 10 years) is a major risk factor. Obesity is not a major factor, since it seldom occurs alone but is usually associated with hypertension, diabetes mellitus, or hyperlipidemia. We have not been particularly impressed with sedentary life or the "Type A" personality as being important risk factors, although they are usually listed. Gout is not a useful risk factor. Based on the history alone, including the history of the chest discomfort and risk factors, you should be able to correctly diagnose angina pectoris in most of your patients.

Recently, there has been considerable interest in Prinzmetal's variant angina. Prinzmetal first described this form of angina in 1959. It includes the following unusual features:

> The pain is not brought on by increased cardiac work, it is usually more severe and of longer duration, often waxes and wanes in cyclic fashion, often occurs at about the same time each day, and is not relieved by rest.*

The electrocardiogram shows ST-segment elevation with the pain. In addition, arrhythmias, which are often ventricular, occur frequently, and conduction defects may occur. Sudden death frequently results. The mechanism of Prinzmetal's variant angina, and of some other rest anginas, has clearly been shown to involve spasm of the epicardial coronary arteries. This may occur with what appears to be a normal coronary artery, or it may occur on a lesion in the coronary artery. Because of the impressive incidence of sudden death, this condition, when identified, requires hospitalization, coronary angiography, and intensive therapy.

PHYSICAL EXAMINATION

As we have said, the diagnosis of angina pectoris can usually be made on the basis of a careful history; as always, this is the most important single tool available. The physical examination is of only limited value in the diagnosis of angina pectoris. During an episode of angina, the patient's systemic blood pressure may rise. Angina may also be associated with the appearance or increase in intensity of an S_4 sound. In some patients, an S_3 sound or a systolic murmur from ischemic papillary dysfunction my become audible during the anginal attack. Occasionally a dyskinetic precordial impulse may be seen or palpated during an attack of angina. However, it is important to emphasize that patients may have an impressively normal physical examination before, during, or after the time when they are having the angina.

ELECTROCARDIOGRAM

The resting electrocardiogram is often perfectly normal in patients with angina. Obviously, if the electrocardiogram shows an old myocardial infarction, the diagnosis of angina would be much more secure. During anginal episodes,

* Prinzmetal M, Kennamer R, Merliss R et al: A variant form of angina pectoris. Am J Med 27: 359, 1959

changes in the ST segment and the T wave in one or more of the electrocardio-graphic leads may be noted, but great care should be taken not to overempha-size the diagnostic importance of this. We have seen patients with classical an-gina who have normal EKGs during their anginal episodes, and we have seen patients with impressive changes in the ST segment and T wave who have nor-mal coronary arteries. The ST-segment elevation which occurs with Prinzme-tal's angina has already been mentioned.

EXERCISE TESTING

Exercise testing has become an extremely important tool in evaluating patients with chest pain and often helps in the diagnosis of angina pectoris. A 1-mm horizontal or downsloping depression of the ST segment at the J point, particu-larly if it occurs during typical chest discomfort, is strong evidence in favor of the diagnosis. Many different protocols are used for exercise testing. We prefer the standard Bruce protocol, where the speed and grade of the treadmill are in-creased every 3 min until the patient reaches a predicted heart rate based on age, which is approximately 85% of the maximal heart rate. The test is stopped if the patient complains of chest discomfort or if there is significant (more than 4 mm) depression of the ST segment, arrhythmias, or hypotension. Obviously, motivation and physical conditioning may affect the test. As with any diagnostic test, there are false positive and false negative results. The likelihood of obtain-ing false positive results increases if stress testing is applied to a population with a low prevalence of coronary artery disease. The probability of an apparently positive exercise test being truly positive is greater if the subject is a middle-aged, cigarette-smoking male than if the subject is a young female. Remember, an asymptomatic young man should not be diagnosed as having angina pectoris on the basis of a positive treadmill test alone; at most, this might be considered an additional risk factor.

Besides serving as a tool to establish the diagnosis of angina pectoris, exer-cise testing is an excellent means of determining the functional capacity of pa-tients with known or suspected coronary artery disease. By measuring the pa-tient's performance during the standardized exercise protocol, an assessment can be made of the daily activities that the patient can tolerate in comfort and safety.

RADIONUCLEAR STUDIES

Recently, radionuclear studies using Thallium ^{201}T1, which is not taken up by ischemic myocardium, have been used to supplement the results of treadmill testing. No doubt with the further development of external counting techniques and better isotopes, radionuclear studies will provide a powerful tool to help in the establishment of the diagnosis of coronary artery disease. The use of ra-dionuclear techniques is discussed further in Chapter 20.

CORONARY ANGIOGRAPHY

The most reliable method for determining whether or not coronary artery disease is present is coronary angiography. This has been discussed in some detail in Chapter 6. Coronary angiography has developed to the point where it can be carried out with a mortality of less than one-tenth of a percent and where it yields highly reliable diagnostic information. This has been one of the major advances in cardiology during the last 10 years. In addition to its usefulness in establishing the diagnosis of coronary artery disease, it is used to determine prognosis and the feasibility of coronary artery bypass grafting. Coronary angiography is indicated to resolve diagnostic problems, such as that presented by the patient with atypical chest pain, and to evaluate patients for possible surgery who have unstable or incapacitating angina. Coronary angiography is not normally indicated for the patient with stable angina which is being well controlled on a medical program. However, because the prognosis of angina is related to anatomy, some patients may undergo angiography for prognosis alone.

TREATMENT

Turning to therapy, once the diagnosis has been established, treatment should be started. Patients with stable angina can have their tests and treatment as outpatients, while patients with a new onset of angina, or unstable angina, may require hospitalization. Treatment is started first with nitroglycerin, which is an effective tool. By dilating the systemic veins, it reduces venous return (preload) and blood pressure (afterload). While it may not cause vasodilatation in the arterioles in the systemic circulation, it clearly does lower the blood pressure. The decrease in ventricular size and blood pressure, in turn, decreases myocardial oxygen needs. In addition, there is increasing evidence that nitroglycerin does improve blood flow to the ischemic myocardium, possibly by dilating collateral coronary vessels or shifting flow to the subendocardium. However, it is important to remember that nitroglycerin could reduce coronary flow by lowering the blood pressure. Therefore, patients should be cautioned to take nitroglycerin either sitting or lying down, when they first start it, and to lie down if they feel lightheaded after taking it. In addition, nitroglycerin does increase the heart rate, which could increase the oxygen needs, and a rare patient will state that nitroglycerin makes the pain worse.

Nitroglycerin is given sublingually. Many patients experience headaches from it at first, but they can be reassured that this side effect will eventually disappear. We have had success with advising that patients take nitroglycerin prophylactically before engaging in strenuous activities. Patients should be told that if their angina persists for more than 30 minutes after they have taken three nitroglycerine tablets, they should go to the nearest hospital emergency room, since the pain may no longer be angina and may represent a myocardial infarction. Many patients are reluctant to take nitroglycerin for fear of tolerance or headache and because the pain subsides promptly with rest. Tolerance has never been demonstrated. We do not insist that they take it, but we do insist that they carry it wherever they go. They must have nitroglycerin available if the pain does not promptly subside with rest. Nitroglycerin loses its potency with time, and the supply should be renewed every 2 months. Long-acting nitrates, such as isosorbide dinitrate, taken sublingually, do appear to be valuable when given on a regular basis, every 3 to 4 hours. The longer duration of action provides sustained effects. Recently we have used nitroglycerin paste applied to the skin, which gives a more sustained action, and it is very effective at bedtime as a prophylaxis against nocturnal angina.

Another group of drugs which are enormously useful in the treatment of angina are the beta adrenergic blocking agents. Beta blockade appears to exert its beneficial effect by reducing myocardial oxygen needs through decreasing heart rate, blood pressure, and contractility. However, beta blockade can also worsen congestive failure, produce bradyarrhythmias, and potentiate bronchospasm in patients with chronic lung disease. Fatigue, mental depression, and cold hands are three very common side effects. There is great individual variation in the dose necessary to produce significant blockade; secondary to differences in hepatic metabolism. Therefore, rather than prescribing an arbitrary dose, one should continue to give the blocking agents until the patient's pulse rate has been reduced both at rest and exercise, if possible. Usually, we start propranolol at 10 mg 4 times a day and increase the dose until either the angina symptoms are controlled or the heart rate is significantly reduced below 55. Recently there has been suggestive evidence in patients treated with beta blockade after a myocardial infarction that suvival may be improved. This may be true for patients with angina pectoris as well, although no studies are yet available. Currently, 3 beta adrenergic blocking agents are available in the United States. However, several excellent ones are available in Europe and should be marketed in this country sometime in the near future.

In addition to drug therapy, every possible effort should be made to alter the risk factors. The factor that can most clearly be eliminated is smoking. Patients with angina should not smoke. Not all patients will stop, but every one should be urged to do so. There is general agreement among epidemiologists that smoking clearly accelerates coronary artery disease. There is also statistical evidence that if the patient does stop, mortality can be modified, although it takes up to 10 years after cessation of smoking. Obviously the other risk factors should be minimized as much as possible, with attention to diet, blood pressure control, and control of diabetes mellitus.

The role of exercise training in angina is controversial. After training, the heart rate for any given workload will be less, and the patient should be able to exercise more before developing symptoms or perform the same workload without symptoms. Training a patient with angina requires initial treadmill stress testing to determine the proper load, and subsequent close supervision.

The patient should be started either on a bicycle or a treadmill training program where supervision is available. In order to assure proper supervision, we feel that this should be done in a hospital setting, although it can be done on an outpatient basis. It has been demonstrated, that patients with angina can get a training effect in 6 weeks of training. However, we feel that exercise training has a very limited role in management of angina pectoris, and that its value has not been proved.

If the patient's angina becomes unstable so that the pattern of his angina changes, coming on with less exertion or at rest, we recommend hospitalization. By placing the patient in a monitored unit at bed rest and administering nitrates and beta adrenergic blocking agents, the unstable pattern can be stabilized, and we believe that we may actually prevent myocardial infarction.

Nowhere in the field of cardiology is there more controversy than in discussions concerning the role of surgery in the management of angina pectoris. We feel that there is a definite place for surgery, but the precise indications remain to be clarified. The indicated surgery is the coronary artery bypass graft developed in 1967 by Favaloro and Effler. In this procedure, obstructive lesions in one or more of the coronary arteries are bypassed, using either the saphenous vein or the internal mammary artery. With an experienced team, bypass grafting can be carried out with a mortality of less than 2% in patients who are good risks. Similarly, relief of pain, while not absolutely complete in all patients, occurs in about 80% to 90%. The graft patency rate has now been shown to be approximately 80%, and it would appear that grafts which remain patent for the first few months will remain so for several years. There is general agreement that the operation is only palliative. The grafts themselves develop intimal changes, and the native coronary artery disease progresses. The major controversy revolves around whether or not the operation prolongs life or prevents myocardial infarction. Since there is an appreciable incidence of intraoperative infarction (5%–9%) and a definite, although small, surgical mortality, the operation is not indicated in all patients with angina. Nor will it be indicated in patients with asymptomatic coronary artery disease until a salutary effect on longevity can be shown. There have been four randomized studies comparing a medical and a surgical program. There appears to be little difference in mortality, although pain relief is better in the surgical program. The current thinking, and our recommendations for surgery, are those presented in an editorial in *Circulation,* March, 1978, by MacIntosh. If the patient has incapacitating angina, he should be considered for surgery. However, the definition of incapacitation varies from patient to patient and from physician to physician. The definition should be flexible, and the individual circumstances of different patients should be considered. For example, the patient who is unable to work is not necessarily incapacitated. A working patient who cannot engage in activities which he otherwise would enjoy on the other hand might be considered incapacitated. While the operation is primarily intended for relief of pain, there are anatomical considerations which modify that indication. Lesions of the main left coronary artery before it branches into the circumflex and left anterior descending arteries are usually considered to be life-threatening and indicate surgery irrespective of symptoms. Similarly, lesions in the left anterior descending artery with an occlusion of the right coronary artery may be considered as indicating surgery even without incapacitating pain. The presence of collaterals and of viable myocardium beyond the obstruction also play a role in the decision for or against surgery. In summary, the current recommendations are that surgery should be performed for relief of pain, with some allowance for anatomy.

Finally, the patient with angina is at an increased risk not only for myocardial infarction but for sudden death. The problem is how to detect the patient predisposed to sudden death. There is no definitive answer, but there is considerable information obtained from detecting arrhythmias on stress testing and 24-hour ambulatory EKG monitoring. Patients who have significant ventricular arrhythmias with either test should be considered for an antiarrhythmic drug program. While we have no definitive answers yet, we hope that during the next 10 years a clearer definition of the high-risk group for sudden death can be obtained in patients with angina and that better information can be obtained about the effect of antiarrhythmic therapy on survival.

TACHYCARDIA AND SUDDEN DEATH

11

Robert H. Eich

Tachycardia may be either supraventricular or ventricular; the two different forms have different etiologies and treatment. Tachycardias may occur in young people who have no heart disease and in older people with severe heart disease; obviously management and prognosis in these two cases will be different. Supraventricular tachycardias will be discussed first. These can be divided into **sinus tachycardia** and **paroxysmal supraventricular tachycardia,** which includes **paroxysmal atrial tachycardia, paroxysmal atrial tachycardia with block, paroxysmal junctional tachycardia,** and **junctional tachycardia.** Two other supraventricular tachycardias are **atrial fibrillation** and **atrial flutter.**

SUPRAVENTRICULAR TACHYCARDIA

SINUS TACHYCARDIA

Sinus tachycardia, defined as a heart rate over 100 beats per minute, is common. It can have multiple causes, including exertion, excitement, fever, anemia, hypoxia, hypovolemia, congestive heart failure, thyrotoxicosis, and sympathomimetic drugs. It is important to remember that sinus tachycardia is a secondary phenomenon resulting from increased sympathetic tone. Treatment must be aimed at the causes of the augmented sympathetic activity rather than directly at the tachycardia. The increased rate may be compensatory, helping to maintain blood pressure, and if the heart rate is deliberately slowed with a drug, such as one of the beta adrenergic blocking agents, the consequences could be disastrous. Blood pressure may fall to critical levels, and the patient may go into shock. That is why one should always find the cause for the sinus tachycardia and treat this.

145

Sinus tachycardia can vary between 100 and 160 beats per minute, and it may be extremely difficult to distinguish from paroxysmal atrial tachycardia. Here, and in all of the supraventricular tachycardias, pressure on the sinus of the carotid artery will be useful. The aim of this is to increase vagal tone by pressing on the carotid sinus and thus setting off a reflex rise in vagal tone and slowing of the heart rate. This must be carefully done in any patient. First one should listen over the carotid arteries for a bruit; if one is present, carotid compression should not be used. The patient's heart rate should be monitored and a continuous ECG recorded. Under no circumstances should the carotid massage be carried out unless the heart rate is at least being determined by auscultation. The patient should be supine, with the neck extended and head turned slightly to the side opposite the physician. First, the right carotid sinus at the bifurcation of the common carotid is compressed or massaged for 15 to 20 seconds. If there is no effect, the left carotid sinus should be compressed for the same period of time after a 2 to 3 minute pause. Bilateral compression should be avoided. Sinus tachycardia will slow gradually and then come back once the massage is stopped. There will be no evidence of atrioventricular block on the electrocardiogram; all of the P waves will be conducted. With carotid compression, paroxysmal atrial tachycardia will either break or not be affected, and in flutter and atrial fibrillation there will be some slowing of the ventricular response as a result of increased atrioventricular block. Carotid sinus pressure will often produce enough block in atrial flutter so that the rapid atrial response, with the P waves going at a rate of 220 to 260, can be seen.

PAROXYSMAL ATRIAL TACHYCARDIA AND PAROXYSMAL JUNCTIONAL TACHYCARDIA

The other supraventricular tachycardias which can occur in normal subjects are paroxysmal atrial tachycardia and paroxysmal junctional tachycardia. These have been clearly shown in most cases to be reentry arrhythmias, which pass through either the atrioventricular node or the sinus node. In these patients, the atrioventricular node can be dissociated into two pathways. In the subjects, who have paroxysmal atrial tachycardia without Wolff-Parkinson-White syndrome, both pathways activate the ventricle normally, and thus, the familiar preexcitation, or delta, waves cannot be seen. The dual pathways likewise occur in Wolff-Parkinson-White Syndrome, and in some patients the presence of the accessory pathway can be demonstrated by premature activation of the ventricle by way of the accessory path. In Wolff-Parkinson-White syndrome, the retrograde path is usually the accessory bundle, however, so that the paroxysmal atrial tachycardia has a normal QRS configuration. In any case, because of the dual pathways, it is possible for a premature atrial beat to go down one pathway and come back by the other, thus setting up a reentrant arrhythmia. Classically, paroxysmal atrial tachycardia occurs in subjects with no heart disease and is a benign arrhythmia in that it is well tolerated for hours. The heart rate is between 140 and 180 and is extremely regular. Carotid sinus pressure either does not affect the rhythm or abolishes it by altering the properties of the atrioventricular conduction system and breaking the reentry circuit. If carotid pressure does not work, other measures to increase vagal tone should be used. These include raising systolic pressure with alpha adrenergic drugs such as phenylephrine or methoxamine. Edrophonium chloride (Tensilon) can be used to increase vagal tone and may result in conversion. Digitalization, if the physician is sure that the rhythm is paroxysmal atrial tachycardia, will often help convert the patient, and in only a small group of patients will cardioversion be necessary.

Paroxysmal junctional tachycardia is managed in the same way as paroxysmal atrial tachycardia. It is important to note that junctional tachycardia may be a manifestation of digitalis toxicity as it is a very uncommon rhythm otherwise.

PAROXYSMAL ATRIAL TACHYCARDIA WITH BLOCK

Paroxysmal atrial tachycardia with block is an entirely different arrhythmia. Presumably it is the result of an ectopic focus (firing as a pacemaker) rather than of reentry, and it is always associated with organic heart disease. In 50% to 60% of all cases, it is due to digitalis toxicity, either from an increased blood level of digitalis or a low level of potassium. The atrial rate is 160 to 200. The block may be in varying combinations of mobitz I or mobitz II. Pressure on the carotid sinus will increase the block and may be helpful in distinguishing this tachycardia from the others. The treatment is to check the blood level of digitalis and the serum potassium level; obviously, if the rhythm is the result of digitalis toxicity, the digitalis should be withheld and hypokalemia corrected. In general, if the ventricular response is satisfactory (an atrial rate of 160 but—because of block—a ventricular response of 80), then one need do nothing else except observe the patient.

A rhythm that is seen only in heart disease, and especially in heart disease secondary to lung diesease, is **multifocal atrial tachycardia, or chaotic atrial mechanism.** This may be difficult to tell from paroxysmal atrial tachycardia with block, but it consists of sinus tachycardia and premature atrial contractions from three different foci. The treatment is very difficult. Beta blockade occasionally will work but should be used with great caution because the patients often have both heart disease and lung disease. Digitalis is seldom effective, but it certainly may be tried.

ATRIAL FIBRILLATION AND ATRIAL FLUTTER

Atrial fibrillation and atrial flutter are almost invariably associated with organic heart disease. In both of these arrhythmias, the atrial contribution is lost, and this may jeopardize cardiac output. Especially in atrial flutter, the patients may become hypotensive or go into heart failure. Atrial flutter is a difficult arrhythmia to treat. Commonly it is seen in chronic lung disease with an enlarged right atrium, arteriosclerotic heart disease, hypertensive cardiovascular disease, and rheumatic valvular heart disease with an enlarged left atrium. It is the result of a circus movement within the atrium and does not involve reentry through the atrioventricular node. Therefore, vagal maneuvers do not break the rhythm, although they may increase the atrioventricular block.

Fundamentally, management depends on the clinical status of the patient. If the flutter has an atrial to ventricular block in a ratio of 4:1, so that, for example, the atrial rate is 240 and the ventricular response is 60, one would do nothing except observe the patient. If the flutter has a response in a ratio of 1:1, then it is an emergency, and one must employ cardioversion as quickly as possible. Management involves either breaking the arrhythmia with electric cardioversion or increasing the atrioventricular block with digitalis and propranolol. Drug therapy will take time, so that if there is any urgency in the management, cardioversion should be carried out. Occasionally digitalis will correct atrial flutter to atrial fibrillation, which is a much more benign condition.

Atrial fibrillation is undoubtedly the most common of the supraventricular arrhythmias, next to sinus tachycardia. It can occur in patients with normal hearts, but usually it represents evidence of organic heart disease, with some enlargement and fibrosis of the atrium. In normal subjects, paroxysmal atrial fibrillation usually occurs after times when the patient has been under considerable stress, perhaps smoking, staying up late, and drinking a fair amount; following this, atrial fibrillation may develop abruptly. It is supposedly characterized by a relatively slow ventricular response and is in itself a benign rhythm. Treatment is merely supportive.

However, most atrial fibrillation occurs in the setting of organic heart disease. The physician should always be alerted to the fact that possible causes for new atrial fibrillation are thyrotoxicosis, the sick sinus syndrome (tachycardia-brachycardia syndrome), and unsuspected mitral valve disease. Often patients with rheumatic heart disease develop symptoms for the first time with the onset of atrial fibrillation, as cardiac output is impaired owing to loss of the atrial contribution and inability to control the heart rate with exercise.

Clinically, atrial fibrillation is relatively easy to diagnose, the important thing being that it is a totally irregular heart rhythm. Pressure on the carotid sinus increases the block and slows the ventricular response. On the electrocardiogram, no two beats have exactly the same R-R interval sequentially, and no atrial activity can be seen.

Atrial fibrillation should have a certain standard workup. Besides the history and physical examination, patients should have blood tests for thyroid function and an echocardiogram for valvular heart disease. In some patients, a Holter monitor to document the presence of the sick sinus syndrome will be very useful in demonstrating both tachyarrhythmias and bradyarrhythmias.

Treatment primarily involves controlling the ventricular response with digitalis. Often the use of the beta adrenergic blocking agents will help increase the atrioventricular block and control the ventricular response. Occasionally quinidine or procainamide will be useful to prevent the atrial fibrillation but normally the patient should be on digitalis as well. We rarely, if ever, use cardioversion, except for new atrial fibrillation in selected patients with rheumatic heart disease.

The major risk with atrial fibrillation in valvular heart disease is the risk of an embolus. In that situation, primarily with mitral stenosis, the onset of atrial fibrillation is a medical emergency: the patient should be promptly put on anticoagulants, kept on them for 6 weeks, and then cardioversion should be carried out if indicated.

WOLFF-PARKINSON-WHITE SYNDROME

Wolff-Parkinson-White syndrome is a part of any discussion of supraventricular tachycardias. We have referred to this in our discussion of paroxysmal atrial tachycardia. The classical form of ventricular preexcitation is seen in the electrocardiogram as a short PR interval (<0.12 sec) and a wide QRS interval (0.11 or greater) with a slurred upstroke (delta wave in some leads). These findings may be persistent, intermittent, or phasic, so that they need not necessarily be present on every EKG. The incidence for Wolff-Parkinson-White syndrome ranges from 0.1:1000 to 3:1000 adults, and 40% to 80% have tachycardias; of these, 70% to 80% are paroxysmal supraventricular tachycardias, while 20% to 30% are said to have atrial fibrillation or flutter. Paroxysmal supraventricular tachycardias occur when a premature atrial impulse is blocked on one pathway, goes down antegrade on the other one, and back up, retrograde, on the previously blocked pathway. As we have said, usually the antegrade impulse passes through the atrioventricular node and the QRS interval is thus normal. However, occasionally, the antegrade impulse may pass down the aberrant bundle, which will produce a wide, bizarre QRS interval resembling that of ventricular tachycardia. Atrial fibrillation is a much more dangerous arrhythmia if Wolff-Parkinson-White syndrome is also present, since the impulses may go down the accessory bundle, which has such a short refractory period that it can respond to 300 impulses a minute; thus atrial fibrillation can give a ventricular response that is incompatible with survival for any period of time. Digitalis does not interrupt this pathway and can actually speed conduction, so that the use of digitalis for atrial fibrillation with Wolff-Parkinson-White syndrome is dangerous. The drug of choice would be procainamide or propranolol. Cardioversion may be necessary. If in doubt whether the condition is ventricular tachycardia or supraventricular tachycardia with aberrancy, lidocaine is a safe drug to use.

VENTRICULAR ARRHYTHMIAS

Ventricular arrhythmias leading to ventricular tachycardia and ventricular fibrillation remain one of the major health problems in the United States. Of the 800,000 deaths per year from coronary artery disease, half are sudden and are the result in most cases of ventricular fibrillation. Overwhelming experimental and clinical evidence has shown that ventricular tachycardia and ventricular fibrillation are set off by a premature ventricular contraction. Similarly, there is overwhelming evidence that ventricular tachycardia and ventricular fibrillation can be easily treated if they are promptly recognized and the proper equipment is available. Finally, prevention of the premature ventricular contraction would appear to prevent ventricular fibrillation. Much of our discussion of ventricular arrhythmias will deal with premature ventricular contractions, but we will start first with ventricular fibrillation and ventricular tachycardia.

VENTRICULAR FIBRILLATION

Ventricular fibrillation is an emergency, and if untreated, it will almost never revert spontaneously. This is a totally chaotic mechanism in which there is no effective myocardial contraction. Ventricular fibrillation must be treated by direct-current defibrillation. With the development of the external defibrillator, this can be done across the intact chest. Once ventricular fibrillation has been identified, the sooner one defibrillates, the better. Use 300 to 400 watt seconds for an adult. If the first attempt at defribrillation is not successful, one should go on to a full-scale resuscitation attempt, unless the patient has obviously been without a blood pressure for some period of time or has terminal disease. Cardiopulmonary resuscitation should be started as a team effort, using external cardiac compression, intubation, and ventilation, and starting with the basic drugs: 3 cc of 1:10,000 adrenalin, either intracardiac or given in the vein and worked around by external compression; calcium and sodium bicarbonate are also given.

While what follows is not intended as a text for cardiopulmonary resuscitation, certain points must be emphasized. First, the physician will need help. The patient must be intubated, an intravenous drip started, and closed-chest cardiac compression carried out. Second, the senior physician will have to take charge and make the decision about the drugs and the therapy to be carried out. Third, one should remember that if the patient has been defibrillated in time and has a blood pressure, the team should keep going, because there are many well-documented resuscitations which occurred after up to 2 hours of cardiopulmonary resuscitation.

VENTRICULAR TACHYCARDIA

Ventricular tachycardia is an emergency, since it may result in ventricular fibrillation. Patients must be placed in the coronary care unit or in a monitored setting in an intensive care unit. Ventricular tachycardia occasionally may be difficult to separate from supraventricular tachycardia with aberrant conduction. The important features are in the electrocardiogram, where the P waves are not related to the QRS complex, the rhythm is not affected by pressure on the carotid artery, and the QRS interval is usually more bizarre than that seen with bundle-branch block.

The treatment of ventricular tachycardia depends upon the patient. With slow ventricular tachycardia, with a rate of 110 and a good blood pressure, one would use lidocaine intravenously and other antiarrhythmics. If the rate is rapid and the patient is deteriorating, cardioversion or defibrillation should be carried out. A thump version, using a blow to the chest to break the reentrant arrhythmia of the ventricular tachycardia, will occasionally be successful.

PREMATURE VENTRICULAR CONTRACTIONS

Premature ventricular contractions (ventricular premature beats) remain one of the major problems in cardiology today. On the one hand, the premature ventricular contractions which occur in 30% to 40% of normal subjects are benign, but on the other hand, sudden death from coronary artery disease appears to be most often the result of ventricular tachycardia and ventricular fibrillation set off by a premature ventricular contraction. In an acute myocardial infarction, the evidence, while circumstantial, is overwhelming, that preventing the premature ventricular contraction will prevent the lethal arrhythmia. In theory, at least, this should also be true for chronic coronary artery disease in general and it is the approach currently being used to lower the mortality from sudden death in coronary artery disease. Major problem areas include lack of knowledge of the mechanism responsible for the premature ventricular contractions; treatment at present is empirical. We also need proof that in chronic coronary artery disease premature ventricular contractions can either be successfully suppressed or, more important, sudden death as a result of them prevented.

Two mechanisms are responsible for the electrophysiology of the premature ventricular contraction: reentrant arrhythmia and ectopic focus. With an ectopic focus, some part of the ventricle has altered electrical properties, and this is responsible for the premature ventricular contraction. A reentrant arrhythmia involves localized block in the Purkinje network, so that an electrical impulse comes down, is blocked, goes through the ventricular muscle, and then is able to go retrograde up the Purkinje fiber and produce the premature ventricular contraction. The essential conditions for the reentrant arrhythmia are a localized block and a long enough pathway for the impulse to reach the Purkinje fiber again after it has recovered its excitability. The reentrant arrhythmia and ectopic focus might require different treatment. For example, a drug which prolongs ventricular conduction might control an ectopic focus but enhance a reentrant arrhythmia. It is likely that in the same heart both mechanisms operate at different times or even at the same time, and certainly different mechanisms may be responsible for premature ventricular contractions in different patients. Since we cannot, with our current techniques, determine the mechanism, treatment is empirical. It should be emphasized that ventricular tachycardia and ventricular fibrillation will not occur unless an abnormal ventricle with a decreased threshold for ventricular fibrillation is present, and enhanced sympathetic tone may also be necessary. Thus, with a normal ventricle and normal sympathetic tone, a premature ventricular contraction, whatever the mechanism, would be benign.

In the setting of an acute myocardial infarction, management of premature ventricular contractions is well standardized. In some cardiac care units, antiarrhythmic drugs are used prophylactically in patients suspected of having a myocardial infarction, while in other units, premature ventricular contractions are suppressed only when they appear. If the latter approach is used, indicators for the use of antiarrhythmic agents are: more than three premature ventricular contractions per minute, runs of two in a row, multifocal premature ventricular contractions, and one which occurs on top of the T wave. The effects of the currently available antiarrhythmic drugs are outlined in Tables 11-1 and 11-2. The tables are somewhat empirical and are based, in part, on our own personal experience. All of the drugs can produce different effects according to variations in the situation and in dosages. For example, while lidocaine does not usually decrease blood pressure, in a high enough dose, with a bad left ventricle and liver disease, it might have this effect.

All of the currently available antiarrhythmic drugs follow first-order kinetics, and a loading dose is necessary in order to rapidly reach a therapeutic level. Without a loading dose, starting with the maintenance dose, four half-lives are necessary before a therapeutic blood level is reached. In the setting of acute myocardial infarction, there is general agreement that for either prophylaxis or treatment of premature ventricular contractions, the initial drug of choice is lidocaine. This is given intravenously as a bolus for loading, followed by constant infusion. The drug is relatively safe, since the difference between a toxic and a therapeutic dose is high, being twice therapeutic before central nervous system toxicity appears. In addition, the drug is rapidly metabolized in the liver, with a half-life of 20 to 40 min if liver function is normal. The bolus should be about 1 mg/kg given intravenously, followed by a drip of 3 to 4 mg/min. The bolus can then be repeated in 3 to 5 min but should not exceed a total of 200 mg. The infusion should be rapidly slowed from 4, to 3, to 2 mg/min as soon as the premature ventricular contractions are controlled. Symptoms of toxicity include convulsions; heart block, in the presence of impaired conduction; and some myocardial depression effects if the myocardial disease is severe. However, minor toxic effects occur in almost everyone, primarily related to central nervous system stimulation, and most patients complain of a rather unpleasant sensation of slight nausea or dizziness related to receiving the drug. If the physician explains that the strange feeling is caused by the drug, it is very reassuring to the patient.

If the premature ventricular contractions cannot be controlled with lidocaine, procainamide should be used in addition, keeping the lidocaine at the same infusion rate. Lidocaine is continued and procainamide started. The procainamide should be given by bolus, first starting with 100 mg given over 3 to 5

Table 11-1. Antiarrhythmic Drugs

Drug	Effect on Blood Pressure	Effect on Cardiac Output	Effect on Conduction	Effect on Refractory Period	Effect on Automaticity	Metabolism
Lidocaine (Xylocaine)	↑	↑	None, if normal	None on A; prolongs in V	2+	Hepatic
Procainamide (Pronestyl)	↑→↑→	↑→↑→	Prolongs	Prolongs in A and V	4+	Hepatic and renal
Quinidine	↑→↑→	↑→↑→	Prolongs	Prolongs in A and V	4+	Hepatic and renal
Propranolol (Inderal)	→	→	Prolongs PR; no change in QRS	Prolongs in A and V	2+	Hepatic
Disopyramide (Norpace)	↑	→	Prolongs	Prolongs in A and V	4+	Renal and hepatic
Phenytoin (Dilantin)	↑	↑←	Little	Little	2+	Hepatic
Bretylium (Bretylol)	→	↑	May speed	Prolongs	2+ Raises fibrillation threshold	Renal

Key:
→ = unchanged
↓ = depressed
↑ = increased
A = Atrium
V = Ventricle

[153]

Table 11-2. Antiarrhythmic Drugs: Side Effects

Drug	Dose	Side Effects	Therapeutic Plasma Levels
Lidocaine	IV only Loading: 50–75 mg IV over 2 min; repeat every 3 min to total 200 mg Maintenance: 2–4 mg/min	Confusion, agitation, seizures, paresthesias; rarely, respiratory and cardiac depression	2–6 µg/ml
Procainamide	IV loading: 500–800 mg (slowly 100 mg over 3–5 min) Maintenance: 2–6 mg/min Oral loading: 750 mg Maintenance: 250–500 mg q 3–6 hours	Hypotension, GI symptoms, confusion, long-term lupuslike syndrome; arrhythmias may develop	4–10 µg/ml
Quinidine	Oral or IM, not IV Loading: 600 mg Maintenance: 200 mg q 6 hours	GI symptoms, cinchonism, thrombocytopenia, hypotension, heart block; ventricular fibrillation and other arrhythmias may occur	2–7 µg/ml
Propranolol	IV: 1–5 mg (0.5 mgs/min) Orally: 10–60 mg q 6 hours	Heart block, congestive failure, asthma, hypotension	?50–100 ng/ml
Disopyramide	Oral only Loading: 200–300 mg Maintenance: 100–150 mg q 6 hours	Hypotension, heart block, congestive failure, impressive anticolinergic effects	2–4 µg/ml
Phenytoin	IV loading: 300 mg (100 mg over 3–5 min) Maintenance: 300–400 mg/day Oral loading: 700 mg Maintenance: 300 mg/day	Ataxia, drowsiness, blood dyscrasias	5–20 µg/ml
Bretylium	IV only Loading: 5 mg/kg up to 30 mg/kg Maintenance 5–10 mg/kg q 6 hours	Hypotension, nausea and vomiting, initial increase in arrhythmias, increased sensitivity to catecholamine	Not established

min and increasing this 100 mg at a time up to as much as 800 mg. It is important to note that the rapid administration of procainamide decreases cardiac output and blood pressure; therefore, it must be given *slowly*, each 100 mg over 3 to 5 min. Once the patient has received the boluses, the procainamide should be given by drip at a rate of 2 to 6 mg per minute. The patient should be carefully watched for changes in hemodynamics and evidence of prolongation in conduction in the EKG. An increased PR, QT, or QRS interval should be taken as evidence of toxicity. The prolongation of the QRS or QT interval increases the possibility that the drug itself can produce reentrant ventricular arrhythmias and ventricular fibrillation. If the QRS interval is prolonged over 50%, the drug should usually be decreased unless the premature ventricular contractions have been very successfully abolished, in which case the prolonged QRS interval might be viewed with less concern.

Quinidine is similar in action to procainamide. It should not normally be given intravenously because of its alpha blockade effect, which will impressively lower the blood pressure. For acute myocardial infarction, quinidine should only be given orally and usually would not be useful in an emergency setting. If it is used intramuscularly, it will significantly elevate the creatine phosphokinase. Other drugs which may be used if procainamide fails are propranolol, phenytoin and, more recently, bretylium. Disopyramide is probably not indicated in an acute infarction, since it has not been tested extensively for that condition and, in addition, it cannot be given intravenously. The ventricular arrhythmias in an acute infarction tend to be self-limiting, and if one can control them, they will usually subside in 2 to 3 days.

Late arrhythmias which occur with an acute myocardial infarction are a much harder problem. They may be extremely difficult to treat. First, the late arrhythmias are associated with big infarcts and bad left-ventricular function. Second, one will need to establish an oral drug program, which can be continued out of the hospital, and it may take a great deal of trial and error before control can be achieved. Very often, more than one drug will be required before the premature contractions can be successfully controlled. The patient should be monitored and possibly put back in the coronary care unit. With the late arrhythmias, lidocaine may be used (intravenously, as always) but of course it is still necessary to get the patient on a program of oral drugs. For oral therapy as well as intravenous therapy, both a loading dose and a maintenance dose are needed. For procainamide, the loading dose is 750 mg orally, with a maintenance dose starting at 375 mg orally every 4 hours and careful monitoring of the blood level. For quinidine, the loading dose is 600 mg, with a maintenance dose of 200 mg every 6 hours. For disopyramide, use a 200 to 300-mg loading dose and a maintenance dose of 100 mg every 6 hours, as a starter.

All of the drugs which have been mentioned have drawbacks and side effects (see Table 11-2). Procainamide is reasonably well tolerated early in therapy, but a significant number of patients will develop a positive lupus erythematosus serology and a lupuslike syndrome over the first 6 months. Also, procainamide will have to be given through the night, and so the patient will have to wake up to take the dose at 3 to 4 hour intervals. Quinidine, while it can be taken every 6 hours, has a 30% incidence of serious gastrointestinal symptoms requiring changes in the drug. Disopyramide has atropinelike effects that may be very unpleasant for some patients, and loss of visual accommodation and urinary retention are common problems.

SUDDEN DEATH

The major problem in cardiology today is sudden death, resulting not from acute infarction but from ventricular fibrillation in coronary artery disease. It is estimated that of the 800,000 deaths which occur yearly in the United States from coronary artery disease, half are sudden. Sudden death from cardiac disease is the leading cause of death among men between the ages of 20 and 64 in the United States. There is an enormous amount of experience to demonstrate that these deaths are not inevitable and are not the final expression of terminal heart disease. The expression, "This heart's too good to die!" is valid, that is, the heart muscle is still good. The deaths are caused by ventricular fibrillations set off by a premature ventricular contraction, and there is good evidence that if the patient is properly defibrillated, some can go on to lead a normal life for some time, in some cases even for years.

The approach to the problem of sudden death from coronary artery disease which has been followed in recent years has been guided by the experience gained in coronary care units. The first strategy has been to provide training and facilities for cardiopulmonary resuscitation outside of the hospital. The mobile coronary care unit ambulance, training of emergency personnel, and the location of monitors and defibrillators in areas with large populations are all examples of this approach. While highly effective, when it can be given, in individual cases, the resuscitation approach does not appear to have substantially reduced mortality, in general due to insufficient equipment and personnel.

The second strategy has been to identify a high-risk population prone to such death and to prevent sudden death by using chronic antiarrhythmic drugs as regular therapy. The population at risk for sudden death from heart disease can readily be identified. This population includes patients who have had myocardial infarctions and who demonstrated complex ventricular arrhythmias during their late hospital phase or in the first 6 months after the infarction occurred. Other high-risk patients include those with angina and complex arrhythmias, patients successfully resuscitated from ventricular fibrillation who have not had myocardial infarctions, and patients with congestive failure from coronary artery disease.

However, in about 25% of patients with coronary artery disease, the first manifestation of the disease is sudden death itself. While these patients can be tentatively identified as having the risk factors for coronary artery disease, very little can be done for this group at present. The strategy here has been to monitor the established high-risk population for premature ventricular contractions by Holter monitoring and possibly by stress testing. The bulk of our experience has been with patients who have complex arrhythmias after a myocardial infarction. Once patients who manifest these complex arrhythmias, based on the number of premature ventricular contractions (two or more in a row or multifocal) are identified, they should be treated. The treatment is to administer the antiarrhythmic agent, and determine the response of the premature ventricular contraction to the drug, and correlate this with the blood level.

While promising, many problems remain in this therapy. First, the premature ventricular contraction has been used as the marker for the patient in need of this treatment, but most people with coronary disease have premature ventricular contractions. In addition, as we have said, 30 to 40% of the normal population also have them, so that the premature ventricular contraction alone may not be an adequate marker. What we really need is a method for determining when a decreased fibrillation threshold has been reached in the left ventricle, so that premature ventricular contractions have become dangerous. Second, even in a single patient, premature ventricular contractions are extremely variable, and what really constitutes a satisfactory response to the antiarrhythmic program is not clear. Thus, while we certainly have identified the problem now, much remains to be done in determining how to properly identify and manage the high-risk patient.

One of the things that is desperately needed today is new and more effective antiarrhythmic drugs. Currently it is certainly safe to say that the ones available at present may not work, either alone or in combination, in some patients. Several new drugs are under investigation, including aprindine, amiodorone, mexiletine and tocainide. As these become available they will certainly have a place in the management of premature ventricular contractions. As a long range goal, probably the important object will be not so much to suppress premature ventricular contractions as to alter the ventricular fibrillation threshold, so that even if premature ventricular contractions do occur, they will not result in ventricular fibrillation.

BRADYARRHYTHMIAS

12

C. *Thomas Fruehan*

The term **bradyarrhythmias** refers to all cardiac rhythms with a ventricular rate slower than 60/min. Some rhythms with rates slower than 60 are perfectly normal variants frequently found in healthy people; other bradyarrhythmias are found only in patients with heart disease or in disorders such as advanced heart block, sick sinus syndrome, or drug intoxication. In order to decide whether the bradycardia is a normal or abnormal condition and whether or not treatment is necessary, it is essential that the rhythm be properly identified and correlated with the patient's clinical condition.

BENIGN ARRHYTHMIAS

SINUS BRADYCARDIA

It cannot be overemphasized that several rhythms with a ventricular rate below 60/min may normally occur in healthy persons. Sinus bradycardia—sinus rhythm at a rate below 60—is extremely common in the resting, physically conditioned young person. Resting heart rates in the 30s are not rare in distance runners and other athletes, and resting sinus rates in the 40s are not unusual in nonathletic healthy individuals. If a resting sinus rate below 60 is found in an asymptomatic person without evidence of heart disease, there is no cause for concern or further investigation.

Under certain circumstances, such as when it is clinically inappropriate, sinus bradycardia may *not* be normal (see the section on "sick sinus syndrome" later in this chapter).

158

ATRIOVENTRICULAR JUNCTIONAL RHYTHM

Another bradyarrhythmia which may be found in healthy young persons is a junctional (atrioventricular-nodal) escape rhythm, at a rate in the upper 30s or 40s, resulting from an intrinsic sinus rate below the intrinsic escape rate of the atrioventricular junctional pacemaker. This may produce **isorhythmic dissociation** (known also as **isochronic dissociation**), in which the rhythm originates part of the time from the sinus mode and part of the time from the atrioventricular junctional pacemaker, as the sinus rate fluctuates above and below the more uniform junctional rate. In asymptomatic individuals without evidence of heart disease who are capable of faster sinus rates when appropriate, this is probably a normal variant, and it is not rare in healthy young persons.

SINUS ARRHYTHMIA

Special mention is made at this point of sinus arrhythmia, a rhythm which may intermittently have cycles exceeding 1 sec or transiently have a rate slower than 60 per min. In general, sinus arrhythmia is a sinus rhythm with exaggerated variation in cycle lengths. There is no uniform standard definition of how much cycle variation is needed before a rhythm should be called **sinus arrhythmia** rather than (ordinary) **sinus rhythm.** Published limits of cycle variation for the sinus arrhythmia label include:

1. Greater than 10% variation in cycle lengths anywhere within a standard ECG
2. Greater than 0.12 sec variation between consecutive cycles
3. Greater than 0.16 sec variation among cycles anywhere in the tracing.

My personal preference is to label as sinus arrhythmia any otherwise normal sinus rhythm which *looks* grossly irregular on ECG or which might be perceived as an irregular pulse upon palpation.

Sinus arrhythmia is believed to be usually the result of momentary variation in parasympathetic and sympathetic tone, as with respiration, for example. It is the rule rather than the exception in children and adolescents, and also very common in young adults. Presumably, the sinus node of young persons is "more labile" than that of adults or has greater sensitivity to variation in parasympathetic tone. Sinus arrhythmia is entirely normal in young adults.

Sinus arrhythmia may also be seen in the elderly, in whom its normality is not so firmly established. In the elderly, sinus arrhythmia should probably be considered a normal variant so long as:

1. The overall average heart rate is appropriate to the subject's clinical state.
2. the longest cycles do not cause symptoms because of their length. In general, single cycles shorter than 2 sec are asymptomatic.

PATHOLOGIC BRADYARRHYTHMIAS

As a rule, all abnormally slow heart rhythms occur because of either a defect in impulse formation—failure of the intrinsic cardiac pacemaker cells to initiate a heartbeat—or a defect in conduction of impulses from one portion of the heart to another. Either of these two conditions may occur because of intrinsic heart disease or becuase of extracardiac influences, such as drugs, central nervous system factors, or electrolyte abnormalities. Either condition may be temporary or permanent, depending on cause.

DISORDERS OF CONDUCTION

In the generation of every normal heartbeat, the pacemaking impulse must be conducted through a number of cardiac structures before the ventricles are stimulated to contract. This sequential process may be interrupted at any level. The site of interruption can usually be determined from the electrocardiogram. For a listing of some of these sites and their ECG manifestations, see Table 12-1.

Table 12-1. Localization of Conduction Disorders

STRUCTURE	BLOCK	EKG RHYTHM POSSIBLE
Pacemaker cells of sinus node		
Perinodal fibers	Sinoatrial block (SA block)	SA block; periods of sinus arrest; atrial asystole
Atria	Intraatrial conduction delay	Extremely broad P waves
AV node	Atrioventricular block (AV block)	1° AV block 2° AV block, Mobitz Type I (with Wenckebach's phenomenon) 3° AV block (with supraventricular escape rhythm)
Common bundle of His	AV block	1° AV block 2° AV block Mobitz Type II 3° AV block (with supraventricular [AV junctional] escape rhythm)
Left and right bundle branches	AV block (left or right bundle-branch block)	Sinus rhythm with bundle branch block 2° AV block, Mobitz II 3° AV block (with idioventricular escape rhythm)
Ventricular myocardium	Intraventricular block (IV block)	Extremely prolonged IV conduction time (longer than 0.12–0.14 sec, the IV conduction time of simple bundle-branch block)

All conduction disorders may be classified in terms of their completeness. The classifications employed are first-, second-, and third-degree block, and simple definitions of them follow:

1. First-degree block: all impulses are conducted, but with an abnormally long conduction time.
2. Second-degree block: some impulses are conducted, others are blocked.
3. Third-degree block (or "complete" block): all impulses are blocked; none are conducted.

These degrees of block most commonly refer to conduction between atria and ventricles (atrioventricular block), but have also been used to describe conduction through any part of the cardiac conduction system.

SINOATRIAL BLOCK

Sinoatrial block occurs when impulses are not conducted from the pacemaker cells of the sinus node to the surrounding atrial myocardium. This results in an ECG with one or more P waves (and following QRS-T complexes) *completely missing* where they were expected. This, in turn, produces long cycles, almost exactly twice as long as the usual sinus cycle length.

The ECG diagnosis of sinoatrial block is by inference only, because we do not have a practical method for recording potentials of the human sinoatrial node to confirm the diagnosis. It is assumed that the unusually long cycles are due to exit block from pacemaker cells which continue to fire regularly.

Sinoatrial block may occur in the following clinical settings:

1. Sick sinus syndrome (discussed later)
2. Drug toxicity (digitalis, quinidine)
3. Hyperkalemia
4. Greatly increased parasympathetic (vagal) tone

Treatment may not be required if the sinoatrial block is infrequent and the patient asymptomatic. If it is caused by drug toxicity, obviously the drug should be withheld. If temporary therapy is needed, either atropine or isoproterenol is useful; atropine is usually the choice because it has fewer side effects, and fewer problems are associated with its use. Temporary pacemaking may be required in severely symptomatic patients while further evaluation proceeds. Such severe symptoms might include transient loss of consciousness or dizzy spells.

When sinoatrial block is chronic, not the result of a reversible cause, and severe enough to cause symptoms, it should be considered as part of the "sick sinus syndrome" which is discussed later in this chapter.

INTRAATRIAL BLOCK

This is primarily an electrocardiographic peculiarity, in which P-wave duration greatly exceeds 0.12 sec. When the P waves range between 0.12 and approximately 0.16/sec, the intraatrial block is indistinguishable from that of the much more common left-atrial enlargement. In extreme cases, P-wave duration may exceed 0.20/sec. Such P waves may have multiple peaks.

The only clinical significance of intraatrial conduction delay is its ECG similarity to left-atrial enlargement and its suggestion of atrial pathology or possible more widespread depression of conductivity.

ATRIOVENTRICULAR BLOCK

The term **atrioventricular block** encompasses a broad clinical spectrum. To put it in the simplest terms, atrioventricular block refers to any conduction abnormality between the onset of atrial activation (shown on the ECG as the beginning of the P wave) and the onset of ventricular activation (shown as the beginning of the QRS complex). In first-degree atrioventricular block, all atrial beats are conducted to the ventricles, but the ECG shows an abnormally long PR-interval. In second- and third-degree atrioventricular block, some or all of the atrial beats are not conducted to the ventricles. On the ECG, second- and third-degree atrioventricular block have P waves which are not followed by QRS complexes. The anatomic location of the conduction disorder in atrioventricular block may be in the atrioventricular node, the common bundle of His, the bundle-branch system, or in any combination of these structures. The causes of atrioventricular block are outlined below.

Causes of Atrioventricular Block
   I. Congenital
  II. Calcific disease of cardiac skeleton with associated valvular calcification (Lev's disease)
 III. Idiopathic degenerative disease of cardiac conduction system (Lenegre's disease)
  IV. Myocardial infarction
   V. Drug Toxicity:
       A. Digitalis
       B. Cardiosuppressive agents, such as quinidine, procainamide, disopyramide, propranolol, and others
  VI. Infectious diseases
       A. Bacterial
          1. Syphilis
          2. Bacterial endocarditis
          3. Rheumatic fever
          4. Tuberculosis
          5. Diphtheria
       B. Parasitic—especially Chagas' disease, where extant
       C. Viral, fungal, rickettsial
 VII. Hyperkalemia, other gross acid-base and electrolyte disorders
VIII. Atrial tachyarrhythmias
  IX. Space-occupying or inflammatory cardiac lesions, such as sarcoid lesions, those which result from hemochromatosis and myocarditis, and others

X. Cardiomyopathies
XI. Increased parasympathetic (vagal) tone
   A. Visceral distension, nausea/vomiting, etc.
   B. Hypersensitive carotid sinus syndrome
XII. Surgery
XIII. Trauma

First-degree Atrioventricular Block

As described previously, first-degree atrioventricular block is shown on the ECG as an abnormally long PR-interval, with all atrial beats being conducted to the ventricles. In the adult, the PR interval is normally 0.20 sec or less; at rates below 60/min, the PR interval may normally be 0.21 or 0.22 sec.

First-degree atrioventricular block itself causes no major problem. However, it can point to two other possible causes of concern. First, the cause of the block should be considered. It may be an early sign of drug toxicity. It may also be the first manifestation of coronary artery disease or of heart disease resulting from a systemic disorder.

Second, the possibility should be considered that first-degree atrioventricular block is the first stage of progression to a higher and more dangerous degree of atrioventricular block. In an acutely ill patient, such as one with acute myocardial infarction, continuous ECG monitoring should be considered until the clinical picture is clarified.

Second-degree Atrioventricular Block

In second-degree atrioventricular block, some atrial beats are conducted to the ventricles and others are blocked. (It is usually understood in the definition that the atrial rhythm is regular, as in sinus rhythm, atrial tachycardia, or the like. The name is not applied to premature atrial beats, which may be physiologically blocked.)

Second-degree atrioventricular block is classified into two distinct types, Mobitz Type I, also called Wenckebach second-degree atrioventricular block, and Mobitz Type II second-degree atrioventricular block. These are named after the men who first described them.

Second-degree atrioventricular block may also be described in terms of the ratio of atrial beats to ventricular beats. For example, an established conduction pattern of: three conducted atrial beats followed by a blocked atrial beat; and then again, three conducted atrial beats, followed by a blocked atrial beat (and so on) is called 4:3 second-degree atrioventricular block, because there are 4 P waves for every 3 QRS complexes. Similarly, an established rhythm in which each conducted atrial beat is followed by two blocked atrial beats is called 3:1 atrioventricular block. This ratio designation is an estimate of the severity of the conduction disorder and is useful descriptively; it has no implication as to the mechanism (Mobitz I or II), localization, or cause of the atrioventricular block.

Mobitz Type I or Wenckebach Atrioventricular Block. In this type of atrioventricular block, consecutive PR intervals become progressively longer until an atrial beat is completely blocked. The next PR interval is relatively short, and the process of increasing PR intervals begins again on successive beats.

The *increment* by which the PR interval increases usually decreases with successive beats. Thus, the R-R interval of successive beats gradually shortens slightly. Also, if many atrial beats conduct before one is blocked, there may be little difference between the PR intervals of the last few conducted beats. Thus, Wenckebach's phenomenon of gradually increasing PR intervals is most noticeable in the first few conducted beats after a blocked atrial beat.

The clinical significance of Wenckebach second degree atrioventricular block is that it is characteristic of conduction difficulty in the atrioventricular node. Other portions of the cardiac conduction system may rarely display Wenckebach's phenomenon, but not typically; its presence in atrioventricular block is almost a guarantee of localization of the block in the atrioventricular node. Atrioventricular block from *any* cause typically produces Wenckebach's phenomenon when it causes second-degree block at the atrioventricular-node level.

This localization to the atrioventricular node has important implications about prognosis and management. Block in the atrioventricular node is often transient and reversible. If it progresses to higher degrees of block, this usually happens gradually. Conduction block in the atrioventricular node can usually be improved with atropine or isoproterenol.

Even in the event that Wenckebach second degree atrioventricular block worsens to complete atrioventricular block, the next lower latent pacemaker site below the atrioventricular node is in the lower atrioventricular junctional tissues or the common bundle of His, so that the next available escape pacemaker site is usually supraventricular, has a dependable rate in the 30s or 40s (sufficient to sustain life), and, if located in the atrioventricular junction, can often be accelerated with atropine. These characteristics of Wenckebach atrioventricular block are summarized in Table 12-2.

Wenckebach atrioventricular block is quite common in acute *inferior-wall* myocardial infarction, occurring in an estimated 10% to 25% of such infarctions. In this setting, it is usually transient, so that normal atrioventricular conduction returns by the time of hospital discharge, and this type of block is not associated with significantly higher mortality. Management will be discussed later in the chapter.

Mobitz Type II Second-Degree Atrioventricular Block. In contrast to the Mobitz Type I (Wenckebach) atrioventricular block, in Mobitz Type II atrioventricular block, the PR interval of successive beats is *constant* until an atrial beat is blocked. There is no change in R-R intevals on successive conducted beats either. From this description, it is apparent that second-degree atrioventricular block may be categorized as Mobitz I or Mobitz II *only* when there are at least two consecutive conducting atrial beats.

**Table 12-2. Comparison of Mobitz I (Wenckebach)
and Mobitz II Atrioventricular Block**

FEATURES	MOBITZ I (WENCKEBACH)	MOBITZ II
Site of Defect	Atrioventricular Node	Infranodal—Usually Bilateral Bundle-Branch Block
Onset	Gradual	Sudden
Permanence	Often Transient	Usually permanent conduction disorder
ECG Features:		
PR Interval	Variable	Constant
R-R Interval of consecutive beats	Variable	Constant
QRS of conducted beats	Normal Duration (usually)	Bundle-Branch Block (usually)
Escape Rhythm	Supraventricular	Idioventricular
Onset of Complete Block	Gradual	Sudden
Effect of Atropine	Improvement	None
Effect of Isoproterenol	Improvement of atrioventricular block	Occasionally, decrease in atrioventricular block; more likely, accelerated ventricular escape rhythm
Treatment	Observation Atropine Temporary pacer if needed permanent pacer rarely needed	Permanent pacing usually required Isoproterenol may speed up escape pacemaker while awaiting electronic pacing
Association with Myocardial Infarction:		
Mortality	Inferior wall—common Not increased	Anterior wall—uncommon Approximately 80%
Treatment	As above	Immediate pacing

Mobitz II block is characteristic of conduction disturbance *below* the atrioventricular node, in the common bundle of His and the intraventricular conduction system (left and right bundle branches). Although Mobitz II block has been reported in atrioventricular-nodal disease, this is uncommon, and Mobitz II block almost guarantees infranodal localization of atrioventricular block. Since lesions of the common bundle of His are an uncommon cause of atrioventricular block, Mobitz II atrioventricular block usually results from disease in both the left and right bundle branches.

The clinical significance of Mobitz II atrioventricular block lies in this usual localization of the conduction defect to the bundle-branch system.

In contrast to Mobitz I (Wenckebach) second-degree atrioventricular block, the onset of Mobitz II block may be sudden. Mobitz II block may suddenly progress to complete atrioventricular block with little or no warning. If it does, the only remaining latent pacemaker sites below the interrupted bundle-branch system are in the peripheral ventricular Purkinje network. Such escape pacemakers may not be reliable, may have slow rates in the teens or 20s inadequate to sustain life with a diseased heart, and cannot be accelerated with parasympathetic blockade. Neither Mobitz II block nor its succeeding complete (third-degree) block is commonly spontaneously reversible; both usually indicate permanent structural defects in the cardiac conduction system.

Mobitz II atrioventricular block is an uncommon but serious complication of myocardial infarction. It is more common in anterior-wall infarction than in inferior-wall infarction. It usually follows infarction of the interventricular septum and bundle branches, and, because the infarction is often extensive, is associated with a mortality rate of approximately 80%, regardless of treatment.

Third-degree Atrioventricular Block

In third-degree (complete) atrioventricular block, *no* atrial beats are conducted to the ventricles. The ventricles thus have no activity except for that initiated by lower pacemakers below the area of blocked conduction. Were it not for these "escape" pacemakers, there would be ventricular asystole. Portions of the previous discussion about second-degree atrioventricular block—related to possible sites of conduction defects, suddenness of onset, latent pacemakers which may take over, and association with myocardial infarction—apply to third-degree atrioventricular block also.

When faced with a patient with complete atrioventricular block, there are two immediate questions: 1) does the atrioventricular block require immediate intervention? 2) is the atrioventricular block the result of a reversible condition (such as digitalis toxicity, for example)?

If the patient is in distress because of extreme bradycardia, immediate temporary pacing is generally undertaken while the patient's condition is further evaluated. While arrangements for pacing are in progress, the heart rate may be increased with atropine or isoproterenol, according to whether the escape rhythm is supraventricular or idioventricular.

The usual starting dose for atropine administration is 0.5 mg given intravenously. If there is to be a response, it will occur within 2 to 3 min. If there is an inadequate response, the dosage of 0.5 mg given intravenously can be repeated up to a total of 2 mg.

When the escape rhythm is idioventricular, with the implied conduction defect below the atrioventricular node, the cholinergic blockade of atropine is not useful. Catecholamines may be used to accelerate the escape pacemaker rate or, less commonly, improve conduction. Isoproterenol, a pure beta adrenergic stimulator, is the agent of choice. It is given intravenously at an infusion rate of 1 to 8 μg/min. A solution can be prepared with 2 mg isoproterenol in 500 cc dextrose and water; this can be begun at ½ cc/min (2 μg/min), and the infusion rate titrated to the effect on heart rate. Problems associated with isoproterenol infusion include increased ventricular irritability (premature ventricular contractions) and hypotension owing to vasodilation; these problems may limit the usefulness of isoproterenol infusion. If the atrioventricular block is caused by a reversible problem, this may be all the therapy required until normal atrioventricular conduction resumes. If the atrioventricular block is permanent, a "permanent" electronic pacemaker can be implanted electively once the patient's condition has stabilized.

In contrast, some patients will present with established, chronic, complete atrioventricular block and may show remarkably few symptoms if they have an adequate escape rhythm. In the past, such patients may have received "permanent" pacemakers only if they were symptomatic. With the reliability and longevity of modern "permanent" pacemakers, permanent pacing is now considered advisable for all patients with established *or* transient complete atrioventricular block which is not the result of a reversible condition. The patient with established chronic complete atrioventricular block, few or no symptoms, and an adequate escape rhythm, and who is clinically stable, can probably safely await elective surgical implantation of a permanent pacemaker.

Escape Rhythms

Previous paragraphs have referred frequently to escape rhythms. These are rhythms originating in lower, ordinarily latent, subsidiary pacemaker areas of the heart when the higher pacemaker's impulses are blocked or otherwise fail. By definition, an escape beat or escape rhythm must have a cycle length longer than the higher pacemaker it replaces; for example, given an atrial rhythm in sinus rhythm at rate 80, followed by complete atrioventricular block, there might be an escape rhythm, originating in the atrioventricular junction, at rate 50. These subsidiary lower pacemakers are ordinarily suppressed by passive depolarization from the higher pacemaker (in sinus rhythm, for example). Failure of the higher pacemaker impulses to arrive permits the subsidiary pacemaker cells to "escape" and initiate their own beats.

Potential escape pacemaker cells are located almost throughout the cardiac conduction system. They have been found in the region near the coronary sinus, in junctional tissues between the atria and the atrioventricular node, in junctional fibers between the atrioventricular node and the common bundle of His, in the common bundle of His itself, in the left and right bundle branches, and in the peripheral Purkinje network. Two locations which probably do *not* contain latent pacemaker cells are the main body of the atrioventricular node and ordinary contractile ventricular myocardium. Escape rhythms thus may have ECG forms indicating an origin in an ectopic area of the atrium, the atrioventricular junction, or the ventricle itself.

Established escape rhythms are characterized by their regularity. Any gross irregularity in an escape rhythm suggests that either the predominant upper pacemaker may have conducted through to the escape locus or a second escape pacemaker may be operative. Intermittent irregularity of the escape rhythm is one of the best clues that one has an occasional conducted atrial beat, and thus a high degree of second-degree atrioventricular block, rather than complete atrioventricular block.

SINUS-NODE DYSFUNCTION, (SICK SINUS SYNDROME)

Cause and Diagnosis

Sick sinus syndrome is a relatively "new" disease. The name is applied to the general condition of failure of the sinus node to initiate a reliable rhythm and sufficiently fast heart rate. The name "sick sinus syndrome" was coined by Lown, who used it to refer to patients who failed to begin a satisfactory sinus rhythm after direct-current cardioversion. Ferrer recognized sick sinus node failure as a distinct, widespread clinical entity in 1968. Since then the disorder has been recognized with increasing frequency, perhaps because of the increased zeal with which it has been sought.

The clinical significance of sick sinus syndrome is that it is an eminently treatable form of heart disease, with good prognosis; and that it is a fairly common disorder; in some centers, up to 50% of all initial artificial pacemaker implantations are for the sick sinus syndrome or its variants.

Sick sinus syndrome is a collective term which includes several different bradyarrhythmias, all resulting from failure of the normal sinus-node pacemaker either to initiate beats or to propagate impulses to the surrounding atria. These rhythms include:

1. Profound sinus bradycardia, inappropriate for the patient's clinical state, causing symptoms
2. Sinus arrest
3. Sinoatrial block, with symptoms
4. Failure of sinus rhythm to begin after cardioversion
5. Escape rhythms when the sinus mechanism fails

In addition to one or more of the above bradyarrhythmias, many patients with sick sinus syndrome have paroxysmal supraventricular tachyarrhythmias—atrial flutter, atrial tachycardia, atrial fibrillation, or regular supraventricular tachycardia. These paroxysmal tachyarrhythmias are a frequent, but not essential, part of the syndrome. When tachyarrhythmias alternate with inappropriate bradyarrhythmias, the condition may be called the **tachycardia-bradycardia syndrome.**

The mechanism of these inappropriately slow sinus rates is not clear. It may include any or all of the following:

1. Failure of sinus-node pacemaker cells
   a. Pacemaker cells dead or replaced by fibrous tissue
   b. Pacemaker cells present, but "defective"
2. Sinoatrial block
3. Reentry of sinus-node impulses from the atrium back into the sinus node, depolarizing the sinus node passively

Although there have been few autopsy studies of patients with this syndrome, a wide variety of cardiac diseases has been associated with it. Some patients have coronary disease affecting the sinoatrial-node artery, with secondary destruction of the sinoatrial node. Other associated diseases include amyloidosis, hemochromatosis, and cardiomyopathy. In several reported cases, there has been no evidence of any other cardiac disease; the sinus-node tissue has been replaced by fibrous tissue.

The symptoms of sick sinus syndrome are palpitations, syncopal episodes or dizzy spells, and fatigue or weakness, in descending order of frequency. Occasional patients with this syndrome will present with congestive heart failure or chest pain. The symptoms may be present for years before the diagnosis is suspected or demonstrated.

The diagnosis of sick sinus syndrome depends on demonstrating the appropriate bradyarrhythmia on the electrocardiogram at the time of symptoms, and exclusion of other, extracardiac factors which can slow intrinsic sinus-node rates. These are summarized in the following list.

Extracardiac Causes of Slow Sinus-Node Rate

1. Altered autonomic tone
   a. Central nervous system injury
   b. Increased vagal tone
      (1) Visceral distension
      (2) Nausea/vomiting
      (3) Reflex to increased sympathetic tone
   c. Carotid sinus hypersensitivity
2. Acute inferior-wall myocardial infarction
3. Drugs
   a. Digitalis
   b. Antiarrhythmic agents
      (1) Quinidine
      (2) Procainamide
      (3) Lidocaine
      (4) Amiodarone
   c. Propranolol, other beta blockade agents
   d. Verapamil, other calcium blockade agents
   e. Antihypertensive agents
      (1) Reserpine
      (2) Guanethidine
      (3) Methyldopa
   f. Anticholinesterase drugs
4. Metabolic and electrolyte abnormalities
   a. Hyperkalemia
   b. Hypothyroidism
   c. Hypothermia

Because sinus-node dysfunction is often a transient event, frequent standard ECGs may not show the diagnostic bradyarrhythmia. In such cases, sick sinus syndrome may be demonstrated by continuous monitoring, either in a coronary care unit or by means of a Holter recording, a continuous 24-hour tape recording of the ambulatory ECG. Even this procedure may have to be repeated many times to demonstrate the diagnostic slowing of the rate at the time of symptoms.

Because continuous monitoring and tape recording are expensive and time-consuming, a number of provocative tests have been developed to demonstrate sinus node-dysfunction in the suspected patient. These include:

1. Isometric exercise
2. Response to atropine
3. Response to isoproterenol

These tests are all based on the fact that the normal sinus node will usually speed up appropriately in response to the test stimulus, whereas the faulty sinus node will not. Unfortunately, these tests are neither very sensitive nor specific for sinus-node dysfunction, so that two invasive provocative tests have been developed: the sinoatrial conduction time test and Mandel's sinus-node overdrive suppression test.

The *sinoatrial conduction time* is determined by introducing pacer-induced premature atrial beats and measuring the time by which the sinus-node rhythm is reset. The first sinus cycle after a premature atrial beat is usually longer than the basic sinus cycle. The longer cycle after the premature beat is considered to be the result of the conduction time required for an impulse to pass retrograde into the sinus node, added to the usual conduction time from the sinus node into the atria. Many patients with sick sinus syndrome have abnormally long sinoatrial conduction time.

In *Mandel's sinus-node overdrive suppression test* the atria are paced by an artificial temporary pacemaker at rapid rates for sustained periods. After pacing is stopped, there is a pause before sinus rhythm resumes. This is the result of the physiologic suppression of automaticity in pacemaker cells when they are passively depolarized. In patients with sick sinus syndrome, this pause after pacing is often exaggerated. In Mandel's original paper on the test, all of his sick sinus syndrome patients had pauses of at least 4 sec before resumption of sinus rhythm. Unfortunately, a number of false positive and false negative responses to this test have been reported. Further, there is much disagreement among cardiologists as to how long a pause before resumption of sinus rhythm is considered pathologic. Despite these shortcomings, the overdrive suppression test of Mandel remains the best of the available provocative tests. We feel that demonstration of a rhythm disorder at the time of symptoms is more conclusive evidence supporting the diagnosis than a positive result of any of the provocative tests described above.

Treatment and Prognosis

Some patients with minimal sinus-node dysfunction who are asymptomatic, or nearly so, may require no specific treatment and merely frequent observation. If treatment is indicated for control of symptoms, medical therapy is unsatisfactory. The only satisfactory treatment is permanent electronic pacing. Some of those patients with the tachycardia-bradycardia variant may have a reduction in the frequency of their tachycardias; others with paroxysmal tachyarrhythmias may require drug treatment of their tachyarrhythmias in addition to pacing.

Patients with sick sinus syndrome are reported to have a significantly higher mortality rate than "normal" control patients, up to 40% per year. Many of the deaths have been attributed to thromboembolic phenomena. However, our own series of 42 paced sick sinus syndrome patients followed for an average of 2 years showed that this syndrome, when treated with a pacemaker, did *not* increase mortality; deaths in these patients were related to other conditions, often other severe heart disease. If there was no other evidence of heart disease, our sick sinus syndrome patients had normal longevity during the study period.

PACEMAKERS

Temporary or Permanent Pacing

It should be apparent from the preceding paragraphs that in many instances appropriate therapy of bradyarrhythmias consists of artificial pacing, on either a temporary or permanent basis. Since the introduction of the implantable cardiac pacemaker in 1959 and the introduction of temporary cardiac pacing in the succeeding decade, cardiac pacing has assumed a large role in the management of certain acute and chronic cardiac disorders. The indications for permanent pacemaker implantation or for temporary pacing, are summarized as follows:

Indications for Permanent Pacemaker

1. Atrioventricular block, second- or third-degree, chronic or recurrent
2. Sick sinus syndrome (sinus-node dysfunction, "tachycardia-bradycardia syndrome")
3. Carotid sinus hypersensitivity
4. Aid in ventricular arrhythmia suppression
5. Used prophylactically in patients surviving anterior-wall myocardial infarction with transient high-degree atrioventricular block
6. Permit use of drugs which cause unacceptably slow heart rate

Indications for Temporary Pacing

1. As adjunct to permanent pacer implantation
2. New second- or third-degree atrioventricular block, while reversibility and patient's condition are assessed
3. In myocardial infarction:
   a. Inferior wall complicated by:
      1) Symptomatic second- or third-degree atrioventricular block, not easily treated with atropine

    2) Symptomatic profound sinus bradycardia, not easily treated with atropine
- b. Anterior wall complicated by:
  1) Bundle-branch block (usually indicated)
  2) Bilateral bundle-branch disease (*e.g.*, right bundle-branch block, abnormal QRS axis); (almost always indicated)
  3) Mobitz Type II or third-degree atrioventricular block (always indicated immediately)
4. For cardioversion of supraventricular or ventricular tachyarrhythmias by competitive pacing
5. During and after cardiac surgery, especially valve replacement

In general, permanent pacing is the treatment of choice for chronic or recurrent second- or third-degree atrioventricular block. Formerly, it was a requirement that patients show symptoms from the block; however, with today's technology, permanent pacing should be considered for all patients with this condition, provided it does not have readily reversible causes.

The sick sinus syndrome and its variants are now a major indication for permanent pacemaker implantation. In many centers, this is now the leading indication for initial implantation of a pacemaker. In our own institution, sinus-node dysfunction is the indication for almost 50% of initial permanent pacemaker implants.

Carotid sinus hypersensitivity is a rare indication for permanent artificial pacing. The disorder itself is uncommon; many afflicted patients are treated by denervation of the carotid sinus. Permanent pacing should be considered for patients in whom carotid sinus denervation is inappropriate.

In unusual circumstances, permanent pacing may serve as an adjunct in the suppression of ventricular arrhythmias. For example, a patient with recurrent ventricular tachycardia and a resting sinus rate of 60 may have fewer episodes of ventricular tachycardia if the heart is pacer-driven at a higher rate. The paced rate need not be as fast as the rate of the recurrent ventricular tachycardia. Such pacing at faster rates has been called **overdrive suppression.**

The value of permanent pacing in patients surviving anterior wall myocardial infarction complicated by transient second- or third-degree atrioventricular block is still under investigation. It has been our experience, and that of others, that patients who recover from anterior-wall myocardial infarction complicated by second- or third-degree atrioventricular block and residual bundle-branch block have a rather high incidence of sudden death within the next several months. It is thought that this occurs because the surviving bundle branch is adjacent to an area of infarcted tissue and is in jeopardy of necrosis in the event of slight extension of the original infarction. Therefore, it is the practice in many centers to implant permanent pacemakers in such patients who survive their infarction. Because this group of patients is necessarily small, the benefits of prophylactic pacing are still not definitely known.

Types of Pacemakers

A great many different types of electronic pacemakers are now available, some designed for special purposes or special modes of operation. However, the vast majority of permanent and temporary electronic pacemakers are of the "R-wave inhibited" or "ventricular inhibited" type. Such a pacemaker will deliver stimuli at a preset, fixed rate, until the pacemaker senses a spontaneous QRS complex. When the pacemaker senses a QRS complex, it does not fire the stimulus which ordinarily would have occurred next; instead, it resets its timing mechanism from the instant of sensing. Thus, a patient with a faster spontaneous rhythm than the preset rate of the pacemaker would continuously inhibit the pacemaker and the pacemaker would deliver no stimuli, permitting the heart to go on beating at the faster spontaneous rate, but never permitting it to beat too slowly.

Until very recently, all permanent pacemakers were powered by mercury-zinc batteries, which had a life span of 2 to 4 years. At the time of this writing (1980), many of these pacemakers are still in use. More recently, however, nearly all implanted pacemakers have been powered by lithium iodine batteries which have a life span of from 4 to 12 years, depending upon the battery size and other factors.

Most permanent pacemakers are preset to a rate of approximately 70 impulses per min; they deliver stimuli of approximately 9 ma at approximately 5 volts. The duration of the stimulus, depending upon the model, may range from 0.5 msec to 2 msec. The pacemakers will sense a QRS complex of 2 mv, or greater, amplitude. In the temporary pacemakers, with external pulse generators, the stimulus current and its rate can be adjustable. A typical range of stimulus currents is from 0.5 to 20 ma, and rates of from 30 to 150 are routinely available. Some special-purpose external pacemakers can generate rates up to 800/min, as for atrial pacing.

A recent development is the programmable permanent pacemaker, in which an external signal can change one or more parameters of the implanted pacemaker. This may be done with radio-frequency signals or coded magnetic pulses. Implanted pacemakers are now available which can be programmed for different rates, duration of stimulus, output current, or even a change in mode from an R-wave inhibited to fixed-rate operation.

All electronic pacemakers need an electrode system to deliver the stimuli to the heart. The electrode may be *bipolar*, in which both anode and cathode are applied to the heart, or *unipolar*, in which the cathode is applied to the heart, current returns through the body tissues, and the anode is located on the body of the pulse generator itself. Neither arrangement is necessarily superior; unipolar electrode systems probably are slightly more reliable in sensing the heart's own ventricular beats but they are more prone to inappropriate sensing of external electronic noise.

Electrode systems may further be categorized as myocardial or endocardial. The implanting surgeon usually chooses the electrode system with which he is most familiar and skilled. With the exception of temporary pacing electrodes implanted at the time of cardiac surgery, all temporary pacing employs transvenous endocardial electrodes. Endocardial electrodes are passed through a peripheral vein, which may be an antecubital vein, an external jugular vein, or a subclavian vein. The electrode is next passed through the superior vena cava under fluoroscopic control, then through the right atrium and the tricuspid valve, and finally into the right ventricle. The electrode catheter is then put under very slight compression to fix the location of the catheter tip at the apex of the right ventricle. Ideally, with the permanent pacer, the tip becomes embedded beneath the trabeculae carnae of the right ventricle and will not become dislodged. Within 2 to 3 weeks, an ingrowth of fibrous tissue envelops the catheter tip which holds the entire electrode firmly in place during the remainder of its life.

After implantation of a transvenous pacing electrode, a lateral chest film should be obtained to insure that the catheter tip is in the right ventricle. It is (unfortunately) quite easy to place the catheter tip in the coronary sinus, which may appear very similar to the apex of the right ventricle on a PA chest film. However, the lateral chest film will clearly show a catheter tip correctly placed in the apex of the right ventricle in an anterior position, whereas the catheter tip placed in the coronary sinus position is shown to be directed posteriorly.

The electrocardiogram may also be useful in determining proper location of the electrode. A pacemaker driving the right ventricle should produce ECG-wave forms roughly comparable to those of left bundle-branch block: driven beats with predominantly upright QRS forms in standard lead I and mostly downward driven QRS complexes in lead V-1.

Myocardial electrodes are sutured directly to the ventricular myocardium. These require open chest surgery. A "screw-in" myocardial lead is available, which permits a myocardial electrode insertion with very limited thoracotomy; it is very literally screwed into the left-ventricular muscle, usually with two to three turns, and is then tacked down with a suture. There is no overriding advantage of one form of electrode over the other. Transvenous endocardial electrodes have an increased risk of dislodgement, but obviate the need for thoracotomy.

Pacemaker Follow-up

In follow-up of patients with implanted pacemakers, it is essential to check pacemaker function at periodic intervals. These intervals should become more frequent as the pacemaker nears the end of its expected life. Except for one little-used brand, all pacemakers manufactured in the United States are designed to slow their intrinsic pacing rate as the batteries become depleted and near the end of their useful life. Slowing of 6 to 8 beats/min, or 10% of the original pacing rate, is sufficient evidence to diagnose battery depletion and cause for prompt replacement of the pulse generator and batteries. Other indications for replacement of the pulse generator are failure of a pacing stimulus to drive the ventricles and failure of the pacemaker appropriately to sense a spontaneous QRS. These two problems require an ECG for diagnostic certainty.

Monitoring of the pacemaker rate may be done by ECG rhythm strip—a recording of a single ECG lead—at the time of a patient's revisit. It is also possible to follow pacemaker rate and function by means of an ECG rhythm strip transmitted by telephone. The patient may attach himself to a device which transmits his rhythm strip by means of a transducer which changes the patient's ECG to an audible tone, which is then transmitted by telephone; on the receiving end, another transducer changes the audible tone from the telephone back into the ECG-wave form. By this means, close pacemaker follow-up is possible without the need for frequent revisits.

With some patients, it may be helpful to instruct the patient or his family on how to check the pulse. A pulse rate clearly slower than the original pacing rate may be an indication of battery depletion in the pacemaker and calls for investigation. A pulse rate faster than the pacemaker rate may indicate merely that the patient is having spontaneous beats of his own at a rate faster than the pacemaker rate and is not necessarily cause for alarm.

Other means have also been used to check pacemaker function. Some clinics have found electronic analysis of the pacemaker stimulus to be of value. In such wave-form analysis, the amplitude, duration, and decay characteristics of the pacemaker stimulus are analyzed. It is felt by some that such analysis can predict impending pacemaker failure before it becomes apparent by a change in pacer rate; however, several studies have demonstrated that the occasional early detection of pacemaker depletion does not warrant the expense and trouble of such analysis. Parameters such as the roentgenographic appearance of the batteries and amplitude of the stimulus artifact in ECG lead I, were once used but are not sufficiently reliable to be depended on. There is no substitute for regular determination of pacer function and rate, which has proven quite reliable for all pacemakers built in this country in the past 8 years.

SUGGESTED READING

Chung EK: Principles of Cardiac Arrhythmias, ed. 2. Baltimore, Williams & Wilkins, 1977

Ferrer MI: The Sick Sinus Syndrome. Mount Kisco, N.Y., Futura Publishing Co., 1974

McAnulty JH et al: A prospective study of sudden death in "high rish" bundle-branch block. N Eng J Med 299: 209, 1978

Varriale P, Naclerio EA: Cardiac Pacing. Philadelphia, Lea & Febiger, 1979

HYPERTENSION

Harold Smulyan

Essential hypertension is probably the commonest major illness in the United States today. It was estimated in the early 1970s that there were 22 million hypertensive individuals, half of whom did not know they had the disease, and half of the remainder of whom were inadequately treated. Since 1972, the National High Blood Pressure Education Program has made significant inroads in improving public awareness and understanding of the disease. Because of the complications which can result from hypertension, such as stroke, congestive heart failure, myocardial infarction, peripheral vascular disease, aortic dissection, and renal failure, hypertension ranks as one of our most serious medical problems. Since the complication rate can be significantly reduced by medical control of the blood pressure, identification of afflicted patients and their optimal treatment can clearly reduce the morbidity and mortality from vascular disease in a significant portion of the population.

DEFINITION OF HYPERTENSION

When the level of blood pressure is plotted against its frequency in any population of American adults (see Figs. 13-1A, B), it can be seen that there is no sharp dividing line separating hypertensive from normal individuals. Since there is no clear separation between normal and hypertensive subjects, an arbitrary division has been established at 150/90 torr. This is based on insurance statistics, which suggest that above a diastolic pressure of 90 torr, there is an increasing mortality. For example, if the blood pressure of a 35-year-old man is above 140/90 torr, his lifespan will be reduced by 9 years, while if it is above 150/100

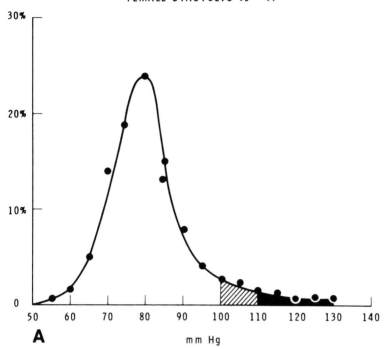

A

FIG. 13-1(A).
Frequency distribution of diastolic pressure in females aged 40–49 in a
London population sample (Hamilton and others, 1954a). The black
area shows patients who are known to be at risk and known to benefit
from treatment. The shaded area, comprising pressures of 100–110
torr, represents subjects who are also at risk, but it is not yet known if
they would benefit from hypotensive therapy. Subjects in the
remaining white area are those with 'normal' blood pressures.
(Pickering GW: Hypertension. ed 2. Edinburgh and London, Churchill
Livingstone, 1974)

torr, his lifespan will be 17 years shorter than that of a man the same age with a
blood pressure under 130/90 torr. The Framingham study showed that between
the ages of 30 to 39, people whose diastolic blood pressures were between 85
and 94 torr had 5 times the number of coronary events as a group whose diastolic pressure was under 85 torr. The stroke incidence varies almost directly
with systolic and diastolic pressures. Also, with any elevation of systolic
pressure over 140 torr, the incidence of congestive failure is 6 times that of a
population whose systolic blood pressure is less than 140 torr. In the black population, hypertension represents a very special problem, since the death rate in
this group is 3 times that of the white hypertensive population. This suggests

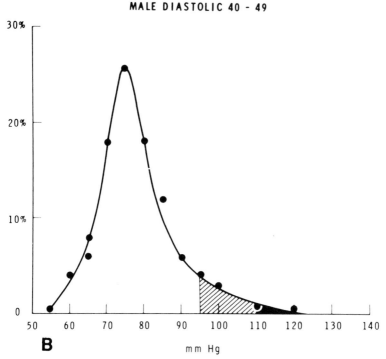

B

FIG. 13-1(B).
As Fig 13-1(A) but for males. The shaded area comprises pressures
between 95–100 torr. (Pickering GW: Hypertension. ed 2. Edinburgh
and London, Churchill Livingstone, 1974)

that the upper normal limit for the black population should be set lower than
for others. All of these statistics are provided to illustrate the increasing complication rate which accompanies increasing blood pressure at all levels, and the
weakness of any level chosen to separate the normal from the abnormal.

The arbitrary definition of hypertension is complicated by the variability of
the blood pressure from moment to moment during any given day or week.
This lability is seen in normal subjects to some extent, but it is exaggerated in
hypertensives. Early in the course of essential hypertension, the blood pressure
may vary between normal and elevated ranges. Such individuals have been said
to have labile blood pressure, and in follow-up studies, 20% to 25% of them
have developed fixed hypertension. It is important to measure the blood
pressure after 10 to 20 min of rest and on several different occasions before the
diagnosis of essential hypertension is made. The best first treatment for high
blood pressure is to measure the blood pressure again. On occasion, it will be
valuable to teach the patient to take his own blood pressure and to establish the
daytime variability outside of the doctor's office. Only when repeated blood
pressure measurements are elevated above 150/90 torr should the patient be

considered hypertensive. Those patients with labile blood pressure should be reevaluated frequently, since they are at an increased risk of developing fixed hypertension. There is some tendency for the blood pressure to rise normally with age, so that for patients age 60 or more, 160/95 is a good dividing line between normality and hypertension.

The technique for blood pressure measurement has been described in the chapter on the physical examination (Chap. 2). Since the accuracy of the measurement is dependent on the care and time taken, nurses, physician's assistants, and technicians are often more precise in making this measurement than busy physicians. As mentioned in Chapter 2, cuff width is extremely important. In a patient with an obese arm, spuriously high values will be obtained unless a cuff is used which is wider than standard and is long enough to completely encircle the arm. It is also now apparent that with advancing years and rigid arteries, the systolic pressure measured by cuff may be 20 to 30 torr higher than the actual intraarterial pressure. There is agreement that the systolic pressure should be measured with the onset of the Korotkoff sounds, but controversy remains regarding the criterion for measuring the diastolic pressure. We recommend, despite random error, that the disappearance of the Korotkoff sounds be used as the standard.

CAUSES OF HYPERTENSION

Once the diagnosis of hypertension has been established, the patient should be evaluated to determine whether or not one of the disorders known to raise blood pressure is present. Correction of such a secondary form of hypertension can potentially normalize the blood pressure and cure the disease.

CURABLE FORMS

Probably less than 5% of the entire hypertensive population have hypertension of a curable type. Some of these patients with hypertension accompanying thyrotoxicosis, pheochromocytoma, or aortic insufficiency are relatively easy to recognize clinically and are seldom mistaken for those with primary hypertension. Other secondary forms of hypertension may be more difficult to recognize and include primary aldosteronism, renovascular hypertension, and coarctation of the aorta. In the following discussion of the history, physical examination, and laboratory evaluation, some attention will be directed toward methods of identifying patients with curable hypertension.

ESSENTIAL HYPERTENSION

The best that can be said for the causes of essential hypertension is that the disease is the result of derangements involving multiple factors. One factor may be more important than another in a particular patient, but the multifactorial approach to etiology is still the best available for understanding hypertension. Much time and effort has been spent in trying to classify patients with essential hypertension into various groups based upon each of these factors. The role of hemodynamics, catecholamines, the sympathetic nervous system, and the renin-angiotensin system have all been extensively studied in an effort to understand the disease, but no single unifying etiology or concept has been established. A discussion of some of the relevant factors follows. However, this brief presentation of the subject cannot do justice to the time and effort put into the field by many investigators.

Familial and Racial Factors

Observations of large numbers of hypertensive patients leave little doubt that the disease tends to occur in families and that heredity plays an important role. Pickering and others have studied the blood pressure correlation in twins and siblings, and investigated the relationship between parent's and children's blood pressure. Children of hypertensive parents have blood pressures generally higher (though within normal limits) than children of normotensive parents. A positive family history is sufficiently common in essential hypertension that one should suspect curable hypertension in a young hypertensive patient without it. Similarly, there are racial factors in hypertension. The average blood pressure of the American black population is several torr higher than that of the white population, and hypertension of severe degree is 6 to 7 times more common in American blacks than whites. The fact that hypertension has not been described as a major problem in black Africans suggests that the origin is not entirely genetic. Therefore, race and environment may play a combined role.

Hemodynamics

One of the approaches that we have found most useful in understanding the pathophysiology of essential hypertension has been the study of hemodynamics. Reduced to its elements, blood pressure is dependent on cardiac output and systemic vascular resistance. Systemic vascular resistance, calculated as the ratio of mean arterial pressure to cardiac output, is roughly related to the cross-sectional area of the arteriolar bed. Most patients with fixed essential hypertension have a normal cardiac output and an elevated systemic vascular resistance. Many investigations have centered about determining the mechanisms for the increased resistance, such as increased sodium and water in the vascular walls, which narrows arteriolar lumens or makes the arterioles hyperreactive to normal endogenous pressor substances. On the other hand, about 10% of patients with essential hypertension have an elevated cardiac output and a normal, or nearly normal, peripheral resistance. An increased cardiac ouput is more common among patients with early labile essential hypertension. Interest in the cause of the high flow rate has focussed attention on the role of the heart in hypertension. Although a primary increase in cardiac contractility could explain the high cardiac output, other initiating factors have been sought. These include increased concentrations, or sensitivity to, circulating catecholamines; an overactive sympathetic nervous system; or incorrect regulation of plasma volume by the kidney. A high flow rate for any cause could induce peripheral autoregulation, raising the peripheral resistance and thus returning the cardiac output to normal. Although autoregulation of many vascular beds in response to artificially increased flow rates has been shown in animals and the gradual return of the cardiac output to normal has been demonstrated in man, the connection remains speculative.

Renal Mechanisms for Plasma Volume and Arterial Pressure Control

One of the postulated defects responsible for the elevated cardiac output has been said to be an error in the renal regulation of intravascular volume. Normally, blood pressure is regulated in part by the renal excretion of sodium and water. An error in volume regulation by the kidney could lead to a high plasma volume, resulting in the elevated cardiac output and elevated blood pressure. This hemodynamic circumstance, in normal individuals, produces a diuresis, which returns pressure and flow to normal. The renal feedback mechanism may be incompletely effective in the hypertensive patient, since the plasma volume remains inappropriately elevated for the level of arterial pressure. Therefore, the "normal" renal function usually described in patients with essential hypertension is, by definition, abnormal, since the necessary diuresis to return blood pressure to normal is absent.

Sodium

An interrelated defect which may play a role in the development of hypertension is an increased amount of dietary sodium, abnormal renal excretion of sodium, or altered vascular responsiveness to sodium. The work establishing the central role of sodium in the development of hypertension has been carried out by Tobian. Epidemiological evidence has also shown an increasing incidence of hypertension which parallels an increasing sodium intake, when the dietary customs of different societies are considered. Northern Japanese, who preserve their fish in salt, have a high salt intake and a hypertension incidence which exceeds that of the rest of Japan, where the sodium intake is lower. Different Solomon Island tribes have differing blood pressures, which also relate to their sodium intake. Although impractical for widespread use, intense restriction of sodium intake alone can be used to treat hypertension and will effectively lower blood pressure. Since not all patients with a high sodium intake develop hypertension, however, there must be other factors which operate to sensitize certain individuals to sodium. This sensitivity has been verified in different strains of rats, some of whom become hypertensive with high sodium intakes while others do not. Tobian has demonstrated that in hypertensive animals and patients, the sodium content of arteries and arterioles is higher than in the blood vessel walls of nonhypertensive animals or patients. The mechanism by which sodium produces hypertension is uncertain, but it may be related to changes in plasma volume, thickness of the arterial wall, or altered reactivity of arterioles to endogenous pressor substances.

Arterial Baroreceptor Function

Normally, a rise in blood pressure stimulates baroreceptor endings in the carotid sinus and aorta, which function reflexly to decrease sympathetic outflow and increase vagal outflow from the brain. This produces vasodilatation and cardiac slowing, and returns the blood pressure toward normal. Baroreceptor function is abnormal in patients with essential hypertension and in animals with experimental hypertension. The work of Gribbin and that of McCubbin is most illustrative of this point. It has never been clear whether the reset baroreceptor reflex causes the blood pressure elevation or occurs because of it. High blood pressure itself can stiffen arterial walls and thereby alter baroreflex function. If this is a factor in sustaining the blood pressure elevation, then effective antihypertensive therapy for a long period might correct the baroreceptor abnormality. Unfortunately, this does not seem to be the case, since withdrawal of previously effective treatment almost always results in a return of the elevated blood pressure. The importance of baroreflex function has been heightened by the recognition that both clonidine and propranolol lower blood pressure, in part by adjusting central nervous system baroreceptor function.

Renin and Angiotension

In recent years, Laragh has pointed out that the hypertensive population can be divided into three groups, based on plasma renin activity relative to urinary sodium excretion (see Fig. 13-2). Patients with low plasma renin activity are generally older and have fewer vascular complications than those with elevated plasma renin activity. Individuals with normal plasma renin activity are between the two in age and in prevalence of complications. The relationship between plasma renin activity and the severity of the disease proposed by Laragh, while a most interesting finding, has not been confirmed by other workers. Plasma renin measurement has also been recommended as a guide to the selection of therapeutic agents, but this, too, is controversial. The connection between the antihypertensive activity of beta blockade and the reduction of renin activity is indirect, since some effective beta blockers do not lower plasma renin activity and others, in low dose, lower the plasma renin activity but with little effect on the blood pressure. It has become apparent that renin grouping for therapy is a relative, rather than an absolute, matter. More patients with high

FIG. 13-2
Relation of noon plasma renin activity to the concurrent daily rate of sodium excretion in 219 patients with essential hypertension. Triangles indicate low, open circles normal, and squares high, renin activity. (Brunner HR, Laragh JH, Baer L et al: Essential hypertension. N Eng J Med 286:444, 1972)

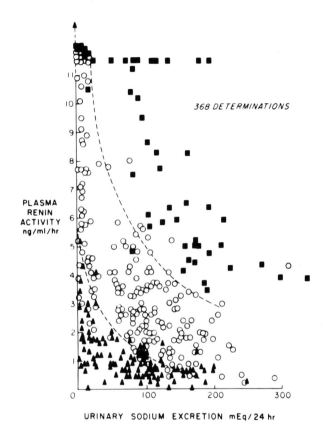

368 DETERMINATIONS

PLASMA RENIN ACTIVITY ng/ml/hr

URINARY SODIUM EXCRETION mEq/24 hr

plasma renin activity respond to beta blockade, but many patients with low plasma renin respond as well. For this reason, it would appear that renin profiling, which is expensive and difficult to do accurately, is not necessary for proper management in the majority of hypertensive patients. It may prove valuable, however, in understanding the nature of the disease.

Sympathetic Nervous System and Catecholamines

Since the sympathetic nervous system functions to support and adjust blood pressure, abnormalities of this system have been considered among the causes of hypertension. Hypertensive patients are known to have excessive pressor reactions to such stresses as cold, pain, or mental activity. The rise in pressure occurs primarily by an increase in central nervous system sympathetic outflow. The fact that many drugs used to treat essential hypertension interfere with sympathetic nervous activity is another reason to suspect an abnormality in this system. The difficulty in defining a role for the sympathetic system lies in the complexity of its role in circulatory control. Sympathetic nerves supply the kidney and influence renin excretion. In turn, renin alters functions controlled by angiotensin and aldosterone. The sympathetic system also controls arteriolar, venous, and venular tone, and cardiac contractility, all of which is further modulated by circulating adrenal epinephrine and norepinephrine, also sympathetically controlled. If it is true that a summary of sympathetic activity can be found in blood and urine levels of catecholamines, such concentrations have not clearly separated hypertensive and normotensive individuals, and a clear demonstration of sympathetic hyperfunction or increased sensitivity to circulating catecholamines has never been made.

THE EVALUATION OF A NEWLY DIAGNOSED
HYPERTENSIVE PATIENT

The purpose of a hypertensive study is, first, to uncover the small number of patients with one of the curable forms of hypertension and, secondly, in those with essential hypertension, to assess the severity of the blood pressure abnormality in terms of damage to target organs. History, physical examination, and laboratory studies are used, as in the investigation of any disease. Because of the large number of patients with essential hypertension, it is important to evaluate patients simply and rapidly and then start a treatment program as quickly as possible. Since in this disease the response to therapy is a measure of the severity of the disease, therapy can be considered as part of the evaluation. If a patient does not respond to a standard therapy program, further study is indicated.

HISTORY

The history is extremely important in establishing the diagnosis and the severity of the disease. Essential hypertension is a disease most often detected in the 30 to the 40 age range, but it is often preceded by a history of labile blood pressure. Patients may recall being told, when they were examined for sports in school, for induction into the service, or for life insurance, of an elevated blood pressure which later returns to normal. Also, in essential hypertension there is often a positive family history which helps in the diagnosis. Sudden severe hypertension in a young man in his middle 20s with no family history of the disease should alert the physician to the possibility of renal-artery stenosis or another secondary form of hypertension. Women will often give a history of having been hypertensive during pregnancy as a forerunner to sustained essential hypertension. Severity of the disease is also influenced by the family history, since a strong family history for vascular disease is predictive of future complications, irrespective of the actual blood pressure levels. Also useful in assessing severity are: diabetes, cigarette smoking, high salt intake, and obesity.

Evidence of target organ symptoms should be searched for in the history, including angina, congestive heart failure, prior stroke or transient ischemic attacks, and intermittent claudication or evidence for renal failure, which may be manifested as nocturia, polyuria, or recurrent urinary tract infections. Headache and epistaxis are commonly listed as symptoms but are rarely related to hypertension. Most headaches in patients with hypertension result from tension, except in those few patients with malignant hypertension in whom headaches may be the presenting complaint. A history of epistaxis is almost worthless, since it is only seldom the result of hypertension.

Historical features associated with curable forms of hypertension include: for pheochromocytoma—tremor, palpitations and sweating; for primary aldosteronism—weakness, muscle cramps, and polyuria; and for aortic coarctation—a history of hypertension since childhood. Occasionally, patients with renal hypertension will have a history of renal trauma.

PHYSICAL EXAMINATION

When a patient comes to a physician's office and is examined for any reason, the blood pressure measurement is most important, because the diagnostic yield is high. Twenty-two million adult Americans have essential hypertension. In young people with hypertension, the blood pressure should also be checked in the leg, using a cuff applied to the thigh and listening for Kortotkoff sounds in the popliteal space. In patients with aortic coarctation, the delay in the arrival of the femoral pulse, when compared to the radial pulse, may be difficult to detect, and a systolic popliteal pressure lower than the brachial is a more reliable measurement. It is also important to check the blood pressure in both arms. Normally, pressure in the right arm may be as much as 10 torr higher than in the left. A greater difference is suggestive of occlusive vascular disease or of a rare aortic coarctation between the origin of the innominate and left subclavian arteries.

Atherosclerosis in the peripheral vessels should be looked for by the absence of palpable carotid, femoral, posterior tibial, and dorsalis pedis pulses. It is useful to listen for a bruit over these vessels as well. In some patients with renal arterial narrowing, a bruit can be heard over the epigastrium or back.

Examination of the heart is carried out to detect enlargement and the presence of an S_3 or S_4 gallop and murmurs. Aortic insufficiency could account for systolic hypertension, while the aortic stenosis murmur, in the presence of hypertension, suggests aortic coarctation. Complicated hypertension is unusual in the presence of aortic stenosis alone. Aortic coarctation produces hypertension, but is also frequently associated with a congenitally abnormal, bicuspid, and often stenotic aortic valve. Therefore hypertension in the presence of an aortic stenosis murmur suggests aortic coarctation. In general, when there is evidence of heart enlargement resulting from essential hypertension, the disease is well along in its course, and the patient is in serious difficulty.

An examination of the optic fundus is extremely important in the evaluation of the hypertensive patient. This helps not only in the diagnosis but also in the assessment of severity. For example, if a 65-year-old patient with systolic hypertension has normal eye grounds and no evidence of any other end-organ damage, one would be reluctant to treat him vigorously, or at all. It is important to become skillful in examining the optic fundus, since the findings classified by Keith, Wagener, and Barker are still used for prognostic purposes. Papilledema is assigned to Grade IV, hemorrhage and exudate to Grade III, while Grades I and II include various degrees of arteriovenous compression. It should be pointed out that such compressions of the retinal veins by their accompanying arteries are normal within one disc diameter of the optic disc but abnormal outside this area. This arteriovenous "nicking" is a physical sign suggestive of atherosclerosis. Arterial spasm can occur in Grades II, III, or IV retinopathy, and is observed when arterial caliber is observed to be reduced when one follows a vessel from distal to proximal or where an artery narrows between branchings.

In addition to the above, a brief neurological examination should be carried out, searching for evidence of neurological deficit. Obviously, one should look for evidence of thyrotoxicosis, hypothyroidism, or the hypermetabolic state of a pheochromocytoma. The last includes tremor, flushing, and excessive sweating.

LABORATORY EVALUATION

If the history and physical examination suggest one of the curable forms of hypertension, then further special laboratory studies should be directed toward the suspected diagnosis. For pheochromocytoma, an uncommon disorder, 24-hour urinary excretion of norepinephrine, metanephrine and vanillylmandelic acid should be used to screen patients for the diagnosis. For primary aldosteronism, which is usually first suspected by the finding of a low potassium level in patients not on any therapy, it is necessary to obtain plasma renin and aldosterone secretion and excretion rates. Recently the hypotensive response to an intravenous infusion of an angiotensin II blocker (saralasin) has been used to identify patients in a high renin-level group. This group would include those with renal hypertension, as well as the small percentage of patients with essential hypertension.

Generally, it is not necessary to measure plasma renin activity in all hypertensive patients, but within the next few years, renin activity measurements and angiotensin blockers should become readily available for use by physicians practicing outside of medical centers. Response of the blood pressure to intravenous infusion of saralasin or blockers of angiotensin I or II could indicate those patients with hyperreninemia and eliminate the need for plasma renin activity measurements. If renovascular disease is suspected (abdominal bruit, severe hypertension of sudden onset, and negative family history), then the patient should have an intravenous pyelogram or nuclear renal scan. If either study is positive or suspicious for renovascular disease, the patient should be referred for aortography and sampling of renal vein blood for measurement of renin activity. The special tests listed above are only required for a small group of patients suspected of secondary forms of hypertension.

The ordinary patient with hypertension will need none of these. The proper extent of the routine laboratory evaluation has been the subject of much debate, weighing the value of information obtained against the cost, when millions of hypertension patients must be considered. The report of the Joint National Committee on Detection Evaluation in Treatment of Hypertension, from the United States Department of Health, Education and Welfare, recommends the following measurements before therapy is started:

1. Hematocrit
2. Urinalysis for protein, blood and glucose (dipstick)
3. Serum creatinine or blood urea nitrogen
4. Serum potassium
5. Electrocardiogram

Most hospitals now offer rapid automated laboratory analyses, which, for the same price as the sodium and potassium tests, will provide a plasma glucose, a blood urea nitrogen, and several other determinations. A chest film, while not particularly sensitive to early cardiomegaly, is a useful baseline study and may screen out those patients with aortic coarctation. It is important to emphasize that the case study in no way requires that the patient be hospitalized or lose more than a half-day from work. It can be done easily on an outpatient basis.

THERAPY

The response to therapy is also used as a part of the evaluation, since those who do not respond to moderately intensive therapy should be more extensively studied. Essential hypertension is a disease without symptoms, especially in its earliest stages. The ordinary American with hypertension feels well and is reluctant to undertake the expense, the inconvenience, and the very possible side effects of chronic drug therapy. The physician will have to "sell" the need for treatment to the patient, since a major therapeutic problem is lack of patient compliance. It is important to emphasize that the seller need not be a physician, but can be a nurse practitioner or a technician; however, it must be someone who can spend time with the patient. The therapist must be certain that the patient understands the reasons for drug treatment, and be available to determine the response after treatment is started. We have found the measurement of blood pressure at home extremely useful, since it allows the spouse or other person in the home to become involved in the program.

In convincing the patient of the need for therapy, the physician must have substantial data to indicate that reduction in blood pressure reduces the complication rate and prolongs life. Such data are available. In 1967, the Veteran's Administration Cooperative Study was carried out on a small number of patients with diastolic pressures between 115 and 129, comparing therapy with placebo. Within 20 months, there were 27 morbid events among the 70 individuals on the placebo contrasted with 2 morbid events in the 73 patients on therapy. In 1970, a larger group of patients with diastolic blood pressures between 90 and 114 were studied, with similar results. Clearly, morbidity is reduced by therapy. The hypertensive complications most effectively prevented included stroke, renal failure, congestive failure, and aortic dissection. There was no statistically significant reduction in the incidence of myocardial infarction. However, many hypertensive patients have other multiple risk factors for atherosclerosis which persist after normal blood pressures are achieved. This may account for the failure of myocardial infarction incidence to fall. How much the pressure should be reduced is a problem, since it is often difficult to bring it absolutely to normal. There is evidence from a similar Veteran's Administration study that reduction of even 10 torr will decrease the incidence of complications. Therefore, drug therapy should not be abandoned if a normal pressure cannot be reached. Recently, the Hypertension Detection and Follow-Up Program from the National Institutes of Health has demonstrated significant reductions in mortality when patients with diastolic blood pressures between 90 and 105 were effectively treated for a 5-year period. This is persuasive evidence that most if not all patients with diastolic pressures greater than 90 torr should have their blood pressure lowered.

The decision to start therapy should not be taken lightly, since at the present state of knowledge it implies pill-taking for a lifetime. Where the blood pressure is high (105 torr diastolic, or greater) and fixed and there is already evidence of target organ damage, the decision to start drug therapy is easily made. In patients whose blood pressure only intermittently exceeds 150/90 and where there is no target organ damage, treatment can be withheld, but follow-up blood pressure measurements should be obtained to determine when and if fixed hypertension develops. Those patients who fall between these guidelines should probably be treated as well. Blacks, males, and those with target organ damage and strong family histories of hypertension are patients whose therapy should be started sooner, rather than later.

Treatment is really quite simple and involves a stepped approach, as developed by the National Institutes of Health. All patients are first started on a thiazide diuretic. These drugs are especially useful for individuals with mild hypertension, since they reliably lower the blood pressure in this group and encourage patient compliance because of the once-daily dosage. There seems to be little difference among the many thiazide diuretics available, except that some of the longer-acting preparations, such as clorthalidone, may be administered every other day. Initially, thiazide diuretics lower the blood pressure by reducing plasma volume and cardiac output. Gradually, the cardiac output returns toward, but not to, normal and the systemic vascular resistance is then reduced. The mechanism of this vasodilation is uncertain and may relate to lower salt and water content of the arterioles, which increases luminal size or reduces their sensitivity to endogenous pressor substances. Thiazide diuretics are usually well tolerated.

Because of their effect on the renal tubule, the serum uric acid is usually elevated, and an occasional case of clinical gout is precipitated. This complication is readily managed by discontinuing the drug or by adding a uricosuric agent such as allopurinol. The most common side effect of thiazide diuretics is renal potassium wasting, and its most frequent symptom is fatigue. Our own experience has been that most patients feel better if they are also given a potassium supplement or spironolactone compound, but not both together.

When control of the blood pressure is not obtained with the use of thiazide diuretics alone, a second agent, either propranolol, reserpine, or methyldopa, is added to the regimen. Propranolol should be given in increasing doses up to approximately 320 mg twice daily, or if methyldopa is chosen, up to 3 g daily may be given. Propranolol is contraindicated or should be used with caution in patients with congestive heart failure, second- or third-degree heart block, chronic lung disease, peripheral vascular disease, or insulin-dependent diabetes. The new subselective beta-1 adrenergic blockers should be valuable in patients with chronic lung disease who require therapy for hypertension. Most patients, however, tolerate beta blockade without significant side effects, the most frequent ones being cold hands and feet, fatigue, drowsiness, loss of libido, and reduced ability to concentrate. The mechanism of action of propranolol involves an initial reduction in cardiac output, following the onset of therapy. This is followed by a return of the cardiac output toward normal and the subsequent reduction of systemic vascular resistance, which is probably central in origin.

Methyldopa lowers cardiac output and systemic vascular resistance. The fall in cardiac output occurs predominantly when the patient is in a standing position; the reduction in systemic vascular resistance is also centrally mediated. The drug also produces side effects such as drowsiness, fatigue, and loss of libido, but its most frequent side effect is orthostatic hypotension. An occasional patient taking methyldopa develops hepatic disease or hemolysis.

Reserpine, which depletes all tissues of norepinephrine, has both peripheral and central actions. These operate to alter pressure and flow in a manner similar to that of methyldopa. The dose of reserpine should be limited to 0.1 to 0.2 mg daily. In this dosage range, the frequency of side effects is minimized. These are similar to the untoward effects of methyldopa, with the addition of depression, bad dreams, and parasympathomimetic effects, such as nasal stuffiness and diarrhea. The increased risks of breast cancer from reserpine is a fear that has been dispelled. Reserpine remains a useful drug in selected patients.

If the combination of two drugs remains ineffective in bringing the blood pressure to normal, hydralazine or guanethedine is added. Hydralazine, which is a direct arteriolar vasodilator, should not be used in doses of greater than 300 mg per day because of the lupuslike syndrome which may occur at higher doses. Hydralazine and propranolol, with or without the thiazide diuretic, make a good combination, since the propranolol blocks the beta adrenergic side effects of hydralazine, predominantly tachycardia. Guanethedine is an antiadrenergic agent which can be used in doses starting with 10 to 25 mg/day and gradually increasing to 75 or 100 mg/day. Since it does not cross the blood-brain barrier, it produces little in the way of central nervous system side effects. Many males refuse to take the drug because of its high incidence of decreased libido. Its other major side effect, shared with methyldopa, is orthostatic hypotension. This symptom is most common on arising from bed in the morning and after strenuous exercise. Patients should be warned about the effects of standing suddenly and their follow-up blood pressures measured in both the standing and supine positions. Clonidine, prazosin, and minoxidil are newer agents which are now available for use should side effects preclude the use of some of the previously discussed drugs.

All antihypertensive agents have side effects and contraindications with which prescribers should be familiar. It is important that patients not be lost to follow-up or allowed to discontinue drug therapy because of side effects. Drug-induced symptoms should therefore warrant a change in the therapeutic program in order to favor patient compliance.

Restricted dietary sodium intake, as the single measure to lower the blood pressure, must be in the range of 200 to 500 mg a day. Such a diet is expensive (salt-free bread, butter, vegetables), unpalatable, induces poor patient compliance, and is generally unsuitable for long-term use. As an adjunct to drug therapy, it is advisable to omit known salty foods and to avoid the addition of salt to cooking or table food, but intense sodium restriction is unnecessary

The therapeutic aim is a blood pressure within the normal range. If this cannot be obtained, any lowering of the blood pressure offers some protection from hypertensive complications. Most patients with essential hypertension can be effectively treated with one of the combinations previously detailed. If a regimen cannot easily be found which is effective in controlling the blood pressure, the patient should be reassessed by an additional search for secondary forms of hypertension.

The results of treatment can often be better followed by blood pressures measured at home, since the patient often tends to be hypertensive near his physician. In uncomplicated cases, nurses or technicians can often supervise the patient better than a physician, because they have more time and can better emphasize the importance of therapy.

To summarize: essential hypertension is a widespread disease of unknown cause, which can be very successfully treated. It is important not to overlook the curable forms of hypertension. Once started on therapy, continuation of the program is essential.

SUGGESTED READING

Effects of treatment on morbidity in hypertension. Results in patients with diastolic blood pressures averaging 115 through 129 mmHg. Veterans Administration Cooperative Study on Antihypertensive Agents. JAMA 202:1028–1034, 1967
Effects of treatment on morbidity in hypertension. Results in patients with diastolic

blood pressures averaging 90 through 114 mmHg. Veterans Administration Co-op-erative Study on Antihypertensive Agents. JAMA 213:1143–1152, 1970

Eich RH, Cuddy RP, Smulyan H, Lyons RH: Hemodynamics in labile hypertension. A follow-up study. Circulation 34:299–307, 1966

Ferriss JB, Beevers DG, Brown JJ et al: Low-renin ("primary") hyperaldosteronism differential diagnosis and distinction of sub-groups within the syndrome. Am Heart J 95:641–658, 1978

Gillum RF, Barsky AJ: Diagnosis and management of patient noncompliance. JAMA 228:1563–1567, 1974

Gribbin B, Pickering TG, Sleight P, Peto R: Effect of age and high blood pressure on baroreflex sensitivity in man. Circ Res 29:424–431, 1971

Guyton AC, Coleman TG, Cowley AW Jr, Scheel KW, Manning RD Jr, Norman RA Jr: Arterial pressure regulation: Overriding dominance of the kidneys in long-term regulation and in hypertension. Am J Med 52:584–594, 1972

Hypertension Detection and Follow-up Program Cooperative Group. Five-Year Findings of the Hypertension Detection and Follow-Up Program I. Reduction in mortality of persons with high blood pressure, including mild hypertension. JAMA 242:2562–2570, 1979.

Kaplan NM: Renin profiles. The unfulfilled promises. JAMA 238:611–613, 1977

Keith NM, Wagener HP, Barker NW: Some different types of essential hypertension. Their course and prognosis. Am J Med Sci 197:332–343, 1939

Laragh JH, Sealy JE: Renin-sodium profiling: why, how, and when in clinical practice. Cardiovasc Med 2:1053–1075, 1977

Littler WA, West MJ, Honour AJ, Sleight P: The variability of arterial pressure. Am Heart J 95:180–186, 1978

McCubbin JW, Green JH, Page IH: Baroreceptor function in chronic renal hypertension. Circ Res 4:205–210, 1956

Mendlowitz M: Neural crest tumors of sympathetic or chromaffin origin (pheochromo-cytoma, ganglioneuroma, and neuroblastoma). In Genest J, Koiw E, Kuchel O (eds): Hypertension: Physiopathology and Treatment, pp 781–789. New York, McGraw-Hill, 1977

Pickering GW: High Blood Pressure. New York, Grune & Stratton, 1968

Report of the Joint National Committee on Detection, Evaluation and Treatment of High Blood Pressure: a cooperative study. JAMA 237:255–261, 1977

Roberts WC: The hypertensive diseases. Evidence that systemic hypertension is a greater risk factor to the development of other cardiovascular diseases than previously suspected. Am J Med 59:523–532, 1975

Streeten DHP, Anderson GH, Freiberg JM, Dalakos TG: Use of an angiotensin II antagonist (Saralasin) in the recognition of "angiotensinogenic" hypertension. N Engl J Med 292:657–662, 1975

Tobian L: Salt and hypertension. In Genest J, Koiw E, Kuchel O (eds): Hypertension: Physiopathology and Treatment, pp 423–433. New York, McGraw-Hill, 1977

ENDOCARDITIS

Harold Smulyan

14

A review of the history of bacterial endocarditis offers a fascinating insight into the effect of medical progress on the natural history of this disease. Medical advances, while improving the prognosis, have not eradicated the disorder and have served to uncover several other unsolved problems. In the preantibiotic era, the ability to diagnose bacterial endocarditis was well developed, but the disease was almost uniformly fatal. It is interesting that the first, nonspontaneous cure of bacterial endocarditis came as a result of surgical closure of an infected patent ductus arteriosus. However, since heart valves, rather than patent ductus, are the most frequently infected sites, surgical closure of a patent ductus arteriosus did not offer a satisfactory form of therapy for most patients with the disease. Most deaths during the preantibiotic era resulted from uncontrolled infection.

The development of potent antibiotics and the techniques of testing them against offending organisms had a significant impact on the disease and lowered the death rate from nearly 100% to between 10% and 15%. Antibiotic treatment of the infection did not eradicate the disease, however, but instead changed the cause of death from sepsis to congestive heart failure. This occurred because of residual deformity of the healed valves and the resultant hemodynamic abnormality which followed cure of the infection.

The next significant advance was the application of cardiac valve replacement surgery to patients with bacterial endocarditis and congestive heart failure. Valve replacement can be accomplished not only in patients in whom the infection has been completely eradicated but also in those whose antibiotic-induced healing is incomplete. The use of surgery in the treatment of bacterial endocarditis completes the cycle of evolution in therapy by returning to the original form of curative treatment for the disease. Although valve replacement surgery has reduced the death rate still further, it cannot eradicate the disease, since it has the potential for producing bacterial endocarditis again, as well as for its cure. The insertion of prosthetic heart valves in patients without bacterial endocarditis provides an increased opportunity for infection both at the time of surgery and at any time thereafter.

Several other recent trends have influenced the behavior of bacterial endocarditis. Larger numbers of elderly people in the population account for a higher incidence of degenerative valvular disease, which is susceptible to bacterial infection. This accounts for the steadily increasing age in the last few decades of patients with bacterial endocarditis. The recent recognition that cardiac infection can complicate the course of abnormalities such as mitral-valve prolapse (click-murmur syndrome) and idiopathic hypertrophic subaortic stenosis has explained some previously puzzling cases. In earlier years, individuals with such conditions would probably have been diagnosed as having infective endocarditis on normal valves.

The other major recent development has been the increasing numbers of young patients with bacterial endocarditis of right-sided heart valves. These cases have been most prevalent in large urban centers where narcotic addition is a major problem. This is due to unsterile intravenous injections of narcotics.

Finally, widespread indiscriminate use of antibiotics for fever, viral respiratory infections, and so forth leads to inadvertent and usually inadequate treatment of unsuspected bacterial endocarditis. Although such therapy is inadequate to effect a cure of bacterial endocarditis, it has led to larger numbers of blood-culture negative cases. When the offending organisms cannot be identified, selection of appropriate antibiotic agents and dosage is more difficult.

PATHOGENESIS

In order for bacteria to grow on cardiac valves or other circulatory endothelial surfaces, organisms must first gain access to the bloodstream and be delivered to the sites where they eventually grow. It is commonly taught that the means by which microorganisms gain access to the bloodstream is through surgical manipulations which disrupt the barrier between the outside and inside environments. Tooth extractions and other dental procedures are associated with bacteremias involving the oral flora, including the streptococcus viridans, while manipulations of the genitourinary tract or lower gastrointestinal tract are associated with infections from the enterococcus. Staphylococcal infections of the skin also relate to endocarditis. However, only 15% to 20% of patients with subacute bacterial endocarditis offer a history which explains the entrance of organisms to the bloodstream. Those with enterococcal infections and staphylococcal infections have a higher (35%–40%) incidence of predisposing events. However, the pathogenetic mechanism of entry is obvious only in a minority of cases. In the remaining majority, the intermittent bacteremia of smaller bacterial inoculums associated with everyday living must be responsible for the infection. Activities known to produce transient bacteremia include chewing hard substances; vigorous teeth-brushing; oral irrigation devices, especially when associated with periodontal disease; barium enemas; and rectal examinations.

We must next consider where the organisms settle, and why. This relates in part to the size of the bacterial inoculum, the pathogenicity of the organism, and the susceptibility of the valvular endothelium. When the numbers of bacteria are small and their invasiveness limited, the normal immunologic and phagocytic mechanisms clear the bloodstream without the development of endocarditis. When bacterial numbers are larger, the organisms more pathogenic, and the heart valve already deformed, the setting is correct for bacterial valvular invasion. It is well accepted that organisms of lower pathogenicity, such as streptococcus viridans, most commonly invade heart valves previously deformed by rheumatic fever. However, such invasion may also occur with other lesions, such as mitral-valve prolapse (click-murmur syndrome), calcific aortic stenosis, idiopathic hypertrophic subaortic stenosis, or any lesion capable of producing trauma to the vascular endothelium. Other sites of predilection besides the valves include the jet lesions produced by aortic coarctation, patent ductus arteriosus, ventricular septal defect, arteriovenous fistulas, or even the endothelial disruption produced by mural clot following myocardial infarction. Such cases involving an organism of low pathogenicity on an abnormal endothelial surface usually follow a subacute clinical course. On the other hand, highly pathogenetic organisms such as the staphylococcus may, in 50% to 60% of the cases, invade normal valves and produce an acute infection with a more acute clinical picture.

Where valve lesions are present, the endocarditis may be more associated with certain characteristics of blood flow than with the valve lesions themselves. In a now classic study, Rodbard has shown *in vitro* why vegetations grow where they do. According to this study, bacterial endocarditis is associated with a high-pressure source driving high-velocity blood flow through a narrow orifice to a low pressure sink. The high-stream velocity beyond the orifice is associated with a decrease in lateral pressure and a related decrease in perfusion of the intima of this segment (see Fig. 14-1). This serves to injure the endothelium and predispose the site for bacterial invasion. The characteristics of flow in the segment just beyond the orifice also favors the deposition of particles in this low-pressure area. Furthermore, the high-velocity flow can also traumatize the endothelium directly in the jet path and produce a second site for bacterial growth.

These *in vitro* formulations provide some explanation for what has been observed clinically. Valves handling high pressures on the left side of the heart are more commonly involved, making mechanical stress a factor in pathogenesis. With mitral regurgitation, the endocarditis lesions are commonly on the atrial side of the leaflets (low-pressure sink) and on the atrial wall (jet). With

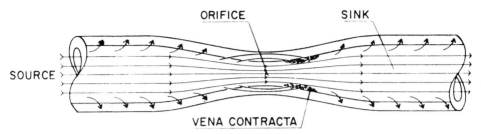

FIG. 14-1.
Flow through a permeable tube. A high pressure source (at left) drives fluid through
an orifice into a low pressure sink. The curved arrows leaving the stream and entering
the wall in the upstream segment represent the normal perfusion of the lining layer.
Velocity is maximal and perfusing pressure is low immediately beyond the orifice
where the momentum of the stream converges the streamlines to form a vena
contracta. The low pressure in this segment results in reduced perfusion and may
cause a retrograde flow from the deeper layers of the vessel into the flowing stream.
(Robard S: Blood velocity and endocarditis. Circulation 27:21, 1963. Used by
permission of the American Heart Association, Inc.)

aortic insufficiency, the vegetations are most commonly on the ventricular surface of the leaflet (low-pressure sink) or on the anterior leaflet of the mitral
valve (jet). In ventricular septal defect, the colonies are most commonly found
on the right-ventricular side of the defect and on the right-ventricular wall opposite the hole. This observation of bacterial colonies on the downstream side
of the jet lesion also holds true for tricuspid insufficiency, arteriovenous fistulas,
aortic coarctation, and patent ductus arteriosus. Lesions associated with low-
flow velocities (large valve areas, absent valvular gradients, or low cardiac output states) are rarely involved with bacterial endocarditis. This principle accounts for the virtual absence of bacterial endocarditis in an atrial septal defect,
in which the velocity of shunt flow is relatively low and steady, when compared
with the higher frequency of endocarditis in ventricular septal defects, especially small ones, in which flow velocity is faster.

   Denuding of the vascular endothelium exposes the underlying collagen,
which induces platelet deposition and aggregation. This is a normal hemostatic
event similar to that which occurs when any blood vessel is interrupted. The
process leads to the formation of a sterile, platelet fibrin thrombus similar to
that in nonbacterial thrombotic endocarditis. Such lesions are not specific for
any particular disease and can be produced by a variety of traumas, including
that of a cardiac catheter. The setting is now appropriate for the appearance of
organisms secondary to a transient bacteremia. If the organisms have been previously "seen" by the reticuloendothelial system from previous bacteremias,
antibody already present may clump the organisms and permit large numbers
to deposit on the platelet fibrin thrombus, thus initiating colonial growth. The
actual mechanism which permits sticking of bacterial clumps onto the valve

thrombus is unknown. Also unknown is the mechanism by which invasive organisms such as the staphylococcus adhere to a normal heart valve.

An animal model has been described by Garrison and Freedman in which the previously described pathogenetic mechanism is demonstrated. Using their technique in rabbits, a cardiac catheter is inserted through the jugular vein and passed across the tricuspid valve, with the tip in the right ventricle. The proximal end is sealed and buried under the skin for 7 to 10 days. At this time, an inoculum of experimental organisms is injected through the catheter and the catheter removed. In applying this method, Durack and Beeson found that control rabbits promptly cleared the organisms from the blood, while those with the implanted catheter had persistent bacteremia, with the subsequent development of vegetations on the injured tricuspid valve. These colonies were protected from phagocytosis by growth of a covering layer of fibrin. This animal model is of great importance, since it allows *in vitro* investigations of treatment and prophylaxis programs against a variety of organisms, studies which cannot be conducted in patients.

Application of the principles outlined above to other special clinical situations can readily be made. With narcotic abusers, the bacterial inoculum is injected intravenously and accounts for the high incidence of right-sided heart valve involvement. In patients with prosthetic heart valves, two mechanisms for endocarditis occur. In the first instance, bacteria gain access to the prosthetic valve at the time of surgery, and infection develops in the immediate postoperative period. The second mechanism accounts for late postoperative infections, which occur in a manner similar to normal or abnormal heart valves. Presumably the prosthetic valve acts as a foreign body with the potential for endothelial injury, forming a locus for bacterial deposition. The final special group at high risk of intracardiac infection are those patients with renal failure who require chronic hemodialysis. Contamination of the hemodialysis equipment leads to the direct introduction of organisms into the bloodstream, providing a pathogenetic mechanism analogous to that of the narcotic abuser, with the addition of an iatrogenic arteriovenous fistula as a possible site for vegetative growth.

BACTERIOLOGY AND PATHOLOGY

The subacute form of the disease is most often caused by the *streptococcus viridans*, which accounts for approximately 40% of all cases. There has been a recent increase in the incidence of microaerophyllic and anaerobic types of organisms similar in pathogenicity to the *streptococcus viridans*. A more fulminating form of the disease is produced by the staphylococcus, which now produces approximately 20% of all bacterial endocarditis. *Staphylococcus aureus* most often arises from the skin, abscesses, or sepsis resulting from contaminated intravenous lines and catheters. In many cases, however, no obvious origin of infection is found. Because of the invasiveness of this organism and its ability to attack normal heart valves, endocarditis should be suspected in every patient with staphylococcal sepsis. *Staphylococcus albus* is somewhat less virulent than *staphylococcus areus*. Midway between the indolent *streptococcus viridans* and virulent staphylococcal infections lie the enterococcal infections, which account for approximately 15% of all cases of infective endocarditis. The pneumococcus and gonococcus account only for a small number of cases. Five to 10% of the cases are caused by gram-negative organisms, fungi (mostly Candida, Aspergillus, and Histoplasma), and rarely by Rickettsia, or possibly even viruses. In approximately 15% of cases, blood cultures are negative, and the causative agent cannot be established. The distribution of offending organisms has been well reviewed by Weinstein and Rubin.

The pathology of the infected valve varies with the invasiveness of the organism. In the subacute type, there is slow progressive activity of the infection, with associated healing which never quite catches up with the destruction. In the acute variety, the vegetations are larger, softer, and more friable. The destruction of the valve or endothelium occurs more rapidly, with little evidence of healing and a tendency toward abscess formation.

The infection can produce tears and perforations of the valve leaflets, aneurysms of valvular rings, and rupture of chorda tendineae and papillary muscles. Myocarditis has also been described, but the cause of this finding is uncertain and may relate to myocardial invasion by organisms, deposition of immune complexes, bacterial toxins, or ischemia caused by emboli.

Serum agglutinating, complement-fixing, and opsonizing antibodies specific for the infecting organisms are commonly present with infections from low-virulence organisms. Patients with such antibodies have increased concentrations of IgM and IgG antibody (rheumatoid factor), both of which decrease following successful antibacterial therapy. High levels of cryoglobulins and microglobulins may be present in the serum as well. These molecules are now thought to be related to the renal lesion which is more common in subacute than in acute bacterial endocarditis. Previously called **focal "embolic" glomerulonephritis,** the lesion is now believed to be a hypersensitivity vasculitis, since antigen-antibody complex deposits have been demonstrated in the glomerular basement membrane. The incidence of renal failure associated with bacterial endocarditis is now approximately 10%.

Embolization of infected material occurs in 15% to 35% of cases. The common sites for embolism are the heart, spleen, brain, and kidneys. The embolism causes ischemia. This ischemic disorder is seldom recognized when the spleen and kidney are involved but is clinically more obvious when emboli lodge in the coronary or cerebral vessels.

Infectious material carried from the heart to other organs can also initiate satellite infections. This is rare with the indolent or subacute variety but more common with more invasive organisms such as staphylococcus. Mycotic arterial aneurysms are usually found only at autopsy and may not develop until months or years after the infection is cured. Weakening of the arterial wall in a given location is probably caused by embolism of the vasa vasorum, direct invasion of the wall by pathogenic organisms, or deposition of immune complexes. The most frequent locations for mycotic aneurysms are the abdominal aorta, sinuses of Valsalva, or cerebral arteries. When located in peripheral vessels, they are usually clinically silent until rupture of the arterial wall occurs. Sinus of Valsalva aneurysms may be associated with ring abscesses which burrow into other cardiac chambers, often the right atrium or right ventricle, producing left-to-right shunts.

Other aspects of the immune vasculitis syndrome include arthritis and arthralgia, which are probably caused by deposition of immune complexes in synovial membranes. Osler nodes, Janeway lesions, Roth spots, splinter hemorrhages, and petechiae are probably all related to immune vasculitis. The immune response initiated by the disease often outlasts the infection.

CLINICAL MANIFESTATIONS

The discussion to this point has included the terms **subacute** or **acute bacterial endocarditis,** but a definition of either has not been offered. In one sense, subacute bacterial endocarditis refers to the infections produced by the less virulent organisms, such as *streptococcus viridans,* while the acute variety refers to those produced by the more pathogenic bacteria, such as the staphylococcus. The less invasive bacteria ordinarily produce a more indolent disease, which is nonetheless fatal if untreated. Organisms such as the staphylococcus produce a disease which is also fatal, but more toxic, more septic, and which runs its course more quickly if untreated. The bacteria which produce the subacute variety rarely grow on normal heart valves, whereas acute endocarditis is caused by organisms which attack normal heart valves in the majority of instances.

The division of infective endocarditis into acute and subacute varieties, however, is not always clear. Should a patient infected with *streptococcal viridans* on the aortic valve develop acute aortic insufficiency from a valvular tear, he could succumb in a very short time to fulminating congestive heart failure, and the term **subacute** would seem inappropriate. On the other hand, the staphylococcus may invade an abnormal valve and in this regard resemble the infection produced by the less virulent organisms. Finally, endocarditis produced by the enterococcus clinically appears to bridge the gap between the acute and subacute varieties by displaying elements of both.

Despite these drawbacks, we believe that such a division is worthwhile, since it draws attention to the rapid progress of the acute type and indicates the urgent need for prompt institution of therapy in patients who have this condition.

The two most common clinical presentations in patients with bacterial endocarditis are fever and heart murmur. Although fever or heart murmur alone are found in many patients with other illnesses, the combination should alert the observer to the possibility of bacterial endocarditis. There is a wide variety of other possible physical findings which are included below for completeness but which are often not present. The most frequent presenting symptoms are nonspecific and so are usually of little help in making the diagnosis. They include fatigue, malaise, backache, arthritis, arthralgia, and intermittent chills. The diagnosis most frequently made on first contact with such patients is influenza or other viral infection.

Some patients may, but most do not, present with more diagnostic physical findings of peripheral embolism, cutaneous petechiae, splenomegaly, clubbing, Roth spots, or Janeway lesions. Splinter hemorrhages are nonspecific findings more often the result of finger trauma than bacterial endocarditis. Rarely, a patient may present with symptoms of a cerebrovascular accident, renal failure, or meningitis.

The importance of early diagnosis is obvious, since proper therapy instituted early in the clinical course preserves valvular tissue. The specific physical findings of the disease outlined above are usually found late in the illness. Hopefully, the diagnosis will have been made before these findings appear.

The mainstay of the early clinical diagnosis is therefore a readiness to suspect this condition even if the suspicion is based on nothing more than fever in the presence of a heart murmur. Fever is absent in only 5% of cases, usually in the elderly, the azotemic, patients with central nervous system disorders, and those unfortunate enough to have the diagnosis of bacterial infection masked by the prior use of antibiotics. Heart murmurs are absent in a slightly higher percentage of cases, often in patients with the acute form of the disease before valvular dysfunction develops. Changing murmurs appear to be of little diagnostic value, since most heart murmurs sound somewhat different on different days, even without endocarditis. The development of a new murmur, however, is of greater significance.

There is a great variety in the types of complications of the disease. Embolization of infected material is most often obvious in the brain but may also be associated with distant infections and abscess formation, especially in the acute form of endocarditis. Various other forms of cardiac disease may be caused by bacterial endocarditis. Myocardial infarction, as the result of coronary embolism, occurs more frequently than was previously appreciated and also may produce myocardial abscesses. The development of sinus of Valsalva aneurysms and aortic ring abscesses may progress to perforation and cardiac tamponade, fistula formation with left-to-right shunts, cardiac arrhythmias, bundle-branch blocks, or even complete atrioventricular block. Pericarditis is a rare complication associated with infections of the aortic valve. Neuropsychiatric syndromes may be the result of meningitis, cerebritis, intracerebral or subarachnoid hemorrages, or toxic encephalopathy of unknown cause. Renal failure occurs in approximately 10% of cases.

However, at present, the most serious complication and the most common cause of death as a consequence of bacterial endocarditis is congestive heart failure. It is precipitated by increasing or abrupt valvular disruption, providing an hemodynamic burden on an unprepared left ventricle. This is most often associated with infections of the aortic valve, aortic insufficiency, and rupture of sinus of Valsalva aneurysms, but may occur with involvement of the mitral apparatus as well. Rarely, both are involved. Contributing factors to congestive heart failure are myocarditis, myocardial infarction, and myocardial abscesses.

Special attention must be given to the clinical manifestations of two particular forms of infective endocarditis. The infections associated with narcotic addiction are estimated as 1½ to 2 cases per 1000 at risk per year. Fever is common, as with other forms of bacterial endocarditis, but heart murmurs, congestive heart failure, or systemic emboli are not. Their absence relates to the frequency (50%) of tricuspid valve involvement, which produces *pulmonary*, rather than systemic, symptoms. The pulmonary symptoms are secondary to multiple pulmonary emboli, often septic. The remaining 50% of bacterial endocarditis cases associated with narcotic addiction also have involvement of the mitral and aortic valves, and these patients present more typically. Narcotic abusers, as a group, have normal hearts resistant to all but highly invasive organisms, causing a higher incidence among narcotic abusers of acute bacterial endocarditis. The staphylococcus is the most common organism, but in different cities, different organisms appear to predominate. These patients are often slow in seeking medical advice and may be unwilling to abide by it.

The second group requiring special attention are patients with prosthetic-valve endocarditis. Those who develop infections on prosthetic valves during the days and weeks immediately following valve replacement present particular diagnostic difficulties, since the symptoms and signs of heart valve infection are easily confused with other, more frequent, postoperative problems. The heart may be infected during surgery by organisms in the operating room or in the cardiopulmonary bypass equipment. Infections may also arise from contaminated equipment used in immediate postoperative care. Late postoperative infections arise from the usual sources, as well as from chronically draining sternal wounds. These infections are similar in presentation to those in patients with natural heart valves, but differences do occur in the increased frequency of valve ring infections and the effect of the infection on prosthetic valve function. In aortic prosthetic valves, the infection tends to detach the valve from the aortic wall, producing aortic insufficiency. Valvular obstruction from bulky vegetations is more common with mitral prostheses, but both problems can obviously occur at either site. Because of the foreign body, infections are more difficult to eradicate with antibiotics, and the survival rate is lower than in patients with infections on natural valves.

LABORATORY DIAGNOSIS

Blood Culture

The most important laboratory aid to diagnosis is the blood culture. Isolation and identification of the causative organism not only confirms the diagnosis of bacterial endocarditis but directs the selection of appropriate antimicrobial therapy. Since this test is crucial, numerous blood cultures must be obtained to increase the likelihood of obtaining a positive result. It appears that all but an occasional case will be properly identified by drawing six blood cultures. The problem of the single positive blood culture is vexing, since an unconfirmed positive culture cannot be readily distinguished from a false positive result owing to contamination. If the entire clinical picture strongly suggests bacterial endocarditis, the single positive culture should be taken as meaningful.

The anticipated venipuncture site and the palpating fingers of the phlebotomist should be prepared with 70% alcohol and 1% to 2% iodine solution. Ten cc of blood should be incubated with approximately 100 cc of culture medium. Cultures should be drawn in pairs, with half being cultured under anaerobic conditions and the other half under aerobic conditions. Three sets of cultures should be drawn within the first 24 hours and the remainder within the next 48 to 72 hours. If fever recurs at regular intervals, there may be some advantage in drawing blood cultures approximately 1 hour prior to the anticipated onset of fever. Most authorities believe there is little advantage in the culture of arterial blood or bone marrow aspirate. If the patient has received penicillinlike antibiotics earlier, penicillinase can be added to the cultures, or cultures can be repeated after an appropriate antibiotic-free interval.

Approximately 15% of patients with suspected bacterial endocarditis have negative blood cultures. It is difficult to decide whether to start antibiotic therapy without an identifiable organism or to obtain more blood cultures while taking the risk of further valvular destruction. When the disease is clinically subacute, treatment can be delayed and more cultures drawn over a 3 to 4-day period. However, in the acute variety, in which valve destruction is accelerated, this interval should be shortened to 1 or 2 days. Negative blood cultures may result from organisms difficult to grow on laboratory media, prior antibiotic use, or right heart valve infections, but most are of unknown cause.

An increased sedimentation rate is a constant but nonspecific finding. Anemia is frequently present, but the white blood cell count may be normal. Monocytes or histiocytes may be present in the peripheral blood, but this, too, is a nonspecific finding. As described earlier, rheumatoid factors are frequently present in the plasma of patients with bacterial endocarditis, especially of the subacute variety.

Echocardiogram

The echocardiogram has made a recent significant contribution to the diagnosis of bacterial endocarditis by making it possible to identify the involved cardiac valves. Two-dimensional echocardiography has been recently found to be more useful in this regard than the M-mode type. The shaggy echoes seen in association with valve leaflets are not specific for endocarditis, are not constantly present in endocarditis, and cannot distinguish acute from healed vegetations. Yet, when positive, this study adds weight to the diagnosis and identifies infection sites. Such information may allow surgical replacement of the offending valve without the risk of cardiac catheterization, since cardiac catheters in contact with left-sided valvular vegetations could produce dislodgement and embolism.

Cardiac Catheterization

In right heart endocarditis, in which negative blood cultures may be a problem, cardiac catheterization is less risky, since embolism would be pulmonary rather than systemic. Samples of blood for culture taken from the pulmonary artery and the right ventricle through a cardiac catheter could permit confirmation of the diagnosis and identification of the offending right heart valve. Right heart catheterization is also useful in detecting left-to-right shunts by the oxygen step-up method. This would facilitate the diagnosis of patent ductus arteriosus, ventricular septal defect, or sinus of Valsalva aneurysms with rupture into the right heart. A retrograde arterial catheter can be safely placed distal to an infected aortic valve and used for the injection of contrast media. This study would permit visualization of the aortic regurgitation, ring abscesses, and aneurysms of the sinuses of Valsalva. Some of these lesions are the primary site of endocarditis, while others are the result of endocarditis, and their identification by catheter techniques cannot make this distinction. These judgments can be made only by review of the entire clinical picture.

TREATMENT

ANTIBIOTICS

The principles of effective therapy are simple. An effective antibiotic agent with the least risk should be chosen and administered to the patient by a route which is most tolerable. The selection of the drug or combination of drugs is determined predominantly by the type of offending organism. It is important to use a bactericidal agent; there is no place for bacteriostatic drugs in the treatment of this disease. The backbone of therapy is penicillin, with or without an aminoglycoside. Average starting doses of antibiotics against the most common organisms are as follows:

> *Streptococcus viridans:* penicillin, 1–2 million units every 2 hours, intravenously
> Group D streptococci (enterococci): penicillin, 2 million units every 2 hours, intravenously
> streptomycin, 500 mg every 12 hours, intramuscularly (4–6 weeks)
> *Staphylococcus aureus:* nafcillin or oxacillin, 1 g every 2 hours, intravenously

If a history of penicillin allergy is present, vancomycin or a cephalosporin such as cephalothin may be used. The type of antibiotics, dosage, and the duration of therapy should be tailored to each patient and to the particular disease. Greater detail regarding drug side effects, alternative antibiotic choices, and modes of administration are beyond the scope of this text. Since the starting doses of antibiotics are determined empirically, it is important that the serum concentration of antibiotic be tested against the offending organism *in vitro* after administration has begun. Prior to a dose of antibiotic, the serum concentration of residual drug should be four times that necessary to kill the offending organism *in vitro*. Conventional sensitivity tests of drugs against organisms will not serve for this purpose, which again emphasizes the need for isolation of the organism by blood culture. The duration of the therapy is also determined empirically; usually, it is 4 to 6 weeks. The risk of longer courses of therapy is superinfection, and the risk of shorter courses is relapse. Fever may not subside, following the institution of effective therapy, for a week or 10 days, and this delay in response should not intimidate the therapist into making frequent changes of drug regimen. Recurrent fever during a course of therapy may not indicate a relapse but may be the result of drug fever, peripheral embolism, or phlebitis.

In general the parenteral routes of drug administration are preferred, although there are reports of successful courses of therapy with oral penicillin against highly susceptible organisms. When blood cultures are sterile and the disease clinically appears subacute, it is advisable to initiate therapy as though the enterococcus was the causative agent. Negative blood cultures are relatively rare in patients with acute bacterial endocarditis, but should this situation arise, the patient should be treated with antistaphylococcal drugs. Blood cultures should be repeated 2, 4, and 6 weeks after the course of therapy is completed to check on the possibility of relapse.

A convenient means of administering large doses of antibiotics intravenously involves the use of a "heparin lock." In this method, a short length of plastic tubing is interposed between a needle inserted into a forearm vein on one end and a rubber dam on the other. The tubing is filled with dilute heparin solution when not in use, allowing the patient freedom from a "keep-open" intravenous drip during the short intervals between nearly constant antibiotic administration.

SURGERY

Effective, targeted antibiotic treatment has reduced the mortality rate of this disease. Acute or residual valvular deformity is now the most frequent killer, causing intractable congestive heart failure. The aortic valve is involved most commonly, and the mitral valve next most frequently, while congestive heart failure is uncommon with infections of the right-sided heart valves. Heart failure often develops before healing is complete, and recent experience has shown that valve replacement surgery can be successfully carried out before the antibiotic course is finished. The risk of valve replacement surgery is lower if it can be delayed, but the risk of death from congestive heart failure is very high if valve replacement is unduly postponed. These considerations have led to the philosophy that when heart failure develops, the patient should be given an initial vigorous trial of antifailure therapy, including digitalis, diuretics, vasodilators, sodium restriction, and bed rest. If this therapeutic trial is ineffective or only minimally effective in relieving the signs and symptoms of congestive heart failure, the patient should then undergo prompt valve replacement. Additional time to arrange for cardiac surgery can be obtained by the use of vasodilators such as intravenous nitroprusside or by the insertion of intraaortic balloon assist devices in patients with mitral valve disease. Left heart valve replacement may be necessary without the benefit of cardiac catheterization, because of its attendant risks and the need for haste. Echocardiography, particularly the two-dimensional type, is useful in this context, since with its aid one may be able to identify vegetations on the cardiac valves and determine which are in need of replacement. In patients with acute severe aortic insufficiency, the echocardiogram can also be of use by demonstrating premature closure of the mitral leaflets because of inordinate increases in left-ventricular end diastolic pressure. If the patient can be managed through the entire course of antibiotic therapy without intractable congestive heart failure, valve replacement can be considered later on an elective basis in the same way as is done for patients without bacterial endocarditis.

Some of the patients who have survived valve replacement during the period of antibiotic administration have developed paravalvular leaks much later in their course. This may be caused by loosening of ring sutures originally placed into infected areas. Even if the patient must return to surgery for correction of the paravalvular leak, the combined risk of two surgical procedures remains lower than the risk of congestive heart failure without a valve replacement. Additional indications for valve replacement include uncontrolled sepsis, repeated embolism, and the need for closure of intracardiac fistulas.

A related but more difficult problem is that of endocarditis therapy in patients who have already had prosthetic valve insertions. Approximately one-half of these patients can be successfully treated with antibiotic therapy alone. Where loosening of the valve ring produces valvular incompetence, or vegetations impede poppet motion, thus inducing valvular stenosis, the valve must be replaced again to prevent death from congestive heart failure. When in doubt in these cases, it is preferable to wait, since the mortality of second valve replacement during the course of antibiotic therapy is considerably higher than that of the first placement of the prosthetic valve. But when hemodynamic intractability becomes evident, surgery should be promptly undertaken.

ANTICOAGULANTS

Many patients with prosthetic heart valves in place are treated with anticoagulants on a long-term basis to minimize the risk of valve thrombosis and peripheral embolism. This situation once again raises the issue of whether the benefits of using anticoagulants in patients with bacterial endocarditis outweigh the risks. The fear of anticoagulation in this disease originated from reports of central nervous system bleeding associated with rupture of cerebral mycotic aneurysms. Since this bleeding would occur with or without anticoagulants and since it is a rare complication, it seems worthwhile to continue anticoagulant use when it is well indicated. The typical embolism which occurs in bacterial endocarditis is not the result of blood-clotting, and the embolism incidence is not reduced by anticoagulation. Where anticoagulants are well indicated, for example in femoral phlebothrombosis, conventional pulmonary embolism, or for prophylaxis in patients with prosthetic heart valves, the risks of anticoagulation are probably no greater than in patients without bacterial endocarditis. A recent study in patients with prosthetic heart valve endocarditis has shown that the complication rate of central nervous system embolism was greater in patients whose anticoagulants were stopped during the course of antibiotic therapy. The question of whether anticoagulants should be discontinued for fear of hemorrhagic cerebral infarction once an embolic stroke has already occurred remains unanswered.

NARCOTIC ABUSERS

Individuals with bacterial endocarditis of the right side of the heart associated with narcotic abuse present a few special problems. Patent peripheral veins for antibiotic administration may be difficult to find, yet the infection is often acute, requiring prompt, vigorous therapy. Fungi are occasionally the offending organisms; they require special therapy and carry a high mortality rate. Narcotic abusers may also have associated hepatic and renal disease, which could influence the selection of antibacterial agents.

PROPHYLAXIS AGAINST BACTERIAL ENDOCARDITIS

The case for prophylactic administration of antibiotics to prevent infective endocarditis is not proved. As discussed earlier in the section on pathogenesis, the majority of patients with bacterial endocarditis give no history of a previous special event during which antibiotics might have been effective in preventing the disease. Since it is not possible to administer therapeutic doses of antibiotics to prevent valvular infection from everyday bacteremias, most of the cases of infective endocarditis therefore cannot be prevented. Probably only 40% to 60% of the patients at risk from bacterial endocarditis are identified at the time when surgery which could induce bacteremia is performed. This reduces even further the number of preventable infections. It is estimated that approximately 1 case in 100,000 dental procedures in patients with predisposing valvular or congenital heart disease will develop bacterial endocarditis.

If one were to design a specific prophylactic regimen, it would be necessary to know a likely bacteriologic diagnosis, the size of the inoculum, and the predisposition of the patient. The last would be important, since patients with prosthetic heart valves would be at greater risk than those with the click-murmur syndrome, for example.

However, the concept of prophylaxis against bacterial endocarditis is sufficiently well entrenched in medical practice that it is prudent to continue it, even if it is effective only occasionally. The American Heart Association Committee on Prevention of Rheumatic Fever and Bacterial Endocarditis regularly updates their recommendations for a variety of surgical procedures. These recommendations should be applied to all patients with predisposing lesions, including rheumatic and degenerative valvular disease, congenital heart disease (except atrial septal defect), the click-murmur syndrome, idiopathic hypertrophic subaortic stenosis, arteriovenous fistula, both physician-constructed and others, and obviously to patients with prosthetic heart valves in place. The use of antibiotics to prevent bacterial endocarditis during the immediate postoperative period in patients with prosthetic valve replacement remains of unproved value. Most surgeons prefer to use antistaphylococcal therapy immediately before and for a few days following heart valve replacement. The incidence of postoperative endocarditis has fallen since the early days of valve replacement, but this effect may be the result of better surgical technique rather than prophylactic postoperative administration of antibiotics.

NONBACTERIAL THROMBOTIC ENDOCARDITIS

Although not an infectious disease, nonbacterial thrombotic endocarditis bears sufficient similarity to infectious endocarditis to warrant inclusion here. The disorder involves the development of sterile platelet fibrin thrombi, most commonly on normal heart valves. Pathologically, these vegetations differ from the infectious variety by the absence of organisms or by a cellular reaction. The mitral and aortic valves are most often involved with rare occurrences on the right-sided heart valves. Although heart murmurs occur, their incidence is far less than with the infectious variety. Otherwise the disorder is quite similar to bacterial endocarditis. Patients have fever, leukocytosis, and petechiae. The most common serious complication of the disorder is systemic embolization. The organs most frequently subject to embolism are the brain, bowel, heart, kidneys, and spleen. Symptoms are more frequent with embolism of the brain, bowel, and heart than the kidneys and spleen. Most patients with nonbacterial thrombotic endocarditis suffer from neoplasm, commonly mucin-secreting adenocarcinomas of the pancreas. Nonbacterial thrombotic endocarditis also occurs, however, in individuals with squamous cell cancer, leukemia, lymphoma, and (rarely) sarcoma. Not all cases of nonbacterial thrombotic endocarditis, however, are associated with malignancy. The condition also occurs with congestive heart failure, pneumonia, pyelonephritis, and glomerulonephritis. There is also an association with venous thromboses, hemorrhage, and disseminated intravascular coagulation, which has led to the speculation that there may be a relation to a hypercoagulable state. It also seems possible that these thrombic valvular lesions are susceptible to infection and could convert from nonbacterial to bacterial endocarditis. Since a bacterial infection has no role in the initiation of nonbacterial thrombotic endocarditis, antibiotics are of no value in prevention. No effective treatment of the disease is known.

SUGGESTED READING

Arnett EN, Roberts WC: Prosthetic valve endocarditis. Clinicopathologic analysis of 22 necropsy patients with comparison of observations in 74 necropsy patients with active infective endocarditis involving natural left-sided cardiac valves. Am J Cardiol 38:281–292, 1976

Belli J, Waisbren BA: The number of blood cultures necessary to diagnose most cases of bacterial endocarditis. Am J Med Sci 232:284–288, 1956

Deppisch LM, Fayemi AO: Non-bacterial thrombotic endocarditis: clinicopathologic correlations. Am Heart J 92:723–729, 1976

Durack DT, Beeson PB: Experimental bacterial endocarditis. I. Colonization of a sterile vegetation. Br J Exp Pathol 53:44–49, 1972

Ferrans VJ, Boyce SW, Billingham ME, Spray TL, Roberts WC: Infection of glutaraldehyde-preserved porcine valve heterografts. Am J Cardiol 43:1123–1136, 1979

Garrison PK, Freedman LR: Experimental endocarditis. I. Staphylococcal endocarditis in rabbits resulting from placement of a polyethylene catheter in the right side of the heart. Yale J Biol Med 42:394–410, 1970

Gutman RA, Striker GE, Gilliland BC, Cutler RE: The immune complex glomerulonephritis of bacterial endocarditis. Medicine (Baltimore) 51:1–25, 1972

Infective endocarditis. American Heart Association Monograph No. 52, 1976

Kaplan EL, Anthony BF, Bisno A: Prevention of bacterial endocarditis. American Heart Association Committee Report. Circulation 56:139A–143A, 1977

Pazin GJ, Peterson KL, Griff FW, Shaver JA, Ho M: Determination of site of infection in endocarditis. Ann Intern Med 82:746–750, 1975

Richardson JV, Karp RB, Kirklin JW, Dismukes WE: Treatment of infective endocarditis: a 10-year comparative analysis. Circulation 58:589–597, 1978

Rodbard S: Blood velocity and endocarditis. Circulation 27:18–28, 1963

Roy P, Tajik AJ, Giuliani ER, Schattenberg TT, Gau GT, Frye RL: Spectrum of echocardiographic findings in bacterial endocarditis. Circulation 53:474–482, 1976

Wann LS, Dillon JC, Weyman AE, Feigenbaum H: Echocardiography in bacterial endocarditis. N Engl J Med 295:135–139, 1976

Weinstein L, Rubin RH: Infective Endocarditis. Prog Cardiovasc Dis 16:239–274, 1973

Weinstein L, Schlesinger J: Treatment of infective endocarditis. Prog Cardiovasc Dis 16:275–302, 1973

Weinstein L, Schlesinger JJ: Pathoanatomic, pathophysiologic and clinical correlations in endocarditis. N Engl J Med 291:832–837; 1122–1126, 1974

Wilson WR, Geraci JE, Danielson GK, Thompson RL, Spittell JA, Washington JA II, Giuliani ER: Anticoagulant therapy and central nervous system complications in patients with prosthetic valve endocarditis. Circulation 57:1004–1007, 1978

PERICARDIAL DISEASE

15

Saktipada Mookherjee

This chapter will emphasize the diagnostic aspects of pericardial disease. The diagnosis of both acute and chronic pericardial disease, which are relatively common conditions in clinical medicine, can be extraordinarily difficult. Acute pericarditis, for example, can mimic acute myocardial infarction or acute pleurisy very closely, and chronic constrictive pericarditis may be difficult to separate from chronic congestive heart failure, particularly that which is caused by a restrictive cardiomyopathy. Once the patient has been diagnosed as having pericardial disease, investigations of the cause can be pursued more aptly.

Normally about 20 to 50 ml of serous fluid is contained in the potential space between the visceral layer of the pericardium (epicardium) and the parietal layer. The fluid helps to minimize friction between the heart and the surrounding structures. The pericardium also prevents displacement of the heart and may play a protective role in preventing overdistension of the heart. In addition, atrial filling may be facilitated by an intact pericardium.

Although the intact pericardium is not essential for survival, and absence of the pericardium is compatible with the maintenance of normal cardiac function in the resting state, changes in the shape of the heart denuded of pericardium may occur progressively, resulting in cardiac dilatation and hypertrophy. Disturbance in cardiac function may follow eventually if the patient engages in continued exertion. Also, infection from adjacent bronchopulmonary regions may occur because the shielding action of the pericardium has been lost.

Inflammation of the pericardium, or *pericarditis,* is a relatively common condition, with multiple causes. It may be acute or chronic and may or may not be associated with a pericardial effusion.

ACUTE PERICARDITIS

Pericarditis is usually secondary to disease elsewhere in the body. Hence it may have many causes. Some of these are as follows:

1. Idiopathic or nonspecific (so-called acute "benign" pericarditis): presumably viral or immunologic
2. Infectious pericarditis:
   a. Viral
   b. Bacterial
      1) Nonspecific
      2) Specific, *i.e.*, TB
   c. Parasitic
   d. Rickettsial
   e. Fungal
3. Pericarditis from disease of adjacent organs
   a. Myocardial infarction
      1) With acute myocardial infarction (after 24–48 hours)
      2) Several days or weeks following the infarction; post-myo-cardial-infarction, or Dressler's syndrome
   b. Pulmonary disease
   c. Esophageal disease
   d. Dissecting aneurysm of the thoracic aorta
4. Pericarditis from immunologic disease
   a. Rheumatic fever
   b. Rheumatoid disease
   c. Systemic lupus erythematosus
   d. Postpericardiotomy syndrome
5. Traumatic pericarditis
   a. Penetrating
   b. Nonpenetrating
6. Uremic pericarditis
7. Neoplastic pericarditis
   a. Primary: rare
   b. Secondary: carcinoma, lymphoma, leukemia
8. Iatrogenic pericarditis
   a. Drugs, *e.g.*, procainamide, hydralazine, and other drugs causing systemic lupus syndrome
   b. Radiation therapy
   c. Surgery, cardiac resuscitation and direct-current countershock
9. Pericarditis associated with diseases like myxedema and gout

RECOGNITION OF ACUTE PERICARDITIS

Symptoms

The important symptom of acute pericarditis is retrosternal or precordial pain. The chest pain is of sudden onset and often of variable intensity, location, radiation, and duration, and may resemble closely the pain of acute myocardial infarction. Referred pain in the muchal region is common in acute pericarditis, following the root distribution of the phrenic nerve, which may be irritated by diaphragmatic pericarditis. Certain other important features of the pain also help to mark its pericardial origin. Associated inflammation or irritation of contiguous structures gives rise to fairly typical symptoms. Thus the pain is often worse on deep inspiration, as a result of adjacent pleural inflammation. As pericardial effusion develops, dull, oppressive so-called protopathic pain may result from stretching of the pericardial sac. The pain of acute pericarditis may be worse on movement of the trunk, quite unlike the pain of acute myocardial infarction. Likewise, the patient with acute pericarditis tends to sit up and often leans forward to obtain relief from the pain.

Bending the head backwards, with stretching of the pretracheal fascia, may sometimes aggravate the chest pain because of the pull on the inflammed pericardial sac. Swallowing may worsen the pain because the pericardium is stretched when food passes through the esophagus. Ventral or dorsal chest pain may result from associated anterior or posterior mediastinitis. Pericoronary nerve involvement from epicardial inflammation or actual coronary arteritis may cause anginalike pain. It is of interest that this type of pericardial pain may be relieved by local anesthetic blockade of the left stellate ganglion. Upper abdominal pain and rigidity may occur, probably in part as a result of irritation of the lower intercostal nerves.

Occasional absence of pain in acute pericarditis can be explained by limitation of the inflammation to an insensitive area of the pericardium. (This explanation, however, does not account for occasional lack of pain in uremic and tuberculous pericarditis, as well as in pericarditis following acute myocardial infarction.) Dyspnea is not a feature of uncomplicated acute pericarditis.

Physical Signs

Sinus tachycardia and fever are very common, although the latter is occasionally absent. However, the most diagnostic sign of acute pericarditis is the pericardial friction rub (Fig. 15-1). The rub is caused not only by mechanical friction of the inflamed pericardial surfaces as a result of cardiac movements but also by a churning motion of the inflammatory exudate in the pericardial sac after effusion develops. The sound of the rub has a superficial, monotonous, and grating or scratchy quality and often sounds close to the ear; it has three distinct phases (see below). The rub may not be heard unless the patient is correctly positioned

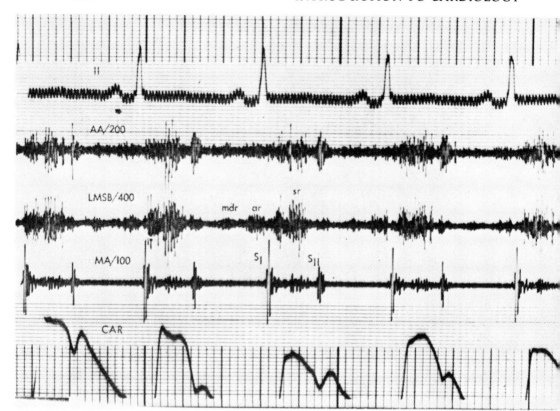

FIG. 15-1.
Typical triphasic pericardial function rub, best recorded in the middle
phonocardiogram, taken at left midsternal border at nominal filter peak of 400 Hz
(**LMSB/400**). The ventricular systolic component (**sr**) has the greatest amplitude, the
atrial systolic component (**ar**) the next, and the middiastolic component (**mdr**) the
least. Top trace: EKG lead II. Bottom trace: carotid pulse. S_I and S_{II}: first and second
heart sounds. (Spodick DH: Acute pericarditis. Prog Cardiovasc Dis 14:197, 1971, by
permission)

and a diligent search made. The patient has to sit up and often to lean forward,
and the diaphragm of the stethoscope should be firmly applied over the left
lower parasternal region, in order to make the rub audible. Often a pleuropericardial rub clearly related to respiration because of adjacent pleurisy becomes
apparent. Sometimes the rub may be confused with murmurs, apical and pulmonary conus rubs, and mediastinal crunches. The scratchy quality of the rub,
and its three phases (namely, atrial systolic, ventricular systolic, and early ventricular diastolic) are helpful in identifying it, although sometimes only two or
(rarely) one of the phases—the ventricular systolic phase—is heard. Contrary to
the common notion, the rub often persists even after the development of pericardial effusion.

With a sizable pericardial effusion (more than 200–250 ml), the cardiac dullness on percussion extends beyond the apical impulse. The heart sounds may be muffled with larger effusions, and dullness on percussion with bronchial breath sound on auscultation may be appreciated over the left infrascapular region from compression of the lower lobe of the left lung (Bamberger-Pin-Ewart sign).

EKG

Saddle-shaped or concave upwards and concordant ST-segment elevation (ST-segment elevation in leads I–III, aVL and aVF, and ST-segment depression in aVR), associated with depression of the PR-segment, is common in acute pericarditis. In lead aVR, the PR-segment is elevated. In acute myocardial infarction the ST-segment displacement is discordant, meaning ST segments are displaced in opposite directions in leads I and III.

Spodick, who has made extensive studies of pericardial diseases, including electrocardiographic changes in pericarditis, has described several stages of evolution in EKG patterns as the disease progresses. In resolving pericarditis, the T waves become isoelectric or inverted when ST- and PR-segments become isoelectric (compare acute myocardial infarction, in which the T waves become inverted before the ST-segments are isoelectric). In contrast to an acute myocardial infarction, Q waves do not appear. Atrial arrhythmias, including transient atrial fibrillation, are not uncommon. Persistent arrhythmias, either atrial or ventricular, may indicate underlying myocarditis.

Chest Film

Enlargement of the cardiac silhouette occurs only after the development of considerable pericardial effusion (more than 200–250 ml). A radiolucent pericardial fat line will be shown on the lateral view between the radioopaque cardiac shadow and overlying pericardial fluid behind the sternum. The typical pear-shaped cardiac silhouette is seen less frequently. The sharp outline of the posterior border of the left ventricle is blurred if a sizable pericardial effusion has developed. This is in contrast to pure left-ventricular enlargement, where the posterior border remains sharp, although it extends backwards as in pericardial effusion.

Echocardiography

Echocardiography is an extremely sensitive noninvasive diagnostic tool for pericardial effusion. Even 15 to 20 ml of pericardial effusion can be detected by this method. In general, a posterior echo-free space between the mobile epicardium and the more densely echogenic, less mobile parietal pericardium, during both systole and diastole, is diagnostic of pericardial effusion (Fig. 15-2). An anterior echo-free space alone, in the absence of a posterior one, is unlikely to be

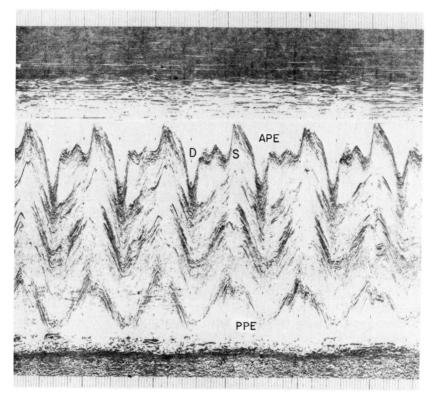

FIG. 15-2. ECHOCARDIOGRAM IN PERICARDIAL EFFUSION.
The whole heart swings forwards with ventricular systole and backward with
diastole. **APE:** Anterior pericardial effusion. **D:** diastole. **S:** systole. **PPE:**
posterior pericardial effusion.

the result of pericardial effusion. It is of interest that the effusion does not
usually extend behind the left atrium and that pseudoprolapse pattern in the
mitral-valve echo and paradoxical septal motion may be observed in the presence of a large pericardial effusion.

Other previously used diagnostic studies, such as contrast radiography or
cardiac blood-pool scan, are less valuable in the diagnosis of pericardial effusion than the echocardiogram.

Confirmation of the diagnosis of effusion may be made by pericardiocentesis. This procedure, which should be done by a physician with technical expertise, is indicated not only in order to investigate the cause of the disease but
also to give immediate relief from cardiac tamponade that might occur from
rapid collection of fluid or blood in the pericardial sac or from a large and tense
pericardial effusion. Sometimes pericardial biopsy is needed for a cytological
diagnosis. Introduction of air into the pericardial space after aspiration of fluid,

followed by the making of a chest film, may outline tumor masses or reveal thickening of the pericardium.

ACUTE CARDIAC TAMPONADE

Acute pericarditis may be complicated occasionally by the development of cardiac tamponade. Acute cardiac compression (tamponade) may result from rapid collection of blood or fluid in the pericardial cavity, limiting the diastolic, and consequently the systolic, function of the heart. The rapidity of collection of intrapericardial fluid, rather than the amount collected, is the important factor, in acute cardiac tamponade. Fast accumulation of 150 to 200 ml of fluid or blood may cause cardiac tamponade, whereas slow collection of several liters over a few months may not do so. In acute tamponade, aspiration of a few milliliters of fluid may alter the intrapericardial pressure volume relationship favorably and cause quick improvement in the hemodynamic state.

Intrapericardial hemorrhage from trauma, rupture of a dissecting aortic aneurysm, cardiac rupture following a recent myocardial infarction, or myocardial tumor can cause acute cardiac tamponade. In common forms of acute pericarditis, tamponade is a relatively rare phenomenon. However, occasional cases of cardiac tamponade following anticoagulant therapy in acute myocardial infarction complicated by pericarditis have been reported. Cardiac tamponade occasionally occurs in uremic pericarditis, even during dialysis, and is rather common in malignant pericardial effusion.

Clinical Features of Cardiac Tamponade

In acute cardiac tamponade, the clinical features are of crucial importance. There is rapid rise in venous pressure, with a fall in arterial pressure and an increase in heart rate. The patient may develop a shocklike condition, with marked lowering of cardiac output, evidenced by cold, often clammy skin; oliguria; and cloudy sensorium. Shortness of breath is also observed. Death may result unless surgical relief is quickly obtained. Although venous pressure is elevated, as evidenced by distension of the neck veins, no prominent x and y descents are observed, and Kussmaul's sign (increase in venous pressure during inspiration, or inspiratory fullness of the neck veins) is noted less often in acute tamponade than in chronic cardiac compression by constrictive pericarditis.

The heart sounds are distant, and, with careful auscultation, wide splitting of the second heart sound is heard. On rare occasions, a diastolic filling sound is audible. The lungs are generally clear, unless complicated by left-ventricular failure, either from preexisting disease or from concurrent myocardial ischemia owing to profound decrease in cardiac output. In the latter situation, long-standing occlusive coronary artery disease is often present, and made worse by compromised coronary blood flow. An acutely tender liver may be felt from systemic venous congestion.

Essential to the diagnosis of acute tamponade is a paradoxical arterial pulse, characterized by a greater than 10 torr fall in systolic blood pressure during inspiration from that on expiration. In severe tamponade, the arterial pulse may be palpable only on expiration, and with extreme reduction in stroke volume, in very severe tamponade, pulsus paradoxus may be absent.

Several mechanisms have been suggested to explain the phenomenon of pulsus paradoxus in cardiac tamponade, but none of them is entirely satisfactory. The normal pulse is somewhat "paradoxical," that is, the amplitude of the arterial pulse is slightly lower during inspiration than that of the expiratory pulse. However, the difference between the systolic blood pressure during inspiration and expiration normally remains under 10 torr. The amount of left-ventricular filling and the stroke volume are normally less during inspiration than those on expiration, as a result of a lag period required to translate the increase in venous return to the right heart which occurs during inspiration into an augmented stroke volume from the left ventricle, which is not achieved until end-inspiration or early expiration. In addition, pooling of blood which occurs in the pulmonary vasculature during inspiration may contribute to the lag period.

Exaggeration of this normal phenomenon constitutes true pulsus paradoxus. This sign is rather nonspecific and may occur not only in tamponade but also in voluntary deep inspiration, obstructive airway disease, tracheal stenosis, obesity, acute pulmonary embolism, constrictive pericarditis, restrictive cardiomyopathy, and advanced congestive heart failure. However, it will be present in virtually all cases of cardiac tamponade to support the diagnosis (Fig. 15-3).

In experimental and clinical cardiac tamponade, flow-meter studies have shown that increase in venous return to the right heart still occurs during inspiration, as it normally does. In tamponade, however, the increase in venous return raises the already elevated intrapericardial pressure further, limiting the filling of the left ventricle. Compromised left-ventricular filling during inspiration then is translated into a reduction in stroke volume, resulting in a drop in systolic arterial pressure and in the amplitude of the arterial pulse—giving rise to the paradoxical pulse. In addition, the decreased stroke volume during inspiration causes early closure of the aortic valve, resulting in the widely split second heart sound.

Laboratory Diagnosis of Cardiac Tamponade

Electrocardiography shows reduction in amplitude of the waveforms with total P, QRS, and T wave alternans, characterized by alternate complexes being relatively large and small. Spodick suggested that the total electrical alternans, and not the QRS alternans alone, is typical of tamponade (Fig. 15-4). Electrical alternans usually does not coexist with pulsus alternans unless associated left-ventricular disease is present.

The mechanism of electrical alternans in cardiac tamponade is based on

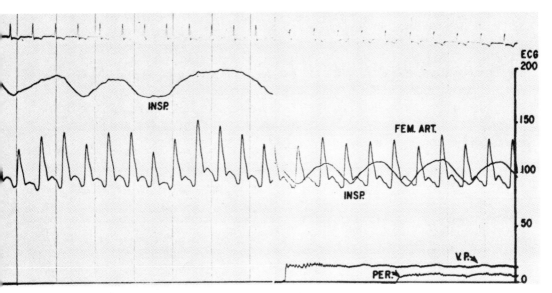

FIG. 15-3. PULSUS PARADOXUS IN ACUTE CARDIAC TAMPONADE FOLLOWING AORTIC DISSECTION.
Prior to removal of 45 ml of blood from pericardium, the femoral arterial pulse is clearly paradoxical. Following pericardiocentesis (right panel), pulsus paradoxus is much less pronounced. (Lange RL, Botticelli JT, Tsagaris TJ, Walker JA, Gani M, Bustamante RA: Diagnostic signs in compressive cardiac disorders. Constrictive pericarditis, pericardial effusion, and tamponade. Circulation 33:769, 1966. Used by permission of the American Heart Association, Inc.)

the shift in the mechanical position of the heart resulting in displacement of the electrical axis. Freed from mediastinal restraints, the heart moves in the fluid-filled pericardium in a rotatory or pendular fashion. When this oscillation bears a 2:1 relationship to the heart rate, electrical alternans is observed. Echocardiography confirms this increased freedom of movement of the cardiac structures within a large pericardial effusion by showing changing position of intracardiac structures synchronous with electrical alternans. If fluid is aspirated, relieving the tamponade, normal cardiac mobility is restored and the electrical alternans is abolished.

Echocardiographic criteria for the diagnosis of cardiac tamponade include widening of the right-ventricular cavity during inspiration with concomitant decrease in left-ventricular diastolic dimension, decrease in amplitude of the motion of the mitral valve and reduction in duration of the opening of the mitral valve during inspiration. Early closure of the aortic valve may also be recorded during inspiration. Recently, marked narrowing of the right-ventricular cavity during expiration has been shown to occur in cardiac tamponade. However, cardiac tamponade is a clinical diagnosis, and the role of echocardiogra-

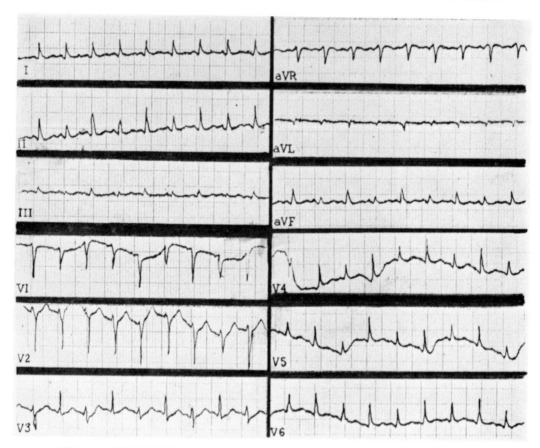

FIG. 15-4. SIMULTANEOUS P-QRS ALTERNANS IN CARDIAC TAMPONADE DURING ACUTE PERICARDITIS.
Alternating configuration of P waves (best seen in **III** and **aVF**) and of QRS (best seen in **II, III, V3**) independent of respiratory phase fluctuations (seen in **V1, V4** and **V5**). (Spodick DH: Acute pericarditis. Prog Cardiovasc Dis 14:196, 1971, by permission)

phy in this setting is a supportive one. It always confirms the presence of pericardial effusion.

The chest film may or may not show a large cardiac silhouette, depending upon the amount of pericardial fluid collected.

Catheterization of the heart for hemodynamic confirmation shows elevation of the right-sided filling pressure, with near equalization of the mean right-atrial pressure, the right-ventricular diastolic pressure, the pulmonary arterial diastolic pressure, and the wedge pressure. With pericardiocentesis and relief of tamponade, there is a significant reduction and separation in these pressures.

Treatment of Cardiac Tamponade

When marked hypotension is present, temporary hemodynamic improvement may occur if intravenous volume can be expanded by infusing fluids or blood or by administering positive inotropic agents such as dopamine. However, early pericardiocentesis is vital. Without it the patient will not survive. Pericardiocentesis should be performed either in an operating room or in an intensive care unit with monitoring facilities by a physician experienced in the technical aspects of the procedure. The preferred site for pericardiocentesis is the angle between the xiphisternum and the left costal arch. To a syringe is fitted an aspirating needle of 16 or 18 gauge size whose proximal end is connected to the V lead of the EKG machine through an alligator clamp. The needle is introduced aseptically under local anesthesia, upwards and backwards in the direction of the right sternoclavicular joint. Gentle suction is applied during this procedure. As soon as the needle enters the pericardial cavity, fluid will be aspirated into the syringe attached to the needle. If the needle happens to touch the myocardium, the monitoring V lead records a current of injury, showing marked elevation of the ST-segment. The needle should then be withdrawn a little until the current of injury subsides, when aspiration can be begun again.

If the echocardiogram is used, the introduction of saline through the needle identifies the position of the needle more accurately by a cloud of echoes in the pericardial cavity or, in the case of myocardial perforation, inside the right ventricle.

Although cardiologists should be familiar with pericardiocentesis, we much prefer to use a surgical pericardial window for treating tamponades. The pericardium is drained through a subxiphoid approach. For chronic tamponade surgical drainage, a pleuropericardial window, or pericardiectomy, may be needed.

INDIVIDUAL FORMS OF PERICARDITIS

Idiopathic Acute "Benign" Pericarditis

This is the most common type of pericarditis, predominantly affecting young individuals; it has an interesting seasonal incidence in spring and fall. Fever and pericardial pain are common. History of cough and upper respiratory infection during the preceding 3 to 6 weeks is obtained in many patients. Pericardial effusion occurs in 50 to 75% of the cases. Recovery in 4 to 6 weeks is the rule, although recurrent attacks occur in about 25%. Constrictive pericarditis has been reported as a sequela, in rare instances.

Viral Pericarditis

Viral pericarditis seems to be a common cause of acute pericarditis. Burch calls this entity **viral myopericarditis,** because of the frequency of underlying myocarditis. Most viruses, particularly those of the Coxsackie B group, have been implicated. In some cases of congestive cardiomyopathy, progression from an acute viral myopericarditis has been suspected. Precise diagnosis is difficult, although every effort should be made to obtain viral cultures from throat washings, blood, urine, and stool. Viral neutralizing antibody titres in the serum should be followed sequentially during the acute stage of the illness and at intervals during the illness and convalescence. Pericardial fluid, when available, should also be studied. Symptomatic therapy with prolonged bed rest in patients showing pericarditis with cardiac enlargement, as confirmed by echocardiography, is recommended.

Bacterial Pericarditis

Pneumococcal, staphylococcal, or streptococcal pericarditis may develop following septicemia or may spread from contiguous structures such as lung, pleura, or the myocardium. Virtually every type of bacterial organism has been associated with pericarditis. For the individual patient, bacteriologic diagnosis is essential for proper therapy. Appropriate blood cultures and chemical, cytologic, immunologic, and bacteriologic studies of the pericardial fluid are necessary.

Tuberculous Pericarditis

Tuberculous pericarditis is now a rare disease. It develops most frequently from direct extension of tuberculous infection from the mediastinal or hilar lymph nodes or occasionally from direct contact with an adjacent pulmonary focus of infection. The pericardium may also be involved, following miliary spread. Recurrent, often bloody, pericardial effusion is common. Unless early chemotherapy is instituted and, if necessary, surgical removal of the pericardium is performed, constrictive pericarditis may develop in a few months.

Fungal Pericarditis

Fungal infections such as histoplasmosis and actinomycosis can cause pericarditis. Appropriate culture of the fluid and biopsy of the pericardium may be needed to establish the diagnosis.

Pericarditis Following Acute Myocardial Infarction

The incidence of pericarditis following an acute myocardial infarction varies from 7% to 16%. The pericardial friction rub is audible 24 hours after the onset of acute myocardial infarction. Detection depends on diligent auscultation and on perseverance by the physician. Complicating pericarditis indicates a full-thickness, or transmural, myocardial infarction, where heart failure, cardiogenic shock, and heart block are common, but the pericarditis itself does not influence the prognosis of the case. In one study, persistence of the pericardial friction rub longer than three days was noted to be associated with a high morality. Anticoagulant therapy should be discontinued if a widespread friction rub is heard, as hemopericardium with tamponade may result. Rare case reports of the development of constrictive pericarditis following acute myocardial infarction have appeared. (Constrictive pericarditis is discussed later in this chapter). The incidence of post-myocardial-infarction syndrome (see below) is about 3%.

Rheumatic Pericarditis

Pericarditis occurs in acute rheumatic fever as a component of pancarditis in children. However, isolated pericarditis without valvulitis may also occur with rheumatic fever in adults. Development of constrictive pericarditis following rheumatic fever is virtually unknown.

Rheumatoid Disease

Pericarditis, often asymptomatic, is common in rheumatoid disease. In 40% to 50% of autopsied patients with rheumatoid disease, fibrinous, adhesive, or even constrictive pericarditis is observed. In most cases, the disease remains clinically silent, although cardiac tamponade has been reported in some. In a small percentage of patients (1%–5%), granulomatous pericarditis, associated with granulomas at the bases of the mitral and aortic valves, occurs. The pericardial fluid has a characteristically low sugar content of less than 12 mg/dl, and rheumatoid arthritis (RA) cells are found in the fluid. In juvenile rheumatoid disease, pericarditis is a frequent finding but does not seem to carry a serious prognosis.

Systemic Lupus Erythematosus

Pericarditis may rarely be the first manifestation of systemic lupus erythematosus. Its overall frequency, however, during the course of the disease, with or without effusion, is about 30%. It may coexist with pleural effusion and pulmonary infiltrates and may indicate concurrent cardiac lesions, particularly Libman-Sacks endocarditis. Lupus erythematosus cells in the fluid are diagnostic. Cardiac tamponade and, rarely, constrictive pericarditis may occur with systemic lupus erythematosus. Lupus nephritis with uremia may be an indirect cause of pericarditis, following systemic lupus erythematosus.

Traumatic Pericarditis

Both penetrating and nonpenetrating cardiac trauma may result in pericarditis, and automobile accidents are common precipitating factors. Tamponade may occur from hemorrhage into the pericardium, and recurrent pericarditis may develop, which in some cases may go on for years (post-pericardial-trauma syndrome).

Postpericardiotomy Syndrome

Postpericardiotomy syndrome, post-myocardial-infarction syndrome (Dressler's syndrome), and **post-pericardial-trauma syndrome** are all clinically identical. Common to all is myoepicardial injury, with or without direct entry into the pericardial sac. Bleeding into the pericardium also seems to be an important determinant. Depending upon the clinical setting, the syndrome occurs in 2 to 6 weeks following cardiac surgery, a transmural myocardial infarction, or trauma. Recurrences are common. The characteristic features include fever; pneumonitis; pleuritis, with or without effusion; and pericarditis, often with an audible friction rub and effusion; anemia; leukocytosis; and high erythrocyte sedimentation rate. Changes in plasma proteins with gammaglobulinemia occur. The course is usually self-limited, averaging 2 to 4 weeks. However, cardiac tamponade may develop occasionally.

The mechanism underlying the syndrome seems to be an immunologic reaction, since high antiheart antibody titers have been found in most cases, particularly in those with increased severity. Antiviral antibody titers have also been high in about 70% of such cases. Engle and her coworkers favor an immunologic response to myopericardial insult, with an associated viral illness, as the cause of the syndrome. Short courses of steroid therapy are indicated in severe cases.

Uremic Pericarditis

Chronic renal failure has become an increasingly common cause (17%) of recurrent pericarditis. Some patients develop pericarditis for the first time during (probably inadequate) dialysis. The patient may complain of precordial pain, but fever and diagnositc ST-segment changes on EKG may not develop. However, acute tamponade with hypotension may occur.

Since the development of acute pericarditis does not correlate well with the magnitude of azotemia, the mechanism of pericardial involvement in chronic renal failure remains unclear. Viral infection has been suspected, because of decreased host resistance in uremia.

Use of indomethacin has been advocated for pain, but early relief of tamponade is imperative by pericardiocentesis. Adequate dialysis and pleuropericardial window have been recommended for chronic and recurrent tamponade. Constrictive pericarditis has been reported as an occasional sequela.

Neoplastic Pericarditis

Primary neoplasms of the pericardium are rare. However, metastatic spread from bronchial or breast carcinomas, as well as lymphomas, are common. Leukemic involvement with pericardial effusion is also well known. In malignant disease, tamponade may occur, with rapid development of pericardial effusion providing the first presenting feature of an underlying malignant neoplasm. Early cytologic study of the pericardial fluid, with or without pericardial biopsy, may be needed to establish the diagnosis.

Iatrogenic Pericarditis

Drugs producing the systemic lupus erythematosus syndrome (hydralazine, procainamide, hydantoins, and other drugs) may cause pericarditis on an immunologic basis.

Postradiation Pericarditis

About one-third of the patients with upper mantle radiotherapy exceeding 4000 rads develop pericardial effusion after an interval ranging from several weeks to 4 years. About 5% of such patients may develop chronic effusion with constriction.

Pericardial Disease in Myxedema

Pericardial effusion, often slowly developing and quite copious, with high cholesterol content, are the usual features of this disease. Thyroid replacement therapy is appropriate. Tamponade is unusual.

SYNDROME OF COMPRESSIVE OR RESTRICTIVE PERICARDIAL DISEASE

Compression of the heart by increased intrapericardial pressure from fluid accumulation or a thick, unyielding, and rigid pericardial shell may cause significant hemodynamic abnormalities, with considerable discomfort to the patient. There are two types of such compressive pericardial disease: the subacute, or *effusive*, constrictive pericarditis, and the chronic, or *noneffusive*, constrictive pericarditis.

CAUSES OF PERICARDIAL CONSTRICTION

Effusive Constrictive Pericarditis

As previously mentioned, subacute pericardial constriction, or effusive constrictive pericarditis, may occur following upper mantle radiation therapy exceeding 4000 rads for malignancies. Other causes include rheumatoid disease, uremia, neoplasia, and infections like tuberculosis; in some cases, the cause is unknown.

The subacute type shows a mixed pathology, with a fibroelastic type of compression. There is a cushion of fluid between the thickened and fibrotic pericardial layers, causing a resilient compression. The peak venous flow to the right atrium occurs during ventricular systole when intrapericardial pressure falls maximally, imparting a prominent x descent to the jugular venous pulse, with the x being larger than the y trough. With progression to chronic constrictive (noneffusive) pericarditis, which usually occurs in less than a year, the y trough tends to be much more conspicuous than the x.

Noneffusive or Chronic Constrictive Pericarditis

Chronic constrictive pericarditis may be idiopathic or tuberculous and occasionally is a sequela of other conditions such as rheumatoid disease or uremia.

In chronic (noneffusive) constrictive pericarditis, usually the whole heart is encased in a thick, rigid, and unyielding fibrous shell, which is often calcified. Thus, the diastolic expansion of the ventricles is restricted, resulting in a high filling pressure. In the jugular venous pulse, both x and y descents may be noted, but the y descent is characteristically more precipitous, with a conspicuous y trough (Friedreich's sign). Immediately after the opening of the atrioventricular valve, ventricular filling is rapid, but it is quickly limited by failure of the ventricle to relax, owing to pericardial compression. Thus, an early diastolic dip followed by a plateau in right-ventricular pressure tracing ("square root" sign) is observed, and a precipitous y descent with a conspicuous y trough in the right-atrial or jugular venous pulse results. A relatively early diastolic pericardial knock is generated in the ventricle, with abrupt termination of the rapid filling by the compressing rigid shell of the constricting pericardium. Dense fibrosis, which may sometimes penetrate the myocardium, and in over 50% of cases is partly calcified, causes this shell.

CONTRASTING CLINICAL FEATURES IN THE TWO GROUPS OF COMPRESSIVE PERICARDIAL DISEASE

Chest pain and pericardial friction rub, though fairly common in the recent past in the subacute compression, are rare in the chronic constrictive form. Both groups present with the symptoms of congestive heart failure. Kussmaul's sign, showing inspiratory fullness of the neck veins or actual rise in jugular venous pressure, is common in chronic constrictive pericarditis but is unusual in subacute constriction. On the other hand, paradoxical arterial pulse is more common in the subacute than in chronic constriction, where pulsus paradoxus occurs in about 15% of the cases. An early diastolic pericardial knock is more usual in the chronic form. An enlarged cardiac silhouette is seen more often in the subacute than in chronic constriction, whereas fairly frequent (50–70%) pericardial calcification is observed in the latter situation. Electrocardiography reveals notched P waves or atrial flutter or fibrillation much more commonly (about 40%) in chronic constriction, and seldom, if ever, in subacute constriction, where sinus rhythm is the rule. The duration of symptoms ranges from several weeks to a few months in subacute constriction and usually spans several years in chronic constrictive (noneffusive) pericarditis.

DIAGNOSIS OF CHRONIC CONSTRICTIVE PERICARDITIS

As chronic constriction is encountered more often than the subacute type, diagnosis of the former condition is discussed in more detail here. Chronic constrictive pericarditis must be distinguished from other causes of congestive heart failure, such as cardiomyopathy. A major diagnostic clue is persistent elevation of venous pressure, even after appropriate diuresis. Examination of the jugular venous pulse, showing prominent x and y descents (with y often more prominent than x), should lead the physician to suspect this condition. If the cardiac silhouette is nearly normal, despite the presence of signs of advanced systemic venous congestion, the suspicion is further strengthened. Presence of pericardial calcification would then strongly support the diagnosis.

Echocardiography may show dense pericardial echoes, but more often a flat diastolic endocardial slope of the left-ventricular posterior wall is observed. Paradoxical septal motion occurs occasionally. Systolic time intervals may indicate a nearly normal, rather than a high (0.4 or more), ratio between the preejection period and the left-ventricular ejection time in a patient with signs of congestive heart failure. Cardiac catheterization would show elevation of right-sided intracardiac pressures, a ratio between pulmonary artery systolic and right-atrial mean pressure of under 3.5, and virtual equalization of the elevated intracardiac diastolic pressures in both right and left ventricles, with nearly identical pulmonary artery diastolic and mean pulmonary capillary wedge pressures. The right-ventricular pressure pulse reveals a characteristic early diastolic dip, followed by a diastolic plateau form, with its level reaching more than one-third of the systolic pressure: the "square root" sign.

In cardiomyopathy, on the other hand, the left-sided filling pressures are almost always higher than those on the right side, more particularly so during exercise, and the ratio between the pulmonary arterial systolic pressure and right-atrial mean pressure remains higher than 3.5.

Right-atrial angiography can be used to detect pericardial thickening. Coronary arteriography may show contrast-filled, nearly immobile coronary vessels positioned within, rather than on the surface of, the cardiac silhouette, a sign of pericardial thickening. These findings are further supportive evidence for the diagnosis of constrictive pericarditis.

Course and therapy

The course of subacute constriction is not influenced by steroid therapy and progression to noneffusive chronic constrictive pericarditis is usual in less than one year. Sooner or later, surgery is needed.

For chronic constrictive pericarditis, a slowly progressive course with features of intractable congestive heart failure is the rule. Occasionally protein-losing gastroenteropathy may result. Surgical removal of the constricting pericardium is the therapy of choice, particularly when continued medical management with diuretics proves no longer effective. Results of surgery are good except in advanced cases with myocardial dysfunction from encroachment of the heart muscle by the constricting and often calcific periocardial fibrosis.

SYNDROME OF RECURRENT PERICARDITIS

Most forms of acute pericarditis are self-limited. However, thre are occasions when an acute relapsing form, occasionally with tamponade, following either a known or presumed viral infection, trauma, or idiopathic pericarditis, may be encountered. Any of the foregoing causes of pericarditis may present as recurrent pericarditis. Considerable discomfort and disability may result, and pericardial constriction may develop. An immunologic, sometimes anamnestic type of response to presumed antigens by the pericardial tissue is suspected. Symptomatic therapy with aspirin or indomethacin is in order. Obviously one would prefer to avoid using steroids because of side-effects on long-term use. However, short courses of intensive steroid therapy, followed by a small maintenance dose may have to be prescribed in many cases. Recently, pericardiocentesis, with instillation of the nonabsorbable topical steroid triamcinolone hexaacetonide, has been noted to prevent recurrences of uremic pericarditis for several years. This form of therapy is now under trial in patients with idiopathic and other forms of recurrent pericarditis with effusion. Pericardiectomy may still be advisable in intractable cases, although recurrence of pain has been reported following surgery.

For recurrent cardiac tamponade from malignant pericardial disease, pericardiocentesis followed by intrapericardial tetracycline therapy has been reported recently to be beneficial.

SUGGESTED READING

Burchell HB: Pericarditis: some current concepts. Cardiovasc Med 2:287–296, 1977

Buselmeier TJ, Simmons RL, Natarajan JS, Mauer SM, Matas AJ, Kjell Strand CM: Uremic pericardial effusion: treatment by catheter drainage and local nonabsorbable steroid administration. Nephron 16:371–380, 1976

Cortes FM: The Pericardium and its Disorders. Springfield, IL, C Thomas, 1971

Fowler N: Physiology of cardiac tamponade and pulsus paradoxus. I. Mechanisms of pulsus paradoxus in cardiac tamponade. Mod Concepts Cardiovasc Dis 47:109–113, 1978

Fowler N: Physiology of cardiac tamponade and pulsus paradoxus. II. Physiological, circulatory, and pharmacological responses in cardiac tamponade. Mod Concepts Cardiovasc Dis 47:115–118, 1978

Hancock EW: Subacute effusive-constrictive pericarditis. Circulation 43:183–192, 1971

Hancock EW: Constrictive pericarditis. JAMA 232:176–177, 1975

Hancock EW: Management of pericardial disease. Mod Concepts Cardiovasc Dis 48:1–6, 1979

Shabetai R: The pericardium. An essay on some recent developments. Am J Cardiol 42:1036–1043, 1978

Spodick DH: Differential diagnosis of acute pericarditis. Prog Cardiovasc Dis 14:192–209, 1971

Spodick DH: Pericardial Diseases, Cardiovascular Clinics. Philadelphia, FA Davis, 1976

Wood P: Chronic constrictive pericarditis. Am J Cardiol 7:48–61, 1961

CARDIOMYOPATHY

16

Saktipada Mookherjee

Myocardial disease may result from disease of the coronary arteries, systemic arterioles (hypertension), pulmonary vessels, cardiac valves, and intrinsic disease of the heart muscle itself. When the primary pathology resides in the heart muscle and does not result from preexisting or coexisting disease of the other structures mentioned, **primary myocardial disease,** or a **cardiomyopathy,** is said to be present. Cardiomyopathy has been defined by Goodwin as a disorder of the heart muscle of unknown cause. He has classified the so-called **secondary cardiomyopathies,** in which the heart is involved as part of a general systemic disease (such as hemochromatosis, connective tissue disease, sarcoidosis, or heredofamilial neuromuscular disease) as specific rare heart muscle diseases. Secondary cardiomyopathies are less common than the so-called primary variety, although the pathophysiological presentation may be quite similar.

CLASSIFICATION OF CARDIOMYOPATHIES

The classification of cardiomyopathies has been attempted from both pathophysiologic and etiologic standpoints. The pathophysiologic, hemodynamic classification developed by Goodwin helps to emphasize the underlying functional derangement, and the etiologic classification deals with the possible cause or causes of the heart muscle disease.

PATHOPHYSIOLOGIC CLASSIFICATION

Congestive Cardiomyopathy

This condition is characterized by failure of the heart as a pump. The heart is enlarged and dilated, with high end diastolic ventricular pressure, often associated with atrioventricular-valve regurgitation, poor ejection fraction, and low cardiac output. Clinically, symptoms and signs of low-output congestive heart failure are the dominant presenting features. Congestive heart failure is often the final outcome of the other varieties of heart muscle disease discussed later.

Hypertrophic Cardiomyopathy

In hypertrophic cardiomyopathy, with or without outflow tract obstruction, there is massive hypertrophy of the interventricular septum (**asymmetric septal hypertrophy**), often associated with hypertrophy of the free wall of the left ventricle. In the obstructive variety (**hypertrophic obstructive cardiomyopathy,** also called **idiopathic hypertrophic subaortic stenosis** in the United States) there is considerable narrowing of the outflow tract of the left ventricle between the hypertrophied septum and the ventrally displaced anterior leaflet of the mitral valve in systole (**systolic anterior motion**), producing a pressure gradient in the subaortic region. The hypertrophied left ventricle is stiff and noncompliant, offering resistance to diastolic filling, but maintains good pump function, at least initially, with an excellent ejection fraction. In over one-third of patients with this type of heart muscle disease, a positive family history is obtained.

Obliterative Cardiomyopathy

In this rare form of cardiomyopathy, the cavity of the left ventricle is progressively obliterated from apex to base, by proliferation of fibrous tissue and endocardium and the development of mural thrombi. In tropical Africa, endomyocardial fibrosis is a typical example of this disease. In temperate zones, Loeffler's fibroplastic eosinophilic endocarditis is the prototype of a similar pathophysiologic entity. Here, in addition to fibrous tissue and mural thrombi, masses of eosinophilic material (with peripheral blood eosinophilia) obliterate the left-ventricular cavity. Mitral regurgitation, pulmonary hypertension, and systemic embolization are particularly common.

Restrictive Cardiomyopathy

In this form of heart muscle disease, ventricular filling is restricted because of limitation in diastolic relaxation of the ventricle, in spite of a high filling pressure, with consequent reduction in diastolic filling and end diastolic volume. The stroke volume may also be reduced, probably as a result of impairment in both diastolic filling and systolic pump function. In many infiltrative cardiomyopathies, including amyloid heart disease, restrictive cardiomyopathy mimicks constrictive pericarditis in symptoms and pathophysiology.

In all of these types of cardiomyopathy, the major coronary arteries are free from significant occlusive atherosclerotic disease. However, the syndrome of ischemic cardiomyopathy with congestive failure, clearly secondary to coronary heart disease, may present with features closely resembling those of congestive cardiomyopathy. In many patients presenting with idiopathic congestive cardiomyopathy, the coronary microcirculation has shown proliferative occlusive disease, with normal extramural vessels. A strong family history is sometimes obtained in such cases. However, a cause-and-effect relationship between the changes in the small coronary vessels and the associated cardiomyopathy has not been proven.

ETIOLOGIC CLASSIFICATION

By definition, *primary* myocardial disease is idiopathic—the cause is unknown. *Secondary* cardiomyopathies are part of a multisystemic disease, the cause or causes of which may or may not be apparent. Any pathophysiologic type of cardiomyopathy may present as a condition of unknown origin. However, certain associations are now well recognized and are probably worth considering when confronted with a given case of cardiomyopathy. Some of these are as follows:

1. Primary Cardiomyopathy
   a. A familial cardiomyopathy (hypertrophic and sometimes congestive cardiomyopathies)
   b. Cardiomyopathy associated with pregnancy and puerperium (peripartal); (congestive cardiomyopathy)
2. Secondary Cardiomyopathy
   a. Cardiomyopathies associated with heredofamilial neuromuscular disorders (often congestive cardiomyopathy)
   b. Nutritional disorders: thiamine deficiency, kwashiorkor
   c. Toxic cardiomyopathy by alcohol, chemicals, and drugs (*e.g.*, doxorubicin, emetine, and phenothiazines)
   d. Infections: diphtheria, chagas' disease
   e. Diseases presumably caused by altered immunologic mechanism (*i.e.*, collagen vascular disease group)
   f. Metabolic and endocrine disorders
      1) Glycogen storage disease
      2) Mucopolysaccharidosis, lipidosis
      3) Hemochromatosis
      4) Thyroid heart disease and acromegaly
      5) Hypokalemia and hypomagnesemia
      6) Hypocalcemia, hypophosphatemia
      7) Catecholamine excess

g. Physical agents: radiation heart disease, heat stroke
h. Sensitivity phenomena: serum sickness, postvaccinal reactions, sulphonamide sensitivity
i. Infiltrative cardiomyopathies:
1) Sarcoidosis
2) Lymphomas, leukemias and tumors
3) Amyloidosis

Many metabolic cardiomyopathies are infiltrative and may present pathophysiologically as the restrictive or congestive type of cardiomyopathy.

CLINICAL DIAGNOSIS

Three steps are required in making a clinical diagnosis of heart muscle disease. The first is to recognize that one is dealing with a cardiomyopathy and to exclude other known causes of heart muscle disease. The second is to identify the *pathophysiologic* type, and the third is to search for a possible *etiologic* factor. A combination of clinical, roentgenologic, electrocardiographic, echocardiographic, radionuclide, and sometimes invasive hemodynamic and angiographic information are needed to make a definite diagnosis. Endomyocardial biopsy is still largely a research tool and not a routine procedure.

A brief discussion of the major pathophysiologic and etiologic types of cardiomyopathy, with comments on diagnosis and management, follows.

PATHOPHYSIOLOGIC TYPES

CONGESTIVE CARDIOMYOPATHY

Characteristics

Most cardiomyopathies are of the congestive type. A cause is sometimes identified. Pregnancy, infections, nutritional, endocrine, and many metabolic diseases, as well as toxic effects (*e.g.,* alcoholic cardiomyopathy) may result in congestive cardiomyopathy. Congestive heart failure, often progressive, along with episodes of supraventricular or ventricular arrhythmias, as well as pulmonary and systemic embolization, are observed. Clinically, symptoms, signs, and the chest film of congestive heart failure are obvious (see Chaps. 7 and 8 on this subject).

The electrocardiogram, in congestive cardiomyopathy, is nonspecific and ranges from low-voltage, patterns resembling those of myocardial infarction, and atrioventricular or intraventricular conduction disturbances, to atrial and ventricular hypertrophy and repolarization abnormalities.

The M-mode echocardiography shows increased diastolic dimension and poor contraction of the left, and sometimes also of the right ventricle, reduced motion of the interventricular septum and posterior wall, poor calculated ejection fraction, attenuated mitral-valve excursion, and a prominent b notching of the mitral valve, indicating an increase in left-ventricular end diastolic pressure. The left atrium may be enlarged and aortic-wall motion decreased, with a reduction in the ejection period reflecting a decrease in left-ventricular stroke volume. Pulmonic valve echogram may show reduction of the diastolic slope, with inconspicuous *a* waves and fast systolic opening, often with a midsystolic notching, all suggesting pulmonary hypertension. With right-ventricular failure, the *a* wave in the pulmonary valve echogram in pulmonary hypertension may become conspicuous.

The systolic time intervals in congestive cardiomyopathy show a prolonged preejection period and an abbreviated left-ventricular ejection time, resulting in an increased ratio between them (normal up to 40%).

Invasive hemodynamic studies are seldom necessary for the diagnosis of congestive cardiomyopathy and may be associated with increased risk. However, when such studies are undertaken, they are done to monitor therapeutic effects of various drugs, including vasodilators, as well as to rule out coronary artery disease as the cause of the condition. Hemodynamic studies confirm the elevated end diastolic pressure in the ventricles (higher in the left than in the right), pulmonary hypertension, and reduction in cardiac output. Left-ventricular angiogram shows generalized poor contraction (hypokinesis) of a large-volume left ventricle and occasional mitral regurgitation. The coronary arteriogram reveals grossly normal, often large, major coronary arteries.

Artrioventricular-valve regurgitation, caused by mitral and tricuspid insufficiency, results from several mechanisms in congestive cardiomyopathy. These include papillary muscle dysfunction from the myopathy itself; altered geometry of the dilated ventricle, disturbing the spatial relationship of the papillary muscles and causing their malfunction; and actual dilatation of the valve ring from massive enlargement of the ventricular chamber. In addition, triscuspid regurgitation may result from pulmonary hypertension and right-ventricular failure.

As mentioned earlier, endomyocardial biopsy is still very much a research tool. However, when a certain diagnosis is absolutely vital for the patient's management (for example, to differentiate between constrictive pericarditis and primary cardiac amyloidosis), transvenous endomyocardial biopsy by an experienced person or an open myocardial biopsy by thoracotomy, if the former is not feasible, is indicated. There are rare case reports of sarcoid heart disease being diagnosed only by endomyocardial biopsy and treated successfully with steroids.

Management

The management of congestive cardiomyopathy is standard. When a specific cause can be identified, appropriate therapy can be planned. When no specific cause is known, therapy for heart failure alone should be carefully pursued. Associated conditions that may aggravate the cardiac failure (*e.g.*, anemia, respiratory or urinary tract infections), should be investigated and thoroughly treated. In suspected alcoholic heart disease, drinking of alcohol should be totally discontinued.

For the heart failure itself, rest, often prolonged bed rest with bathroom privileges, salt restriction, digitalization, and diuretic therapy with adequate potassium supplements, when appropriate, are needed. Vasodilator therapy, using intravenous infusion of sodium nitroprusside for a few days, under appropriate hemodynamic monitoring of left-ventricular filling pressure (using a triple lumen, balloon-tipped floating catheter), and monitoring of arterial pressure and cardiac output, may be required in intractable cases. Oral vasodilator therapy, using nitrates such as isosorbide dinitrate, sometimes with addition of a predominantly arteriolar dilator such as hydralazine, may be instituted and continued indefinitely in such cases.

In view of its deleterious effects on the circulation, cigarette smoking should be forbidden. In patients with severe heart failure, anticoagulant therapy to prevent thromboembolic complications is also appropriate.

Positive inotropic agents such as dopamine, in addition to digitalis therapy, may be useful in patients who are hypotensive and who have a low cardiac output and a high left-ventricular filling pressure. On occasion, judicious combination of vasodilator and positive inotropic agents may tide the patient over a severe crisis of congestive heart failure. Recently, careful administration of beta blocking drugs such as Propanolol has been noted to be beneficial in some patients with severe congestive cardiomyopathy, particularly those with a fast heart rate at rest.

HYPERTROPHIC CARDIOMYOPATHY

Characteristics

Hypertrophic cardiomyopathy is a true primary myocardial disease of unknown cause. The pathologic process ranges from asymmetric hypertrophy of the interventricular septum to generalized hypertrophy, with or without outflow-tract obstruction. In about one-third of the patients, a positive family history of heart murmurs or sudden death is obtained.

Braunwald and others established the dynamic nature of the obstruction and observed the typical pulse wave of the disease. Goodwin and Oakley and their group in England also made extensive studies to clarify the pathophysiology and clinical features of this disease. Shah and his colleagues, using echocardiography in the 1960s, described the systolic anterior motion (SAM) of the mitral valve, which tends to obliterate the left-ventricular outflow tract, and subsequently it was observed that the degree and duration of this motion might correlate with the outflow-tract gradient.

Histologic studies show grossly disorganized myocardial fibers with extreme hypertrophy. The abnormal fibers are collected in circular "whorls" and have a mottled appearance, with bizarrely shaped nuclei and a surrounding perinuclear halo. The haze, or halo, around the nuclei is particularly characteristic and probably results from partial disappearance of myofibrils. Abnormal and normal areas of myocardium might coexist very closely. Gross and extensive myofibrillar disarray showing their orientation either oblique or perpendicular to the long axis of the cells, which also run in abnormal directions instead of parallel, are striking changes on electron microscopy.

The functional abnormality in hypertrophic cardiomyopathy results from increased stiffness and reduced distensibility or compliance of the ventricular myocardium. The ventricular cavity is small and is markedly reduced during systole. Outflow-tract obstruction is not invariable, although it is present in some degree in the majority of patients. It is more marked with a massive septal hypertrophy, with or without severe hypertrophy of the free wall of the left ventricle. The abnormal mitral-valve motion may result from papillary muscle dysfunction or a venturi effect, pulling the anterior leaflet toward the hypertrophied septum in systole. In almost all patients, the left-ventricular end diastolic pressure is raised, and often markedly elevated, during exercise or with infusion of isoproterenol. There is resistance to left-ventricular filling, which is unduly slow. Hence a reduction in diastolic filling time, as may happen with tachycardia, for instance, or withdrawal of atrial transport mechanism (atrial kick at end diastole) such as occurs with atrial fibrillation, would be catastrophic, causing marked elevation of left-atrial and pulmonary venous pressure. Acute pulmonary edema may be precipitated.

Clinical Features

The clinical features of hypertrophic cardiomyopathy include: (1) syncope, either exertional or from arrhythmias; (2) mitral regurgitation, from forward displacement of the anterior mitral-valve leaflet during systole; (3) anginal pain in the presence of normal coronary arteries; (4) dyspnea on exertion.

The common age of presentation is between the fourth and the sixth decade, although the disease may be noted from infancy to very old age. In an asymptomatic individual, a characteristic murmur and arterial pulse (described below) may be observed. The natural history depends on the magnitude of elevation of the left-ventricular end diastolic pressure, particularly during exercise. Outflow-tract obstruction may become progressively more marked in some patients. However, about 20% of patients lose the outflow-tract obstruction over a period of several years, probably as a result of progressive impairment of systolic contractile function without an increase in systolic volume. The systolic murmur (discussed below) may decrease or actually disappear in these patients, but an increase in dyspnea and congestive heart failure may be observed. Tachyarrhythmias, particularly atrial fibrillation, occur in 10% of all cases and, as mentioned, have a catastrophic effect, with development of pulmonary edema, systemic embolization in some of them, and worsening of congestive heart failure in most of them.

The estimated overall mortality in hypertrophic cardiomyopathy is 3.5% per year. The ever-present danger of sudden death is very real and does not seem to be related to the outflow-tract obstruction. In children and young adults, sudden death is commoner (20%) than in older age groups (8%). It is not related to a single factor, but in Goodwin's series it frequently appeared to be associated with a short, but progressively symptomatic history and high left-ventricular end diastolic pressure. A strong family history of sudden deaths is particularly ominous and seems to be an important predictor of the event. However, in isolated cases, sudden death may be the first definitive manifestation of the underlying disease. The relationship of sudden death to exertion is also very striking in this condition.

Although the precise mechanism causing sudden death in hypertrophic cardiomyopathy is not known, ventricular tachyarrhythmias seem to be the terminal event. Ventricular ectopic activity is common in hypertrophic cardiomyopathy both at rest and during exertion, and ventricular fibrillation may be the immediate cause of death. Atrial tachyarrhythmias, with fast ventricular response, may be dangerous in this disease, as mentioned earlier, since they may precipitously lower the cardiac output, with resulting hypotension and cardiac arrest. Rapid transmission of supraventricular impulses through anomalous or accessory pathways (Wolff-Parkinson-White syndrome) may also result in ventricular fibrillation. Such anomalous atrioventricular conduction is not unusual in hypertrophic cardiomyopathy. The interesting common denominators in patients dying suddenly are a distinctly abnormal electrocardiogram and moderate to severe ventricular septal thickening.

Physical Signs

In general, the patients are seldom in overt heart failure. The arterial pulse has a characteristically sharp upstroke, with a jerky quality, caused by the abrupt and forceful contraction of the hypertrophied left-ventricular myocardium. The quality of the arterial pulse simulates the water-hammer pulse of aortic insufficiency. A bisferiens pulse with two upstrokes is often better recorded than felt, although in occasional cases it is easily felt. A bisferiens pulse in this setting indicates partial closure of the aortic valve in systole, because of outflow-tract obstruction.

In idiopathic hypertrophic subaortic stenosis, in contrast to aortic insufficiency, the arterial blood pressure does not show a wide pulse pressure. Following a premature ventricular contraction, the subsequent arterial pulse normally feels stronger and has a larger amplitude. However, in idiopathic hypertrophic subaortic stenosis, the postextrasystolic beat is characteristically weaker (Brockenbrough's sign). This occurs because increased inotropy or contractility of the hypertrophied muscle following the postextrasystolic pause produces further narrowing of the outflow tract, compromising the stroke volume, and a weaker pulse results. However, if the premature ventricular beat occurs later (less premature, or interpolated), this sign may be absent.

In the jugular venous pulse, often prominent a waves from septal hypertrophy on the right side or hypertrophic cardiomyopathy involving the walls of the right ventricle are observed.

Cardiac examination reveals a double or a triple apical impulse on palpation with the patient turned to his left side. Double apical impulse is usual and may be visible on inspection. Powerful atrial contraction is responsible for the first impulse; the second one is caused by the strong apex beat, and the third one, when present, results from abnormal ventricular contraction later in systole. A fourth heart sound is the rule.

The characteristic murmur, when outflow-tract obstruction is present, is a crescendo-decrescendo systolic murmur beginning after the first heart sound and ending before the aortic component of the second heart sound, which is normal. The murmur has the maximum intensity at the left sternal border in the third and fourth interspaces, and occasionally at the apex. It does not radiate into the neck and has poor conduction to the left axilla. The murmur arises from a combination of left-ventricular outflow-tract obstruction and mitral regurgitation.

The systolic murmur of idiopathic hypertrophic subaortic stenosis differs from that of classic mitral regurgitation as well as that of valvular or fixed subvalvular aortic stenosis. In idiopathic hypertrophic subaortic stenosis, the outflow-tract obstruction is dynamic, and the Valsalva maneuver may increase the murmur. Other physical and pharmacologic influences that tend to affect the left-ventricular size modify the murmur. For example, standing, or inhalation of amyl nitrite, increases the murmur by decreasing the ventricular volume, whereas leg-raising in the supine position, prompt squatting, or infusion of phenylephrine, all characteristically decrease the murmur while making the ventricular volume large.

In idiopathic hypertrophic subaortic stenosis, occasionally an ejection sound (a "pseudo-ejection-click"), a third sound, or a short middiastolic rumble (from significant inflow restriction, with delayed ventricular filling) may be heard on auscultation. The early diastolic, high pitched, blowing murmur of aortic insufficiency is rarely heard. A paradoxically split second heart sound in the absence of left bundle-branch block in idiopathic hypertrophic subaortic stenosis would indicate severe left-ventricular disease.

In hypertrophic cardiomyopathy, the chest film and the electrocardiogram, although nonspecific, are seldom normal. Prominent left-ventricular silhouette is commonly noted on the chest film. Abnormal septal Q waves, left-ventricular and left-atrial hypertrophy, intraventricular conduction disturbances, and nonspecific repolarization abnormalities, singly or in combination, are the usual electrocardiographic changes.

On echocardiography, marked thickening and granularity of the ventricular septum, with poor systolic contraction and septal motion, and a ratio between the thickness of the septum and that of the left-ventricular posterior wall in diastole equal to or exceeding 1.3:1.0 is characteristic of asymmetric septal hypertrophy. Shah prefers this ratio as 1.5:1 for more diagnostic specificity of this condition. The ventricular cavity is small, and the thickening of the posterior wall may also be quite marked. In idiopathic hypertrophic subaortic stenosis, the echocardiographic hallmark is the abrupt systolic anterior motion of the anterior mitral leaflet approaching the thickened septum, which tends to obliterate the left-ventricular outflow tract. In diastole, too, the excursion of the mitral-valve leaflet is restricted in the relatively small and muscle-bound ventricular cavity, and the E-F slope may also be reduced. A prominent presystolic a wave in the mitral-valve echo is the rule. The aortic-valve echo may show intra-systolic closing motion, followed by reopening of the leaflets, corresponding to the bisferiens quality of arterial pulse. Left-atrial enlargement or a prominent atrial systolic wave may also be noted.

In idiopathic hypertrophic subaortic stenosis, cardiac catheterization is performed to assess the severity of the obstruction by measuring the gradient, during pull-back of the end-hole catheter, between the outflow tract and the cavity of the left-ventricle, particularly when surgery is contemplated for therapy. The previously mentioned noninvasive studies, however, are usually enough for the diagnosis and medical follow-up of the patient. On occasion, catheterization may show a provokable gradient only after inhalation of amyl nitrite or infusion of isoproterenol. On the other hand, a very high peak-systolic pressure gradient, exceeding 70 torr, across the left-ventricular outflow tract at rest may be noted, and this may decrease with acute intravenous administration of propranolol. The left-ventricular angiogram may show encroachment on the left-ventricular cavity by the hypertrophied septum and free wall, often with cavity obliteration in systole and a high ejection fraction. Outline of the hypertrophied muscles, including papillary muscle, may be visualized. Abnormal mitral-valve motion, narrowing of the outflow tract, and mitral regurgitation may also be appreciated. The coronary arteries, as mentioned previously, are characteristically normal.

Management

Management is both medical and surgical. The beta adrenergic blocking agent, Propranolol, is the mainstay of medical therapy in hypertrophic cardiomyopathy. Its negative inotropic and antiarrhythmic effects are helpful in the management of the angina, syncope, and arrhythmia which may accompany the cardiomyopathy. Patients with only exercise-induced or provokable outflow gradients respond best to Propranolol. However, an occasional patient with marked outflow-tract obstruction and a high systolic pressure gradient even at rest may respond to high doses of Propranolol.

Although symptomatic improvement may occur on long-term oral Propranolol therapy, sudden death still may not be prevented. Furthermore, patients who do not have a variable outflow-tract obstruction may not respond favorably to beta blockade. However, there are recent encouraging reports on the beneficial effects of large dose Propanolol therapy (average 460 mg daily) in hypertrophic cardiomyopathy. In a follow-up period averaging 5 years, Frank and coworkers observed marked symptomatic improvement and no deaths among 22 patients, including 3 without outflow tract obstruction.

More recently, Verapamil, the blocker of the slow channel for entry of calcium into the myocardium, has been shown to improve the myocardial compliance and hemodynamics in hypertrophic cardiomyopathy. Further results from clinical trials are awaited with interest.

Patients with a large outflow tract gradient at rest, who are severely symptomatic and whose symptoms do not respond satisfactorily to medical therapy, are candidates for surgery. Septal myotomy-myectomy is the operation of choice. Deep incision into the hypertrophied septum and, often, wide excision of the abnormal muscle are performed. Mitral-valve replacement is not recommended unless there is severe mitral regurgitation. Long-term follow-up shows symptomatic improvement, with marked reduction in left-ventricular outflow gradient at rest, in about 70% of patients. There is an operation-related mortality of 8%. Of the survivors, 12% continue to deteriorate despite surgery, with an annual mortality of 3.5%. Half of the late postoperative deaths (6 months or longer after surgery) (about 2% per year) are sudden. Atrial fibrillation is more common in patients who died in the late postoperative period than in survivors. Thus, surgery does not seem to influence the natural history of the underlying cardiomyopathy. Furthermore, patients without outflow tract obstruction at rest are not candidates for surgery.

Complications require special expertise in management. These include atrial fibrillation and congestive failure. Because the development of atrial fibrillation signals the beginning of a dramatic downward course, early cardioversion, probably with anticoagulant cover, should be considered. Digitalization is certainly indicated. A combination of propranolol and quinidine therapy in an attempt to maintain sinus rhythm is recommended. Therefore, the patient should be admitted to the hospital when this complication develops. For paroxysmal or established atrial fibrillation, anticoagulant therapy should be maintained indefinitely to prevent systemic embolization.

In 10% to 20% of patients, the disease may progress, with loss of outflow gradient, disappearance of the murmur, and development of congestive cardiac failure, with or without atrial fibrillation. Usual antifailure therapy, with digitalization and diuretics and a smaller dose of Propranolol, should be instituted. Anticoagulant therapy is usuful to help guard against systemic and pulmonary embolism.

For prophylaxis of infective endocarditis usually involving the mitral valve, appropriate antibiotic cover for dental work, instrumentation, labor, or similar procedures should be provided.

RESTRICTIVE CARDIOMYOPATHY

This type of heart muscle disease, in which ventricular filling is limited because of limited relaxation of the ventricle in diastole, is rare and is often secondary to infiltrative diseases of the myocardium. Amyloid heart disease, heart disease in mucopolysaccharidosis, or neoplastic infiltration of the heart may cause a restrictive type of cardiomyopathy. The hemodynamic features may simulate constrictive pericarditis, with high ventricular filling pressures. The cardiac output which may be normal in the early stages decreases progressively. Clinically and radiologically it may be impossible to distinguish it from noncalcific constrictive pericarditis, but attention to details in clinical, noninvasive, and invasive studies may be helpful to better clarify the situation. However, endomyocardial biopsy or an open biopsy of the myopericardium after thoracotomy remains the only definitive test to clinch the diagnosis in such cases. Biopsy may be indicated to separate the potentially surgically curable constrictive pericarditis from restrictive cardiomyopathy.

Clinical features include dyspnea on exertion, fatigue, and dependent edema, often with ascites. Some patients complain of fluttering in the neck, resulting from exaggerated venous pulsations. Both a and v waves are prominent, but a characteristic y descent, simulating that of constrictive pericarditis, may be noted. Heart rate is fast, and the arterial pulse may on occasion be paradoxical. The precordium may show a diastolic impulse. On auscultation, heart sounds may be quiet; a fourth heart sound and a third heart sound may be audible. Murmurs of mitral and tricuspid regurgitation are less common than in congestive or obliterative cardiomyopathy.

Roentgenographic examination shows that the heart is moderately enlarged and that there is no pericardial calcification. Pulmonary venous congestion, Kerley B lines, and dilated pulmonary arteries may be noted.

Low voltage is usual on the electrocardiogram. Abnormal Q waves and intraventricular conduction defects, with or without typical bundle branch-block patterns, and nonspecific repolarization abnormalities are common.

Using echocardiography, a thick-walled ventricle with a relatively small cavity and poor contractions, is usually present. The aortic-valve opening and aortic-wall motion may indicate poor stroke volume. Mitral-valve motion may reflect high left-ventricular end diastolic pressure.

The systolic time-interval studies using simultaneous external phonocardiogram, carotid pulse tracing, and electrocardiogram, show that the ratio of the preejection period to left-ventricular ejection time is abnormally high (0.5 or higher), in contrast to constrictive pericarditis, in which the ratio remains near normal, and less than 0.4.

Hemodynamic studies are often undertaken in restrictive cardiomyopathies to differentiate them from the potentially curable condition of constrictive pericarditis. In restrictive cardiomyopathy, the a waves on atrial pressure tracing are larger than those in constrictive pericarditis. The ratio of the pulmonary artery systolic pressure to the right-atrial mean pressure is greater than 3.5, the pulmonary capillary wedge pressure is also higher than that in constrictive pericarditis, and the difference between the mean left-atrial and right-atrial pressure is usually greater than 6 torr. For a given degree of elevation of venous pressure, the cardiac output is lower in cardiomyopathy than in constrictive pericarditis. The left-ventricular end diastolic pressure, as in the case of left-atrial mean pressure, is higher than the right-ventricular end diastolic pressure, particularly during exercise. This is so because cardiomyopathy is predominantly a left-sided disease, in contrast to constrictive pericarditis, in which the diastolic pressure on the two sides tends to remain about the same, even on exercise. Left-ventricular angiography, in restrictive cardiomyopathy, may show poor ventricular contraction and a reduced ejection fraction; in constrictive pericarditis, ventricular contraction and the ejection fraction may be nearly normal until very late in the course of the disease.

In spite of all of these special studies, myocardial biopsy may at times be needed to arrive at a definite diagnosis. This is not an academic exercise, but may be potentially life-saving in a patient with constrictive pericarditis masquerading as a case of restrictive cardiomyopathy. Surgery, as already emphasized, may be curative in the former condition.

Next we discuss briefly four etiologic types of congestive cardiomyopathies.

ETIOLOGIC TYPES

ALCOHOLIC CARDIOMYOPATHY

Chronic alcohol abuse may be associated with depression of myocardial function and may lead to the development of alcoholic cardiomyopathy. Physiologic studies in animals and in man have shown that left-ventricular function, following chronic use of alcohol, resembles that of a failing heart. Under stress of exercise or angiotensin infusion, the cardiac output fails to increase significantly. In most cases it actually falls, and the left-ventricular end diastolic pressure is elevated, as in cardiac decompensation. Abstinence from alcohol in a patient with presumed alcoholic cardiomyopathy may cause subjective and objective improvement in cardiac function. The heart size may get smaller, with improvement in cardiac output and reduction in ventricular end diastolic pressure. However, challenging such an exalcoholic patient later on with daily administration of a moderately large dose of whisky may put him back into heart failure again, with dilated, hypokinetic left ventricle, fall of cardiac output, and elevation of left-ventricular end diastolic pressure.

Alcoholic cardiomyopathy has been noted in patients (particularly males) who have consumed alcohol heavily for 10 years or longer. It is of interest that drunkenness, peripheral neuropathy, liver cirrhosis, and hepatocellular decompensation are conspicuous by their rarity in patients with alcoholic cardiomyopathy.

Histologic studies, even in alcoholics without overt cardiac disease, have shown interstitial Alcian-positive glycoprotein and collagen in the myocardium, with interstitial fibrosis of variable degrees.

The patient with alcoholic heart disease is usually a male, between 30 to 55 years of age, with a history of more than 10 years of alcoholism (often difficult to elicit), a clinically normal nutrition at the onset, and low-output heart failure. There is often moderate to marked cardiomegaly and both atrial and ventricular arrhythmias, with atrial fibrillation being particularly common. Pulmonary and systemic embolization is more frequent than with other types of congestive heart failure. Ventricular (S_3) and atrial gallop (S_4) sounds, the latter in sinus rhythm, and murmurs of mitral and tricuspid regurgitation are often present. The course of this congestive cardiomyopathy is progressive if alcohol intake is continued. However, the myocardial disease may be reversible if the intake of ethanol is discontinued, provided the disease is not too far advanced. As in all cardiomyopathies, sudden unexpected deaths, presumably from ventricular fibrillation, may occur.

Chest pains are not uncommon in alcoholic cardiomyopathies. In addition, myocardial infarctions have occurred in occasional patients with alcoholic cardiomyopathy despite the absence of occlusive coronary atherosclerosis. Morphologic studies of the myocardium at postmortem, in such cases, revealed concentric periarterial fibrosis. It has been postulated that the fibrosis restricted increments in coronary blood flow during periods of high-flow requirement, precipitating anginal pain and even myocardial infarction.

The high-output heart failure observed in some chronic alcoholic patients with thiamine deficiency does not come under the purview of the low-output congestive alcoholic cardiomyopathy.

PERIPARTAL CARDIOMYOPATHY

About 5% to 10% of cases of idiopathic cardiomyopathy are related to pregnancy, or more commonly the puerperium. Peripartal cardiomyopathy occurs during the last month of pregnancy or in the first 3 months after delivery, more often during the latter period. Relatively elderly multiparous black women or women having twins or toxemia comprise a significant number of cases with peripartal cardiomyopathy. The diagnostic clue for this type of cardiomyopathy lies in the development of congestive heart failure, often with embolic complications, in the last month of pregnancy or first 3 to 5 postpartum months, without evidence of prior demonstrable heart disease. The prognosis depends on whether the heart size returns to normal after the initial episode of peripartal heart failure. Tendency to recurrence in subsequent pregnancies with severe deterioration of cardiac function occurs mainly in those patients whose heart size does not return to normal within 6 months following the initial episode. Such patients, in particular, should be advised against further pregnancies.

DRUG-INDUCED CARDIOMYOPATHY

Many drugs, including digitalis, may cause heart-muscle damage. Recently an antitumor agent, doxorubicin (adriamycin), has been shown to cause a congestive type of cardiomyopathy. There is a dose-related (240 mg or more per square meter of body surface area) increase in myocyte damage observed by serial right-ventricular apical biopsies. Systolic time-intervals show a rise in the ratio of the preejection period to the left-ventricular ejection time, when a total dose of 400 mg/M^2 of body surface area is reached. With more than 600 mg/M^2 dose of andriamycin, congestive cardiomyopathy develops in one third of the patients. Andriamycin cardiomyopathy is often irreversible. Previous mediastinal irradiation, older age (70 years or more), and hypertension are risk factors for congestive cardiomyopathy associated with the drug. Very young children also appear to be susceptible to adriamycin cardiomyopathy.

CARDIOMYOPATHIES ASSOCIATED WITH
HEREDOFAMILIAL NEUROMYOPATHIC DISEASES

Most cardiomyopathies in this subgroup are of the congestive type. Diseases in this category are types of muscular dystrophy, particularly the pseudohypertrophic Duchenne type, myotonia dystrophica (Steinert's disease), and the neuro-muscular disease Friedreich's ataxia. Arrhythmias, abnormal electrocardiograms, and cardiomegaly with congestive heart failure are common, and sudden death frequently occurs. Chest pains and even true angina may occur, and coronary arterial lesions with intimal proliferation, varying from minor to complete luminal obliteration, may be found in many patients with Friedreich's ataxia and the Duchenne type of muscular dystrophy. Cardiac involvement is less marked in other types of muscular dystrophy.

APPROACH TO THE PROBLEM OF
CARDIOMYOPATHY

Unexplained cardiomegaly with gallop rhythms and arrhythmias should suggest a cardiomyopathy. Once the pathophysiologic type is recognized, etiologic possibilities have to be explored. Any pathophysiologic type can be idiopathic. Congestive cardiomyopathy, however, is likely to be toxic, infective, metabolic, or peripartal. Restrictive cardiomyopathy is likely to be infiltrative. Hypertrophic cardiomyopathy, particularly with outflow tract obstruction, is probably familial. A history of recent viral illness—for example, upper respiratory infection—may be responsible for myocarditis and subsequent development of congestive cardiomyopathy. Attempts to recover viruses from throat and stool should be made and appropriate serologic tests ordered. History of chronic ethanolism should be specifically looked for not only from the patient but his close relatives and associates also. Family history of heart disease and sudden deaths are to be inquired into. Dietary habits and drug intake also need a careful historical inquiry.

DIAGNOSTIC PITFALLS

Cardiomyopathy may be mistaken for the usual types of heart disease, for example, rheumatic, hypertensive, coronary, chronic pericardial effusion, and idiopathic pulmonary hypertension. Regurgitant murmurs in congestive cardiomyopathy become less pronounced with improvement in heart failure, in contrast to the organic valvular disease, in which improvement in cardiac function makes the murmurs louder. True diastolic murmurs are rare in cardiomyopathy. Valvular calcification contradicts the diagnosis of cardiomyopathy. Transient hypertension, common during episodes of heart failure in cardiomyopathy, should not be confused with hypertensive heart disease. Chest pains from documented coronary artery disease warns against the diagnosis of cardiomyopathy. However, typical anginal pain can occur in patients with myocardial disease, particularly hypertrophic cardiomyopathy with or without idiopathic hypertrophic subaortic stenosis. Infarction patterns may appear in the electrocardiograms in the absence of chest pains in both coronary heart disease and cardiomyopathies. However, typical electrocardiographic evolution would go against the latter diagnosis. Chest pains in patients with cardiomyopathy may also occur from pulmonary embolism or from pericarditis—a true myopericarditis, at least in the initial stage.

Idiopathic pulmonary hypertension may occasionally be mistaken as a cardiomyopathy with pulmonary hypertension. Measurement of pulmonary capillary wedge pressure should show normal pressure in the idiopathic or primary pulmonary hypertension, whereas in cardiomyopathy the wedge pressure would be high.

When confronted with the development of congestive heart failure or arrhythmias in a patient with a systemic illness that may affect the heart, the possibility of a secondary cardiomyopathy becomes strong. Appropriate diagnostic studies should be undertaken.

When amyloidosis is suspected, rectal or gum biopsies and, on occasion, myocardial biopsy will be diagnostic. Associated diseases such as multiple myeloma should be looked for.

SUGGESTED READING

Braunwald E: Natural history of idiopathic hypertrophic subaortic stenosis. In Wolsten-
  holme GEW, O'Connor M (eds): Hypertrophic Obstructive Cardiomyopathy, pp
  30–49. CIBA Foundation Study Group 37. London, J & A Churchill, 1971
Cohn JN, Franciosa JA: Vasodilator therapy of cardiac failure. N Engl J Med 297:27–31;
  254–258, 1977
Fowler NO: Differential diagnosis of cardiomyopathies. Prog Cardiovasc Dis
  14:113–128, 1971
Frank JM, Abdulla MA, Canedo MI, Saylers RE: Long-term medical management of hy-
  pertrophic obstructive cardiomyopathy. Am J Cardiol 42:933–1001, 1978
Friedberg CK: Symposium on cardiomyopathy. Circulation 44:935–968, 1971
Glancy DL, Epstein SE: Differential diagnosis of type and severity of obstruction to left
  ventricular outflow. Prog Cardiovasc Dis 14:153–191, 1971
Goodwin JF: Classification of the cardiomyopathies. Mod Concepts Cardiovasc Dis
  41:41, 1972
Goodwin JF: Treatment of cardiomyopathies. Am J Cardiol 32:341–351, 1973
Maron BJ, Epstein SE: Hypertrophic cardiomyopathy. Recent observations regarding the
  specificity of three hallmarks of the disease: asymmetric septal hypertrophy, septal
  disorganization, and systolic anterior motion of the anterior mitral leaflet. Am J
  Cardiol 45:141–154, 1980
Maron BJ, Merrill WH, Freier PA, Kent KM, Epstein SE, Morrow AG: Long term clinical
  course and symptomatic status of patients after operation for hypertrophic subaor-
  tic stenosis. Circulation 57:1205–1213, 1978
Oakley CM: Clinical recognition of the cardiomyopathies. Cir Res [Suppl]
  35(2):152–167, 1974
Regan TJ, Haider B, Ahmed S, Lyons MM, Oldewurtel HA, Ettinger PO: Whiskey and
  the heart. Cardiovasc Med 2:165–177, 1977
Stapleton JF, Segal JP, Proctor Harvey W: Clinical pathways of cardiomyopathy. Cir Res
  [Suppl] 35(2):168–178, 1974
Wigle ED, Adelman AG, Felderhof CH: Medical and surgical treatment of the cardio-
  myopathies. Cir Res [Suppl] 35(2):196–207, 1974

VALVULAR HEART DISEASE

Robert H. Eich

17

This discussion of valvular heart disease includes rheumatic valvular heart disease, the syndrome of mitral-valve prolapse, and the congenital bicuspid aortic valve, which is the commonest cause of significant aortic stenosis in the adult population. We will start first with rheumatic valvular heart disease.

RHEUMATIC HEART DISEASE

The number of patients with rheumatic heart disease compared with those with coronary artery disease is small. Mortality from rheumatic heart disease is less than 5000 per year. However, the disease kills and incapacitates men and women in their most productive years, between the ages of 30 and 40. It is a disease for which the proper management is well established, but one in which mismanagement can be disastrous. There are still too many preventable tragedies in the treatment of this disease.

ACUTE RHEUMATIC FEVER

Acute rheumatic fever remains a difficult diagnosis to make, both in children and adults. An antecedent Group A streptococcal infection is necessary, but it often is not recognized at the time when it occurs. In children, the Jones criteria are used for diagnosis. The five major criteria are:

1. Carditis
2. Polyarthritis

3. Chorea
4. Erythema marginatum
5. Subcutaneous nodules

Minor manifestations include prior rheumatic fever or rheumatic heart disease, arthralgia, fever, increased sedimentation rate, an elevated C-reactive protein, leukocytosis, or a prolonged PR interval on the EKG. For the diagnosis of acute rheumatic fever, if one of the major and two of the minor criteria are met, or two of the major, it is highly probable that the rheumatic fever is present. In adults, nodules, rash, and chorea are extremely rare, and one will have to make the diagnosis based on polyarthritis, which may be difficult to distinguish from arthralgia. Only 50% to 60% of patients with rheumatic heart disease have a positive history of having had rheumatic fever as children. However, it is important to ask about this. Rheumatic fever may have been passed over as "growing pains" in the child, and any protracted febrile episode could have been rheumatic fever.

All patients with a history of prior rheumatic fever and carditis should be on lifetime daily penicillin prophylaxis for streptococcus. This will prevent recurrence of the rheumatic fever. In addition to rheumatic fever prophylaxis, patients with known valvular heart disease should have subacute bacterial endocarditis prophylaxis prior to dental procedures, pelvic and rectal surgery, and deliveries.

CHRONIC RHEUMATIC VALVULAR HEART DISEASE

Chronic rheumatic heart disease can cause mitral stenosis, mitral insufficiency, aortic stenosis, aortic insufficiency, tricuspid stenosis, and tricuspid insufficiency. Mitral stenosis alone is always rheumatic. The other valve lesions which may be rheumatic or have other etiologies are indicated where the lesions are discussed. Mitral valve prolapse is given a separate section because it is a common abnormality occurring in 6% of the population. Rarely, it can cause chronic mitral insufficiency, but much more usually it is acute mitral insufficiency, a topic that is dealt within this chapter. We will discuss chronic rheumatic heart disease in terms of the individual valves and their lesions. Obviously, different types of lesions (stenosis or insufficiency) may be mixed in the same valve, and more than one valve may be involved in the same patient. In general, the proximal valve gives the symptoms—that is, in patients with mitral stenosis and aortic insufficiency, the symptoms are those of mitral stenosis. Similarly, in general, where the lesion is mixed, as in mitral stenosis-mitral insufficiency, the symptoms will be those of the predominant lesion. Significant mitral stenosis with some mitral insufficiency will act like mitral stenosis.

Mitral Stenosis

Mitral stenosis is the best understood of the valve lesions. This is due to the fact that beginning in 1947, mitral commissurotomy became available, and we have had 30 years of experience in treating this lesion. Mitral stenosis alone occurs four times more often in women than in men, so that in men with mitral stenosis, one should suspect concomitant mitral insufficiency, aortic disease, or the possibility of an atrial myxoma. The life history of mitral stenosis has been modified by the use of penicillin as prophylaxis against rheumatic fever. However, the natural history remains predictable. The patient will have the first episode of rheumatic fever sometime after age 5, usually in the teens. This will be followed by a 20-year asymptomatic period, although a murmur may be heard during this time. Such patients are totally asymptomatic, but the rheumatic valvulitis continues to develop and eventually produces stenosis and scarring of the mitral valve. Once symptoms of shortness of breath or ease of fatigue develop, the disease continues its inexorable course, and the patients go down one class of the New York Heart Association's ranking of the severity of heart conditions every 2 years, until in 8 years they are totally incapacitated. The inexorable clinical course reflects the continuing progression of the mitral stenosis.

While the rate of progress varies somewhat, the life history is sufficiently well documented so that once patients develop symptoms, they should be evaluated for surgery. Significant mitral stenosis is a surgical, not a medical disease. The only contribution in medical management is penicillin prophylaxis, which may slow the downhill course. Digitalis will improve the patient with atrial fibrillation by slowing the heart rate and lowering the left-atrial pressure. Diuretics will also help to lower the left-atrial pressure. However, no drug will release the obstruction to blood flow at the mitral valve which is the basic defect.

As stated, the two major symptoms of hemodynamically significant mitral stenosis are shortness of breath and ease of fatigue. Patients with rheumatic heart disease, in general, tend to be minimizers. They play down their symptoms out of fear. Patients also voluntarily limit their activity. We have all seen patients with severe mitral stenosis who plan their activities so carefully that they do not get short of breath. One must take time with the history before deciding whether patients are symptomatic or not. An important clue in the history will be the fact that the patient has given up various activities—he no longer climbs stairs, or plays golf, or bowls.

The shortness of breath on exertion has a mechanical basis, as in congestive failure. Whenever cardiac output increases, the left-atrial pressure rises, lung compliance falls, and the patient becomes short of breath. The increase in left-atrial pressure is necessary to drive blood across the stenotic valve. Similarly, factors which decrease left-ventricular filling time will also increase the left-atrial pressure. Thus, exercise not only increases the cardiac output but shortens diastole, which results in an even greater rise in left-atrial pressure. Atrial fibrillation similarly increases left-atrial pressure because of the rapid rate and a loss of the atrial contribution, which can contribute to the transport of blood across the stenotic mitral valve. Patients with mitral stenosis almost invariably become symptomatic after they develop atrial fibrillation.

The other cardinal symptom of significant mitral stenosis is fatigue. This is a difficult symptom to evaluate, of course, since it is nonspecific and very common. The typical patient with mitral stenosis is a housewife in her 30s, caring for small children at home and often working to help support the family. Obviously, she might complain of fatigue without having rheumatic heart disease. However, the fatigue here will be severe and progressive. If one is not sure, one can follow the patient for a few months to evaluate the progression of all of the symptoms which occur with significant mitral stenosis.

While not classically a symptom, the onset of atrial fibrillation is an important point in the life history of the patient. When this occurs, the patient will complain of palpitations occasionally but, more important, he will notice an increase in shortness of breath and fatigue. The onset of atrial fibrillation in the patient with mitral stenosis is a medical emergency, because of the very high risk of systemic emboli once the organized atrial contraction is lost. A clot will form in the left atrium behind the stenotic valve, and the patients have a very high incidence of embolus early after the onset of atrial fibrillation. Seventy percent of the emboli go to the brain and produce a stroke, this results in significant loss of function.

When atrial fibrillation develops, the patient should be hospitalized, given heparin, and then changed to warfarin sodium crystalline (Coumadin). A trial of cardioversion may be carried out after the patient has been on anticoagulants for 6 weeks, if the atrial fibrillation is known to be new and, in addition, if the left-atrial size as measured by the echo is below 45 mm. Contraindications to anticoagulants include a prior history of any kind of abnormal bleeding, an unreliable patient, or an unreliable laboratory. If one cannot use anticoagulants, then one must consider catheterization and valve surgery.

Other important symptoms, although not necessary for the diagnosis, are hemoptysis and recurrent respiratory infections. Hemoptysis will often be the symptom that first brings the patient in to seek medical attention, although it may occur early, before the valve is critically narrowed. The hemoptysis may be the result of recurrent respiratory infections (often called winter bronchitis), pulmonary embolus and infarction, or rupture of a bronchial vein. The bronchial veins drain into the left atrium, are subjected to high pressure, and may rupture into the bronchii. This form of hemoptysis, while rare, can be extremely impressive, and emergency mitral-valve surgery may be required to control it. Recurrent respiratory infection may be a symptom of significant mitral stenosis with pulmonary vascular congestion. The patient will complain of having had a "cold" throughout the entire winter, with a chronic cough; this cough is very often a subtle and early sign of decompensation. Edema, primarily dependent ankle edema, is a late sign, and one should not wait for this to develop before considering catheterization or surgery.

One will suspect significant mitral stenosis on the basis of the history but one must, of course, hear the characteristic murmur of mitral stenosis to be sure of the diagnosis. This is one of the more difficult murmurs to hear, especially late in the course of the disease. The murmur is low-pitched, localized to the apex, and heard best with the bell. Turning the patient on the left side, after he has done a few sit-ups, will raise cardiac output and help bring out the murmur. In some patients, there will be a presystolic accentuation, if they are in sinus rhythm, which is helpful. As the stenosis progresses, the murmur tends to become pandiastolic. Frequently, there will be a systolic murmur, indicating some mitral regurgitation.

There may be other signs that may help one suspect mitral stenosis. A right ventricular lift may be palpable just to the left of the sternum. Typically, the first sound is accentuated, the pulmonic component of the second is increased, and there is an opening snap after the second sound, which is an extremely useful sign, since it is relatively easy to hear.

Although it cannot give precise results, we use the physical examination to estimate the severity of the mitral stenosis. The presence of a right-ventricular lift and a loud P_2 suggests pulmonary hypertension, and a pandiastolic murmur indicates significant mitral stenosis. The interval between the second sound and the opening snap (2-OS) is related to the severity of the mitral stenosis. The shorter the interval, the tighter the stenosis. The mitral opening snap occurs just after the left-ventricular diastolic pressure falls below the left-atrial pressure. The higher the left-atrial pressure, the shorter the time from aortic closure to the crossover of the left-ventricular and left-atrial pressure. However, the 2-OS interval also depends on the stiffness of the valve and on left-ventricular compliance, so that it is not completely reliable.

If the history and physical examination are suggestive of mitral disease, the next step is to obtain a chest film, EKG, and an echocardiogram. The chest film is especially valuable when combined with fluoroscopy and oblique views using the barium-filled esophagus. A completely normal chest film will almost always exclude significant mitral stenosis. Some enlargement of the left atrium should be present in patients with hemodynamically significant mitral stenosis. In addition, as the left-atrial pressure exceeds 18 mmHg, signs of congestive failure develop, with venous redistribution, Kerley B lines, and haziness of the pulmonary vessels. Right-ventricular enlargement may be seen on the chest film, with significant mitral stenosis, but oblique and lateral films must be used, since heart size can appear normal on the PA film.

The echocardiogram has proved a very powerful tool in the diagnosis of mitral-valve disease. It is noninvasive and serves as an excellent screen for significant mitral stenosis. A normal mitral-valve echo excludes significant disease. As the mitral stenosis progresses, the valve is held open in diastole, so that the diastolic closing (E-F) slope becomes flatter. Stenosis can be roughly graded as mild, moderate, and severe by the degree of flattening of the E-F slope. Poor left-ventricular compliance can alter the slope, and in order to be sure that the flat slope is the result of mitral disease, the posterior leaflet should move anteriorly and follow the anterior leaflet during diastole.

The EKG is not particularly useful, since we have seen normal EKGs in patients with significant mitral stenosis; however, usually it will show evidence of both left-atrial and right-ventricular enlargement.

A symptomatic patient should have cardiac catheterization before surgery. The catheterization is needed to:

1. Evaluate the severity of the mitral stenosis by calculating the valve area (under 1.5 cm^2 is significant mitral stenosis)
2. Provide information about the other valves involved
3. Identify associated coronary artery disease, which does occur in older patients
4. Calculate pulmonary vascular resistance and assess left-ventricular function

As mitral stenosis progresses, the pulmonary vascular resistance increases. This is owing to organic change and to some element of vasoconstriction in the pulmonary vasculature, both caused by the high left-atrial pressure. While there is good evidence that pulmonary vascular resistance usually falls following mitral surgery, if it is significantly elevated before surgery, it may not return to normal. Thus, one can get some indication of what to expect from surgery, based on the pulmonary vascular resistance.

As mitral stenosis progresses, cardiac output tends to decrease because of the restricted valve flow and, in some patients, impaired ventricular function. The mechanism for abnormal performance of the left ventricle is not clear, since it does not necessarily return to normal after surgery. Therefore, a combination of high pulmonary vascular resistance and a lower-than-normal cardiac output will result in a poorer surgical result.

Once the decision is made for surgery, most surgeons prefer the mitral commissurotomy. This is done with the patient on cardiopulmonary bypass and the fused commissures opened back up under direct vision. The advantage of the commissurotomy is that the patient retains his own valve and does not require anticoagulants. The disadvantage is that the stenosis tends to recur in 6 to 8 years.

The results of surgery can be predicted with considerable accuracy. Factors include the functional capacity of the patient (that is, a class IV patient will seldom advance again to a class I). Other important factors include calcium in the valve and mitral regurgitation, both of which suggest that the mitral valve will have to be replaced at the time of surgery. Age, pulmonary vascular resistance, cardiac output, and the duration of atrial fibrillation all affect the long-term results. Patients over age 65 do not do as well as younger persons. Atrial fibrillation is an inefficient rhythm and when present for more than 6 months tends to persist after surgery. Finally, involvement of other valves, especially significant tricuspid insufficiency, will result in a less satisfactory result from surgery. After surgery, the patient should be kept on penicillin prophylaxis permanently for streptococci. Also, as previously mentioned, the stenosis can recur following a commissurotomy, and the patient must be followed closely for recurrence of symptoms with history, physical examination, chest film and echocardiogram.

Mitral Insufficiency (Mitral Regurgitation)

In discussing rheumatic mitral insufficiency, or mitral regurgitation, it is important to emphasize that the life history of regurgitant lesions (both mitral and aortic) is much less predictable than that of the stenotic lesions. Chronic mitral insufficiency is thus much more difficult to evaluate than mitral stenosis. The life history is not clearly established; and there are well-documented series in which some patients have done extremely well over many years with good medical management. The basic rule is the same as in mitral stenosis: to wait for symptoms, primarily shortness of breath and ease of fatigue. The disease is not inexorable once symptoms occur, and prognosis depends largely on left-ventricular function. Most cardiologists thus prefer to follow and wait for symptoms to develop despite good medical management. Management includes digitalis, diuretics, salt restriction, decreased activity, and (more recently) the use of vasodilators to reduce afterload and thus decrease the mitral regurgitation.

Both chronic pressure and volume overload on the left ventricle can result in irreversible deterioration in left-ventricular function, as a result of cellular changes and fibrosis. If left-ventricular function deteriorates too badly, the patient's condition may eventually become inoperable. Therefore, while we tend to be conservative in sending patients to surgery, we worry about waiting too long and about the impossibility of returning left-ventricular function once a certain stage of deterioration has been reached. Recently, it has appeared possible to follow left-ventricular function by the noninvasive techniques of the echocardiogram and the radioactive ventriculogram. Cardiac catheterization, while important, may not provide the information necessary for a surgical decision, and one must depend on progressive symptoms, increasing heart size (shown by chest film and EKG), and changes in ventricular function (shown by echocardiogram and radioactive ventriculogram) for the decision about when to intervene and replace the mitral valve.

Physical examination for mitral regurgitation is useful but does not quantitate the degree. There is left-ventricular enlargement, with a point of maximal impulse outside the midclavicular line. The point of maximal impulse is more brisk than that seen in aortic stenosis. A systolic thrill may be present at the apex. Occasionally, with massive regurgitation, the regurgitant jet can be felt as a left-parasternal lift. The P_2 sound is often widely split, because of the vigorous contraction of the left ventricle, and the A_2 sound is early. The murmur is high-pitched, pansystolic, and heard best at the apex, although in acute mitral insufficiency the murmur may decrease before the second sound. The murmur will be widely transmitted, laterally to the apex or at times even to the aortic area. There may be a short diastolic murmur at the apex. A chest film and EKG will show increased size of the left atrium and the left ventricle. The echocardiogram, while not specific for mitral regurgitation, will show the enlarged left atrium and give some measure of left-ventricular function. Cardiac catheterization is necessary, as in mitral stenosis, to assess the other valves, the presence of coronary artery disease, and left-ventricular function. Left-ventricular function is best evaluated by the ventriculogram at catheterization but as previously mentioned, can also be well measured noninvasively, using the radioactive ventriculogram or the echocardiogram. The amount of mitral regurgitation is determined by injecting dye in the left ventricle and measuring the opacification of the left atrium. The decision regarding surgery, as in all valvular heart diseases, is based first on symptoms borne out by the physical examination and noninvasive studies, followed by cardiac catheterization.

Surgery for mitral insufficiency involves valve replacement, using either the tilting-disk prosthesis or the porcine heterograft. The tilting-disk, Lillehei-Kaster or Bjork-Shiley, valve is a durable valve with a good record for mechanical competency. However, it is noisy, permits some gradient across it, and the patient must take anticoagulants during his entire lifetime. The porcine valve is now being used much more commonly for mitral-valve replacement. This valve has excellent hemodynamic characteristics, and the patients do not require anticoagulation if they are in sinus rhythm and have a fairly normal-sized left atrium. However, the durability of the porcine valve is not as good as that of the tilting-disc type, so that in 6 to 10 years the valve may have to be replaced.

Mitral-valve Prolapse

Mitral-valve prolapse is a nonrheumatic, congenital defect in the mitral valve apparatus that may occur in as many as 6% of the normal population. Some 19 different names have been applied to it, including **click-murmur syndrome** and **Barlow's syndrome.** While it can be rheumatic, normally the etiology is either idiopathic or, in some cases, familial. The basic defect is probably an abnormality in the length of the chordae tendineae, which are too long. Most patients are asymptomatic, but the history can include symptoms of atypical chest pain, ease of fatigue, and palpitations. Indications found on physical examination are classical and extremely helpful. Approximately 30% of patients will have associated thoracic skeletal abnormalities, including pectus excavatum, "straight back," with loss of the normal convexity of the thoracic spine, or scoliosis of the thoracic spine. Auscultation will reveal the systolic click, followed by an apical systolic murmur. The *click* occurs as the redundant chordae tendineae snap tight; at that instant a small part of the mitral valve leaflet prolapses into the left atrium and the systolic *murmur* begins.

The click and murmur respond in the classical manner to maneuvers which affect heart size. Standing makes the heart smaller, thus disproportioning the length of the chordae tendineae, so that the prolapse occurs earlier in systole. The click moves toward the first sound, and the murmur becomes louder and moves toward the first sound. Amyl nitrate has the same effect.

The echocardiogram shows the mitral leaflet (posterior alone, or both the posterior and anterior), prolapsing into the atrium. An echocardiogram, if positive, is sufficiently diagnostic of mitral-valve prolapse. However, at times the echocardiogram may miss a small mitral prolapse. Cardiac catheterization is seldom necessary.

The life history is usually benign. However, there is a low incidence of subacute bacterial endocarditis, for which prophylaxis should be carried out prior to dental work and pelvic surgery. There is a 1% incidence of sudden death, presumably resulting from ventricular fibrillation. Patients at risk for this would appear to be those with large numbers of premature ventricular contractions. We have recommended Holter monitoring in those with a history of palpitations, and if they demonstrate complex ventricular arrhythmias, a trial of suppression should be carried out with propranolol or quinidine. Finally, a small percentage will develop significant mitral insufficiency. This may be acute, from ruptured chordae or myxomatous degeneration of the mitral valve, or it may develop gradually.

Acute mitral insufficiency due to a ruptured chordae or ruptured mitral valve is not well tolerated and requires prompt recognition and treatment. Acute mitral insufficiency can occur following endocarditis, from rupture of a chordae rheumatic heart disease, from rupture of a chordae or a valve in the mitral valve prolapse syndrome, or more rarely from rupture of a papillary muscle or severe papillary dysfunction due to a myocardial infarction. Rarely a blunt trauma to the chest can result in a rupture of a corde or a papillary muscle. Acute mitral insufficiency can be suspected by the presence of certain features. The most important is the abrupt onset of a loud systolic murmur often associated with a systolic thrill in the patient to where a murmur had not been heard before. The murmur is pansystolic, although it may be somewhat decrescendo late in systole. Other associated findings that suggest acute mitral insufficiency are based on the normal sized left atrium. Because the insufficiency is acute, the left atrium has not dilated. Thus, there will be sinus rhythm instead of atrial fibrillation, a very loud pulmonic second sound due to the severe pulmonary hypertension resulting from the regurgitation into a small non-compliant left atrium and an S_4. By echocardiogram and by chest film the left atrial size will be normal. While the acute mitral insufficiency can be decreased somewhat by afterload reduction, cardiac catheterization and mitral valve replacement are the treatment of choice.

Aortic Stenosis

Aortic stenosis is the other lesion (besides mitral stenosis) with a well-established life history. Two times as many men as women have the disease, and symptoms classically start in the 50s. While it can be rheumatic in origin, more often aortic stenosis originates as a congenitally bicuspid aortic valve that calcifies in middle life. Rarely, in later years a normal tricuspid valve may calcify. The symptoms include shortness of breath, chest pain, and syncope. Once the patient develops any of these symptoms, there is some incidence of sudden death in aortic stenosis, presumably from both tachyarrhythmias and bradyarrhythmias. The shortness of breath is exertional, as is the chest pain. The pain is indistinguishable from angina, although classically it has been described as longer-lasting and requiring more exertion to set it off. Exertional syncope is related to the cardiac output's being fixed by severe stenosis: exercise results in vasodilatation, the cardiac output cannot rise, the blood pressure falls, and the patient faints. Less severe disease may produce only light-headedness with exertion. Syncope may also be the result of ventricular tachyarrhythmias or bradyarrhythmias secondary to calcium deposited in, and impairing function in, the conducting system. In general, once the symptoms develop, patients should undergo cardiac catheterization, and surgery, if the condition is operable. All of these symptoms carry an ominous prognosis and suggest the need for surgery.

The physical examination is helpful but not diagnostic, because of various pitfalls. First, patients with significant aortic stenosis are usually hypotensive but may be hypertensive because of intense peripheral vasoconstriction. Second, the disease produces concentric hypertrophy, so that the left ventricle may not appear enlarged because it is palpable inside of the mid-clavicular line. The point of maximal impulse will be diffuse and heaving, but not displaced. Third, an aortic systolic thrill is not necessary for the diagnosis and may not be present, although when it is present it suggests a large gradient.

The aortic stenosis murmur is typically an ejection murmur, late-peaking and diamond-shaped, which starts after the first sound and ends before the second. However, with severe aortic stenosis, left-ventricular systole may be prolonged, and the murmur may go through the pulmonic components of S_2 with no aortic component. Thus, it may not be typically an ejection murmur. The murmur is transmitted to the carotid vessels and often to the cardiac apex, making separation from the murmur of mitral regurgitation extremely difficult. One of the most useful signs is the behavior of the murmur after a premature ventricular contraction. Following a premature ventricular contraction, the murmur of aortic stenosis increases, while the mitral insufficiency murmur does not change. Many older patients will have systolic murmurs over the aortic area, owing to a tortuous aorta.

Significant aortic stenosis should be associated with a delayed upslope of the carotid pulse. This is a useful sign, and we rely on it heavily; however, the carotid pulse is modified by several things, including reflected waves, the distensibility of the artery, and the rate of rise of pressure in the left ventricle. Therefore a brisk arterial upslope can occur in severe aortic stenosis, and a prolonged upslope can occur in patients with poor left-ventricular function and very little aortic stenosis.

We have found cardiac fluoroscopy and the echocardiogram to be valuable in determining whether there is hemodynamically significant aortic stenosis. With significant aortic stenosis in the older age group, the aortic valve will be calcified at fluoroscopy. Echocardiography of the aortic valve, while not quantitative, can exclude significant aortic stenosis. A normal aortic valve on echocardiogram excludes significant calcific aortic stenosis.

If history, physical examination, cardiac fluoroscopy, and echocardiography suggest significant aortic stenosis, then cardiac catheterization should be carried out. Again, the purpose of catheterization is not only to determine the area of the aortic orifice but to evaluate the other valves and, especially, to look for mitral regurgitation, to determine the presence of coronary artery disease, and to fully evaluate left-ventricular function. The normal aortic valve is 3 cm^2. Significant aortic stenosis is felt to occur when the valve is narrowed to under 0.75 cm^2.

The mechanism for angina cannot be determined from the history. In evaluating patients for surgery, it is impossible to separate patients with aortic stenosis and normal coronary arteries, whose angina is caused by an increased oxygen need of the hypertrophied ventricle, from those with aortic stenosis and significant coronary atherosclerosis on the basis of the history. Therefore, coronary angiography is necessary. The diagnosis of aortic stenosis accompanied by mitral insufficiency is difficult, and catheterization is again necessary to make the distinction.

Cardiac surgeons are aggressive about operating for aortic stenosis, even in patients with borderline ventricular function, because surgery instantly alleviates the obstruction and permits clinical improvement. However, an ejection fraction below 20% is probably a contraindication to surgery, in that surgery will not improve the patient.

Aortic-valve replacement has been a difficult operation in the past because of the need to cross-clamp and open the aorta to gain access to the aortic valve. Since the development of cold potassium cardioplegia to arrest the heart and reduce myocardial demands, myocardial function is better preserved and surgical results have improved. Surgery involves valve replacement, and several good valves are now available. Among the prosthetic valves, the tilting-disk Lillehei-Kaster or the ball-valve of the Starr-Edwards 2400 series are both excellent and durable. However, if these are used, anticoagulants are a necessity for the lifetime of the patient. Recently, the porcine valves, which do not require the use of anti-coagulants, have been used.

Aortic Insufficiency

Chronic aortic insufficiency or regurgitation, like mitral insufficiency, is difficult to assess, because the life history is somewhat variable. Aortic insufficiency may be caused by congenital aortic valvular disease, rheumatic heart disease, aortic dissection, or endocarditis. Chronic aortic insufficiency is often rheumatic, while the acute type is more often the result of dissection or endocarditis. However, many other uncommon causes can produce significant aortic insufficiency, including myxomatous degeneration of the aortic valve, rheumatoid spondylitis, hypertension, coarctation of the aorta with a bicuspid aortic valve, and ventricular septal defect. As in the mitral valve, chronic aortic insufficiency and acute aortic insufficiency present differently. Acute aortic insufficiency is a

medical emergency, whereas mild chronic aortic insufficiency may be well tolerated for many years with no problems. In fact, patients with rheumatic aortic
insufficiency may have been quite athletic in their teens and twenties.

The important symptoms in significant aortic insufficiency include shortness of breath; which may manifest itself as paroxysmal nocturnal dyspnea; angina; and an occasional patient may complain of syncope or lightheadedness on
exertion. Some patients are aware of the abnormal pulsations produced by the
wide pulse pressure. Again, as in mitral insufficiency, the development of
symptoms depends on the state of the left-ventricular myocardium. However,
because of concern over deterioration of left-ventricular function, we use the
onset of symptoms, rather than the progression of symptoms in spite of good
medical management, as the indication for surgery.

The diagnosis of aortic insufficiency may be first suspected from the blood
pressure. Significant aortic insufficiency is characterized by a wide pulse
pressure, often over 100 mmHg, and a low diastolic pressure, below 60 mmHg.
The systolic pressure may be as high as 180 mmHg because of the large stroke
volume due to the aortic insufficiency. It should be emphasized that part of the
cause of the wide pulse pressure is vasodilatation. As congestive failure develops, the diastolic pressure may rise, owing to both peripheral vasoconstriction
and a very high diastolic pressure in the left ventricle, which reduces the backward flow. Thus a normal diastolic blood pressure of 60 or 70 may be found in
someone who is desperately ill with aortic insufficiency.

Since a wide pulse pressure can be seen in other vasodilated states, such as
thyrotoxicosis and atherosclerosis of the aorta, the diagnosis of aortic insufficiency has to be based on detection of the characteristic murmur. The murmur
may be difficult to hear and learning to hear it often requires a good deal of
practice. The classical murmur of aortic insufficiency is a high-pitched decrescendo murmur, starting immediately after the second sound. It is almost never
loud, and if it is higher than grade III in loudness, one should suspect an unusual etiology for the aortic insufficiency. To hear the murmur best, the patient
should sit up, exhale fully, lean forward, and auscultation should be carried out
in the second left and second right interspaces, using the diaphragm of the
stethoscope. Aortic insufficiency resulting from rheumatic heart disease is classically heard in the left second interspace, whereas that which is heard best in
the right second interspace suggests an unusual etiology for the aortic insufficiency. The aortic insufficiency murmur can be confused with the pulmonic insufficiency murmur, since they are both decrescendo diastolic murmurs, but the
patient with pulmonic insufficiency will almost always have severe heart disease
and pulmonary hypertension.

Other findings on physical examination which result from the wide pulse
pressure have fascinated physicians for years. These include the peripheral
signs of the wide pulse pressure, including systolic nodding of the head (de-
Musset's sign), a bounding pulse (Corrigan's pulse or water-hammer pulse),
capillary pulsations in the nailbed, and finally pistol-shot sounds over the bra-

chial and femoral arteries (Duroziez's sign). Duroziez's sign is elicited by pressure over the femoral artery with the bell of the stethoscope, so that a systolic and diastolic murmur are produced.

Other important physical findings include cardiomegaly, with the heart enlarged downward and outward lateral to the midclavicular line and in the sixth interspace, with a thrusting point of maximal impulse. The biggest hearts of all are seen with aortic insufficiency.

Besides the aortic insufficiency murmur and cardiomegaly, most patients have an aortic systolic murmur, because of the large stroke volume going across a distorted valve, and there may be mitral regurgitation, producing a regurgitant murmur at the apex. Finally, in the presence of significant aortic insufficiency, especially if left-ventricular function is somewhat compromised, the patients may have the Austin Flint murmur, which is a mid-diastolic, rumbling murmur at the apex. The best explanation for the Austin Flint murmur is that it is a combination of transmission of the aortic insufficiency murmur to the apex and fluttering of the mitral valve (caused when the aortic regurgitation produces flow against the mitral valve as it is held open in diastole).

Other important laboratory data include the chest film, which will show a large heart and, very frequently, dilatation of the ascending aorta. The EKG, in significant aortic insufficiency, will show left-ventricular enlargement. The echocardiogram will show a dilated aorta, a possibly thickened aortic valve, and fluttering or chattering of the mitral valve in diastole, which is quite suggestive of significant aortic insufficiency. However, the echo findings are not absolutely quantitative and nothing on the echocardiogram will specifically quantitate the amount of aortic insufficiency.

Because we cannot always predict the life history, and surgery for aortic insufficiency does involve valve replacement, cardiologists in general tend to be conservative about surgery. However, again, as with mitral insufficiency, undue delay can result in irreversible deterioration of left-ventricular function as a result of cellular changes and fibrosis. Therefore, while we still feel that one should usually wait for the development of symptoms (shortness of breath, angina, or syncope), we believe that a patient should be considered for surgery even if he has not developed symptoms, if there is evidence of deteriorating left-ventricular function. There is some preliminary evidence that we may be able to preselect patients likely to become symptomatic and follow these patients closely. The pulse pressure is an important prognostic sign. If the pulse pressure is over 100, the systolic pressure above 140, or the diastolic pressure below 40 mmHg, the patients tend to develop symptoms sooner. Development of left-ventricular enlargement shown by electrocardiogram; increasing heart size, shown by chest film; or deterioration in ventricular function, as judged by the radioactive ventriculogram or the echocardiogram, are now being used as criteria to select patients for catheterization studies and surgery before waiting for severe symptoms to develop.

The patient should have a cardiac catheterization prior to surgery, for the usual reasons. While left-ventricular function may be assessed noninvasively, it is always important to have an angiographic determination of the actual ejection fraction and the severity of the aortic regurgitation. In addition, a measure of the left-ventricular end diastolic pressure can serve as a prognostic indicator. If it is above 20 mmHg the patients will apparently develop problems much sooner, and this finding may help one to determine the need for surgery.

Acute aortic insufficiency can be a very serious condition. The valve leak is usually the result of aortic dissection or endocarditis, although occasionally the cause may be myxomatous degeneration of one of the aortic cusps, with abrupt onset of fulminating aortic insufficiency. The patient can deteriorate extremely rapidly, appearing clinically stable in the morning and terminal by evening. If one suspects acute aortic insufficiency, the patient should be hospitalized in an intensive care setting. Pulmonary artery pressure should be measured, using a Swan-Ganz catheter, and afterload reduction carried out using nitroprusside infusion. Cardiac catheterization should be carried out as quickly as possible, to evaluate the other valves, detect the presence of coronary artery disease, and evaluate left-ventricular function.

Occasionally, however, a patient is too sick to be catheterized and you have to go directly to surgery. In this patient, one should use all the noninvasive techniques that one can to confirm the diagnosis but should also remember that the condition can be a fairly desperate surgical emergency. Sometimes one must operate on patients with acute endocarditis which has been inadequately treated. While one is reluctant to operate in the presence of an infected valve, patients with severe aortic insufficiency will not survive without aortic-valve replacement. It is truly a medical emergency and one which requires early and constant surgical consultation for proper medical management.

Tricuspid Stenosis and Tricuspid Insufficiency

Tricuspid-valve disease is relatively uncommon as an isolated lesion. Tricuspid stenosis is almost always the result of rheumatic heart disease and usually occurs with mitral stenosis. The problem of diagnosing it may be very subtle, since the murmur can sound like that of mitral stenosis. If there is significant mitral stenosis, the clue to the presence of tricuspid stenosis will often be peripheral edema, without a great deal of shortness of breath. The diagnosis of tricuspid stenosis by cardiac catheterization requires a very high index of suspicion and a very careful measurement of pressures. A gradient across the tricuspid valve of 3 or 4 mmHg is significant.

Tricuspid insufficiency commonly occurs in longstanding rheumatic heart disease, especially mitral disease. This can be functional, due to dilatation, or organic. Again, it is an extremely difficult diagnosis to make. Classically, patients will have distended and pulsating neck veins, with a prominent v wave. The murmur of tricuspid insufficiency, heard best adjacent to the sternum in the fifth intercostal space, increases with inspiration (Carvallo's sign). However, in long-standing rheumatic heart disease, it may be difficult to elicit this sign, and the tricuspid valve should be evaluated at the time of catheterization. If this is not done, the valve should be evaluated during surgery. The prosthetic tricuspid valves available are not particularly satisfactory, so that a tricuspid annuloplasty is often carried out, especially when the insufficiency is functional. The presence of significant tricuspid disease alters the results of surgery on other valves. The tricuspid valve may be involved in the mitral-valve prolapse syndrome and occasionally in myxomatous degeneration of the tricuspid valve.

CONGENITAL HEART DISEASE

Robert Warner and Robert H. Eich

18

This chapter will deal with congenital heart disease in the adult. It is not intended to be a complete discussion of the topic. For that, the interested reader is referred to a superb book covering the subject, *The Clinical Recognition of Congenital Heart Disease*, by Joseph K. Perloff.

Congenital heart disease makes up only a small percentage of the heart disease seen in adults. Since congenital heart disease is cared for primarily by pediatric cardiologists, most adult cardiologists have rather limited experience of it. In general, we will limit ourselves to the types of congenital heart disease which are more common and survive to adult life. The case of the complex cyanotic infant is beyond the scope of this book, and we will not discuss such entities as truncus arteriosus or tricuspid atresia.

Common congenital heart diseases seen in the adult include atrial septal defect (which is the most common), ventricular septal defect, patent ductus arteriosus, coarctation of the aorta, pulmonic stenosis, and aortic stenosis. In addition, congenitally corrected transposition of the great vessels, tetralogy of Fallot, and Ebstein's anomaly occasionally will be seen in adults, and obviously a few complex anomalies, as well as those which have been treated surgically will be seen in adults.

The diagnosis in the patient with congenital heart disease can be somewhat bewildering but, as we have said, it is simplified somewhat by the filtering process of the patient's having lived to reach adult life. Starting with the history, there are several important questions. First, is there a history of a murmur dating back to either birth or childhood? This may not always be helpful, since many children have functional murmurs. However, the question is still useful. The presence of a murmur can sometimes be supported by a history of slow growth and development, recurrent respiratory infections, or even the fact that the patient was kept out of gym class in school because of a murmur. Another key point in the history is the presence of cyanosis. A history of cyanosis at birth surviving to adult life is highly suggestive of a tetralogy of Fallot. Cyanosis developing later in life is much more likely to be due to shunt reversal from an elevation in the pulmonary artery pressure, which can occur in atrial septal defects, ventricular septal defects, and patent ductus arteriosus.

The physical examination will also help to establish the diagnosis. First, the presence of cyanosis and the often associated clubbing of the nail beds can be determined. Coarctation of the aorta is recognized by hypertension limited to the upper extremities. Specific chamber enlargement will help to establish whether a valve is stenotic, right-ventricular enlargement obviously being the result of pulmonic stenosis. In atrial septal defects, a very characteristic finding is a wide split, often fixed, of the second sound. Finally, the presence of a murmur, and its location and type, will do much to establish the diagnosis. An ejection murmur is seen with stenotic valves. A regurgitant murmur along the left sternal border is seen with ventricular septal defect. The flow murmur of an atrial septal defect is heard best along the left sternal border into the pulmonary outflow tract.

Noninvasive studies are valuable. The chest film is used to determine chamber enlargement, and the presence of increased pulmonary blood flow, resulting from a left-to-right shunt, may indicate a septal defect or a patent ductus arteriosus. The electrocardiogram is helpful in determining chamber enlargement and in separating ostium secundum atrial septal defect from ostium primum atrial septal defect, which has an abnormal left-axis deviation. Finally, the echocardiogram appears to be developing as a very powerful diagnostic tool, especially in children with complex anomalies. In the infant, because the ribs are not calcified, the echocardiogram can actually be used to determine much of the anatomy. In the adult, the echo will also determine chamber enlargement and be very suggestive of a left-to-right shunt, if there is paradoxical motion of the septum.

Cardiac catheterization is indicated wherever congenital heart disease is suspected in the adult, even if the patient is not being considered for surgery, in order to establish the diagnosis.

The incidence of the various lesions is variable, depending on the age group studied. In brief, Nadas, in his book *Pediatric Cardiology*, states that in the pediatric age group, ventricular septal defect alone or in combination with pulmonic stenosis is the most common of the congenital heart disease abnormalities. The rest is made up of atrial septal defect (10%–15%), patent ductus arteriosus, coarctation of the aorta, aortic stenosis, pulmonic stenosis, and finally, transposition. As we have stated, in patients who survive to adult life, atrial septal defect becomes most common, and patients with uncorrected transposition of the great vessels usually do not survive childhood.

Most classifications of adult congenital heart disease are based on the pres-

Table 18-1. Congenital Heart Disease: Clinical Findings

DEFECT	CYANOSIS	CHAMBER ENLARGEMENT	P₂	MURMUR	CHEST FILM	EKG	ECHOCARDIOGRAM
Valvular Pulmonic Stenosis	0	Right ventricle	Lessened intensity Widesplit	Ejection murmur in the pulmonic area Ejection click	Right-ventricular enlargement Normal pulmonary blood flow Poststenotic dilatation	Right-axis deviation Right-ventricular enlargement	Right ventricular-enlargement; if severe, increased a wave on the pulmonic valve
Ebstein's Anomaly	20%	Quiet precordium	Single	Tricuspid insufficiency	Globular heart Clear lungs Large right atrium	Wolff-Parkinson-White Syndrome (25%) Right-atrial enlargement Atypical right bundle-branch block	Tricuspid valve displaced and abnormal
Atrial Septal Defect (Primum)	0	Right-, and possibly left-ventricle enlargement	Wide and Fixed	Flow murmur, left sternal border Mitral regurgitation murmur	Increased pulmonary blood flow Enlargement of pulmonary artery, right ventricle, and atrium Enlargement of left atrium and ventricle	Incomplete right bundle-branch block Left-axis deviation	Defect in the atrioventricular valves Paradoxical septal motion
Atrial Septal Defect (Secundum)	0	Right-ventricular lift	Wide and fixed	Flow murmur, left sternal border	Increased pulmonary-artery size; Increased pulmonary blood flow Right ventricular-and right-atrial enlargement	Incomplete right bundle-branch block	Right-ventricular enlargement Paradoxical septal motion
Ventricular Septal Defect	0	Thrill, left sternal border Left-ventricle enlargement	Variable	Regurgitant murmur, left sternal border	Increased pulmonary blood flow Enlargement of right and left ventricle	Biatrial and biventricular enlargement	Increased left-atrium size Left-ventricular dilatation Septal defect visualized at times

Table 18-1. Continued

DEFECT	CYANOSIS	CHAMBER ENLARGEMENT	P₂	MURMUR	CHEST FILM	EKG	ECHOCARDIOGRAM
Patent Ductus Arteriosus	0	Wide pulse pressure Left ventricle enlargement	Variable	Continuous murmur, "machinery murmur"	Increased pulmonary blood flow Left-ventricular and left-atrial enlargement	Left ventricular enlargement	Increased left atrium size Left-ventricular dilatation
Tetrology	+	Right ventricle enlargement	Lessened intensity	Ejection murmur	Decreased pulmonary artery size Decreased pulmonary blood flow No specific chamber enlargement Boot-shaped heart	Right ventricular enlargement	Overriding of the aorta Right-ventricular enlargement

ence or absence of cyanosis and the presence of increased, decreased, or normal pulmonary blood flow. A classification modified from Perloff is presented in the accompanying list. Some of the typical findings related to the common lesions are given in Table 18-1.

CLINICAL CLASSIFICATION OF ADULT CONGENITAL HEART DISEASE

1. *Acyanotic without a shunt*
   a. Malformations originating in the left heart
      1) Aortic stenosis: valvular; subvalvular
      2) Coarctation of the aorta
      3) Congenital mitral insufficiency: endocardial cushion defect; corrected transposition; miscellaneous
      4) Congenital obstruction to left-atrial flow
      5) Congenital aortic insufficiency
   b. Malformations originating in the right heart
      1) Pulmonic stenosis: valvular; infundibular
      2) Idiopathic dilatation of the pulmonary artery
      3) Congenital pulmonary-value insufficiency
      4) Primary pulmonary hypertension
      5) Ebstein's anomaly of the tricuspid valve
2. *Acyanotic with a shunt (left-to-right shunt)*
   a. Shunt at the atrial level
      1) Atrial septal defect: osteum secundum; osteum primum; sinus venosus
   b. Shunt at the ventricular level
      1) Ventricular septal defect—isolated: infracristal; supracristal; cushion defect involving the atrioventricular valves
      2) Ventricular septal defect with mild pulmonic stenosis—acyanotic tetralogy; other complicating lesions
   c. Shunt between aortic root and right heart
      1) Coronary areriovenous fistula
      2) Ruptured sinus Valsalva aneurysm
   d. Shunt at more than one level
      1) Complete endocardial cushion defect
3. *Cyanotic with a shunt (right-to-left shunt)*
   a. Normal or decreased pulmonary blood flow
      1) Dominant right ventricle: tetralogy of Fallot
      2) Dominant left ventricle: Ebstein's anomaly with right-to-left shunt at the atrial level
      3) Normal or nearly normal ventricles: pulmonary arteriovenous fistulas
   b. Elevated pulmonary artery pressure
      1) Ventricular septal defect with reversed shunt—Eisenmenger's complex

      2) Atrial septal defect or patent ductus arteriosus with reversed shunt

      3) Complete transposition with high pulmonary vascular resistance

  c. Increased pulmonary blood flow

      1) Complete transposition

      2) Taussig-Bing anomaly—right-ventricular origin of both vessels

      3) Truncus arteriosus

      4) Fallot tetralogy with pulmonary atresia and increased bronchial artery flow

(Modified from Perloff, JK: The Clinical Recognition of Congenital Heart Disease. ed. 2. Philadelphia, W. B. Saunders, 1978)

INTERATRIAL SEPTAL DEFECT

OSTIUM SECUNDUM DEFECT

We will start first with the interatrial septal defect and left-to-right shunt. Atrial septal defect of the secundum variety is the congenital heart disease most commonly found in adults. The patients are asymptomatic, and, while their exercise tolerance may not actually be normal, they are not aware of a reduced exercise tolerance.

The most common site of the interatrial communication in the atrial septal defect is the region of the fossa ovalis. The basic hemodynamic abnormality associated with an atrial septal defect is a left-to-right shunt of oxygenated blood, occurring at the level of the atrium. In defects larger than about 2 cm^2, the right and left atria are in free communication, so that no pressure gradient exists between them. The existence of a left-to-right shunt without such a gradient is the result of the fact that the right ventricle has greater diastolic compliance than the left ventricle. A corollary of this is that in patients with a large atrial septal defect, the magnitude of the shunt is determined by the disparity in the degree of distensibility (that is, compliance) of the two ventricles. For example, as patients with atrial septal defects grow older, they may acquire diseases such as systemic hypertension, which further reduce left-ventricular compliance. Under these circumstances, the magnitude of the left-to-right shunt increases. Conversely, 10% to 15% of patients with secundum atrial septal defects develop pulmonary hypertension as a result of anatomical changes in the pulmonary arteriolar bed. The mechanism for the changes has not been well established, but at some point they became irreversible. The resultant progressive thickening of the right ventricle and fall in its diastolic compliance reduces, and many eventually reverse, the direction of the shunt, so that it finally shifts from right to left and produces cyanosis.

Secundum atrial septal defect is significantly more common in women than in men. Although most patients remain asymptomatic through early adulthood, symptoms begin in the fifth and sixth decades of life, usually because of failure of the right ventricle or pulmonary hypertension. The most common symptoms are exertional dyspnea and fatigue, and there is often a history of frequent respiratory infections. Besides the relative changes in ventricular distensibility discussed above, another factor that may contribute to the hemodynamic deterioration of patients with atrial septal defect is development of atrial tachyarrhythmias, usually atrial fibrillation or flutter. The arrhythmia not only results in a sensation of palpitations but may precipitate or worsen the symptoms of heart failure. In some patients with pulmonary hypertension, chest discomfort indistinguishable from angina pectoris may occur. In addition, some patients may have hemoptysis.

Patients with secundum atrial septal defect are often smaller in stature than their normal siblings. The arterial pulse may be reduced in amplitude, if there is a large left-to-right shunt. Cyanosis is present if there is a significant right-to-left shunt. The abnormalities of the jugular venous pulse in patients with atrial septal defect are variable, depending on the right-ventricular pressure. For example, the development of right-ventricular failure may not be associated with increased systemic venous pressure, because the elevated right-atrial pressure may be directly transmitted to the left atrium. On the other hand, left-ventricular failure may result in an increase in right-atrial and, therefore, jugular venous pressures, because of the communication across the atrial septal defect. A large a wave in the jugular venous pulse may result from the loss of right-ventricular compliance, and a large v wave may result from the development of tricuspid insufficiency. The patient with an uncomplicated atrial septal defect has a vigorous, but brief, right-ventricular impulse, felt to the left of the sternum, and an inconspicuous left-ventricular impulse at the apex. Pulmonary-artery pulsations may be felt over the second left interspace. If pulmonary hypertension is present, the right-ventricular impulse becomes more forceful and sustained, the pulmonary arterial pulsations become more prominent, and the pulmonic-valve closure may be palpable.

The auscultatory findings of atrial septal defect depend, again, on whether or not there is pulmonary hypertension. In an uncomplicated secundum atrial septal defect, the first heart sound is often rather loud. Because of the large volume of blood that the right ventricle must eject, pulmonary closure is delayed, which results in the wide splitting of the pulmonic second sound. The increased volume of blood that returns to the right heart during inspiration is distributed equally between the right and left atria, because of flow across the defect. This results in fixed splitting, which does not vary with respiration. However, a wide split alone should alert the listener to the possibility of an atrial septal defect; the split does not necessarily have to be fixed. Patients with dilatation of the pulmonary artery often have a pulmonic ejection click, heard early in systole.

The large flow across the pulmonic valve results in a crescendo-decrescendo systolic murmur, loudest over the second left interspace but also heard well along the left sternal border. Similarly, the large volume of flow across the tricuspid valve caused by the left-to-right shunt may produce a rumbling diastolic murmur that may mimic the murmur of mitral or tricuspid stenosis. This is heard to the left of the sternum, rather than at the apex, and has a somewhat higher-pitched quality than the murmurs of mitral or tricuspid stenosis. However, at times, differentiating between atrial septal defect and mitral stenosis by auscultation may be very difficult. With very large shunts, systolic murmurs may be audible over the peripheral lung fields from augmented flow through the distal branches of the pulmonary artery.

If pulmonary hypertension supervenes in a patient with secundum atrial septal defect, the pulmonic component of the second heart sound becomes even louder. If the left-to-right shunt is obliterated, the splitting of the second sound becomes normal. With diminished compliance of the right ventricle, a right-sided S_4 sound may appear. As the left-to-right shunt decreases, the pulmonic ejection murmur becomes shorter and softer, and the diastolic tricuspid-flow murmur commonly disappears. If right-ventricular dilatation occurs because of the increased pulmonary-artery pressure, the typical holosystolic murmur of tricuspid regurgitation may be heard. With significant pulmonary hypertension, an early diastolic murmur of pulmonic insufficiency (Graham Steell murmur) may occur.

The electrocardiogram in uncomplicated atrial septal defect characteristically shows a pattern of incomplete right bundle-branch block, best seen in lead V_1. With the development of pulmonary hypertension, changes suggesting right-ventricular enlargement, such as increased amplitude of the R' wave in lead V_1 and right-axis deviation, often occur. The radiologic findings in secundum atrial septal defect can be predicted from the pathophysiology of this disorder. With a significant left-to-right shunt, there is prominence of the pulmonary arteries, hyperemic lung fields, evidence of right-atrial and right-ventricular enlargement, a diminutive aortic shadow, and a normal-sized left atrium and ventricle. In a patient who has developed pulmonary hypertension as a result of increased pulmonary vascular resistance, the right ventricle and the main trunks of the pulmonary artery become even larger, and there is oligemia of the peripheral lung fields.

The echocardiogram in secundum atrial septal defect is helpful and reveals right-ventricular enlargement and paradoxical motion of the interventricular septum. The finding of paradoxical motion of the interventricular septum occurs with left-to-right shunts in which the pulmonic blood flow is 1 to 1½ times that of the systemic flow. Therefore, the absence of paradoxical motion does not completely exclude an atrial septal defect. In as many as 30% of patients with secundum atrial septal defect, there is prolapse of the posterior leaflet of the mitral valve.

If an atrial septal defect is suspected in a patient, cardiac catheterization is indicated to confirm the diagnosis and to identify any associated abnormalities. The presence of the intracardiac shunt can be demonstrated and quantitated using oximetry and dye-dilution curves. With a left-to-right shunt, there is an increase in the oxygen saturation of the venous blood at the level of the right atrium. With a right-to-left shunt, there is desaturation of the systemic arterial blood. The degree of the left-to-right and right-to-left shunt can be calculated using the Fick principle, and, in general, a 2-to-1 left-to-right shunt, in which the pulmonary blood flow is twice that of the systemic, is an indication for surgery.

An atrial septal defect with a significant left-to-right shunt should be closed surgically, even if the patient is not yet symptomatic. The mortality rate associated with closure of an uncomplicated atrial septal defect is extremely low, and the procedure is indicated to prevent the long-term complications of the disorder. The major complication, of course, is the development of pulmonary hypertension.

If the patient already has pulmonary hypertension, with balancing or reversal of the shunt, surgery is contraindicated, and medical management is directed towards preventing a manifestation of right heart failure. Other possible complications of atrial septal defect include paradoxical emboli, a venous embolus crossing the septal defect and producing an arterial embolus, and, as already stated, atrial fibrillation as a late complication. Subacute bacterial endocarditis is a very rare complication of atrial septal defect. In some patients with atrial septal defect, the right pulmonary veins may appear to enter either the right atrium or a systemic vein, directly. This has been called **partial anomalous pulmonary vein** or **pulmonary venous connection.** This abnormality of pulmonary venous drainage almost never occurs alone and usually occurs in association with an atrial septal defect. The abnormality associated with an atrial septal defect is the same whether partial anomalous venous return exists or not.

OSTIUM PRIMUM DEFECT

If the defect is in the lower part of the atrial septum, this may be a part of the ostium primum defect. Although ostium primum defect can occur as an isolated anomaly, it is usually associated with some defect of the atrioventricular valves, part of the so-called endocardial cushion defect. Perloff has used the terms **complete endocardial cushion defect** and **partial** or **incomplete cushion defect.** The incomplete cushion defect is most often the ostium primum defect in association with a cleft mitral valve. Complete cushion defect usually is not compatible with survival to adult life if it remains uncorrected; since it must be dealt with by pediatric cardiologists, we will not discuss it further.

Patients with incomplete cushion defect of the ostium primum and a cleft mitral valve may survive until adult life. The nature of the altered physiology depends on the size of the atrial defect and the amount of mitral insufficiency. Major mitral insufficiency can occur with a very small atrial defect, in which case the pathophysiology will be that of mitral insufficiency. On the other hand, there may be a large atrial septal defect and only minimal mitral insufficiency, in which case the defect will act in the same way as an ostium secundum defect.

In the history, the symptoms of the ostium primum defect usually begin sooner in infancy or childhood, and the patients are much more symptomatic than those with the ostium secundum defect, who are generally asymptomatic in childhood.

On physical examination, the pulmonic second sound is widely split, as in the ostium secundum defect, and the split may be fixed. If there is significant mitral insufficiency, the physical findings will include left-ventricular enlargement, with the point of maximal impulse displaced down and out to the left, and the murmur of mitral insufficiency.

The electrocardiogram is invaluable to separate ostium primum defects from ostium secundum defects. The ostium primum defect will manifest left-axis deviation, which may be extreme. However, the absence of left-axis deviation does not entirely exclude an ostium primum defect, and left-axis deviation can occur in secundum defects.

The chest film, again, will depend on the amount of mitral insufficiency, in conjunction with the amount of shunt from left to right. However, if there is significant mitral insufficency, the chest film will show left-ventricular enlargement and even left-atrial enlargement. If the amount if mitral insufficiency is small, the chest film will resemble that of the ostium secundum defect with pulmonary plethora.

VENTRICULAR SEPTAL DEFECT

In most patients with a ventricular septal defect, the lesion is in the membranous portion of the interventricular septum, below the crista supraventricularis. The direction and magnitude of the shunt in a patient with a ventricular septal defect is a function of the size of the defect and the relative resistances of the systemic and pulmonary arterial systems. If the defect is smaller than 1 cm^2, the pressure on the left side of the defect is greater than that on the right, and the blood, thus, is shunted from left to right along that gradient. With larger defects, however, the ventricles are in free communication. If pulmonary vascular resistance is lower than systemic vascular resistance, a left-to-right shunt will be present, despite the absence of a pressure gradient between the left and right ventricles. If the pulmonary vascular resistance becomes elevated, the shunt will decrease in magnitude and may reverse and become right to left.

In many patients, the size of the ventricular septal defect decreases significantly and may even close completely, spontaneously. This generally occurs in infancy or childhood, but it has been documented on rare occasion in young adults. The pathological changes that tend to restrict right-ventricular emptying and, thus, predispose to the development of a right-to-left shunt, are of two types. The first is narrowing of the pulmonary arterioles, with consequent pulmonary hypertension. The second is narrowing of the right-ventricular outflow track, as a result of infundibular pulmonic stenosis associated with right-ventricular hypertrophy.

The clinical course of patients with ventricular septal defects is largely determined by the size of the defect. With a small ventricular septal defect, there is no functional disturbance, and the defect often closes early in life. With a moderate-sized defect the pulmonary pressures usually remain normal, and the magnitude of the left-to-right shunt tends to decrease with time. With large defects and associated pulmonary hypertension, one of three possibilities will occur. First, there may be a reduction in the magnitude of the left-to-right shunt, either by diminution in the size of the defect or by the development of infundibular pulmonic stenosis, and, as the shunt decreases, the pulmonary hypertension may decrease. Second, the left-to-right shunt may remain large, with continued volume overload of the left ventricle and with the eventual development of left-ventricular failure. Third, there may be a progressive increase in the pulmonary vascular resistance, with eventual reversal of the shunt and the development of right-ventricular failure and cyanosis.

Left-ventricular failure as a result of ventricular septal defect usually occurs in infancy or early childhood. Patients who survive into adulthood without this complication either have an initially small defect, have spontaneous reduction in the size of the defect, or develop obstruction to the right-ventricular outflow as a result of infundibular stenosis. Thus, spontaneous improvement in the manifestations of left-ventricular failure in an adult patient with ventricular septal defect may be associated with a sustained overall hemodynamic improvement or may herald the onset of right-ventricular failure. In patients with ventricular septal defects of any size, there is a risk of bacterial endocarditis at the site of impact of the "jet" lesion associated with a defect.

Patients with a large ventricular septal defect are often of small stature because of retarded growth and development. If a right-to-left shunt is present, cyanosis and clubbing of the fingers are prominent features. Right-ventricular failure may be associated with an elevation of the jugular venous pressure and accentuated a and v waves. A parasternal thrill to the left of the sternum is very common in all but the smallest ventricular septal defect. With a left-to-right shunt, the left-ventricular impulse is hyperdynamic. As pulmonary hypertension develops and the shunt reverses, the left-ventricular impulse becomes quiet, and the right-ventricular impulse is prominent. Under the latter circumstance, the pulmonary artery and the pulmonic-valve closure sound may become readily palpable. The pulmonic second sound is not fixed, so that the split will vary with respiration, but the split may be quite wide, depending on the magnitude of the shunt.

The murmur associated with a ventricular septal defect tends to be maximal in the third and fourth intercostal spaces, just to the left of the sternum. Its characteristics depend upon the size of the defect and the height of the right-ventricular pressure. The murmur of a small ventricular septal defect may occur only early in systole, because the defect tends to close as systole progresses, or, with a larger ventricular septal defect, the murmur may be holosystolic. With a larger defect, not only is the murmur holosystolic, but it is louder and harsher. As the right-ventricular pressure rises and the left-to-right shunt decreases, the murmur occurs earlier in systole and then disappears as the shunt becomes balanced. The typical auscultatory features of pulmonary hypertension, as discussed under atrial septal defects, may now appear.

The electrocardiogram of a patient with a ventricular septal defect depends upon the hemodynamic status. It may be perfectly normal in a small defect, or it may show evidence of left, right, or biventricular enlargement. The appearance of the chest film, similarly, depends upon the size of defect and the direction and magnitude of the shunt. The radiologic findings are similar to those described with an atrial septal defect in the evidence for increased pulmonary blood flow. However, the existence of left-atrial and left-ventricular enlargement helps to identify the ventricular septal defect, since these features are very unusual in atrial septal defects. At cardiac catheterization, the shunt can be demonstrated at the ventricular level by oximetry and dye-dilution curves. In addition, left-ventriculography reveals the contrast material shunting into the right ventricle via the defect.

Most patients with symptomatic ventricular septal defects undergo surgical repair in early childhood. Operation at any age should be advised if the shunt is above 1.4:1.0 and the pulmonary vascular resistance is not elevated. The risk of the operation is low, and the patient then is protected against possible development of pulmonary hypertension. In patients with a balanced or reversed shunt resulting from pulmonary hypertension, surgery is contraindicated. All patients with an uncorrected ventricular septal defect should receive antibiotic prophylaxis against bacterial endocarditis for dental procedures or pelvic surgery.

PATENT DUCTUS ARTERIOSUS

Patent ductus arteriosus represents persistence of the fetal communication between the aorta and the pulmonary artery. With a small-caliber communication, there are no significant hemodynamic changes. As the size of the ductus (and, thus, the magnitude of the left-to-right shunt) increases, there is volume overload of the left ventricle, often with resultant left-ventricular failure. With large shunts through a patent ductus arteriosus, pulmonary hypertension frequently occurs. If the pulmonary vascular resistance exceeds the systemic vascular resistance, then the shunt will reverse and go from right to left. The development of pulmonary hypertension in a patient with a large patent ductus arteriosus results from any of the following factors: direct transmission of aortic pressure to the pulmonary artery, increased pulmonary blood flow, pulmonary venous hypertension secondary to left-ventricular failure, and a pathological narrowing of the pulmonary arterioles, resulting in a high pulmonary-vascular resistance. Right-ventricular failure commonly results from the increased afterload imposed upon it by pulmonary hypertension.

Patent ductus arteriosus is significantly more common in women than men, often occurs in siblings, and may be associated with a history of maternal rubella in the first trimester. Symptoms of left or right heart failure can occur at any age, depending upon the hemodynamics associated with the individual lesion. Patients with a patent ductus arteriosus of any size are at risk of bacterial endocarditis resulting from the jet lesions striking the intima of the pulmonary artery at the site of the ductus.

Cyanosis is an important physical finding in patients with patent ductus ateriosus and a right-to-left shunt. Because the site of the ductus in the aorta is distal to the left subclavian artery, cyanosis (and clubbing) are characteristically confined to the lower extremities. However, more rarely because of the proximity of the ductus to the left subclavian artery, there may be some cyanosis and clubbing of the left, but not of the right, hand.

Patients with a patent ductus arteriosus with a large left-to-right shunt characteristically have a bounding pulse and a wide pulse pressure similar to that found in aortic insufficiency. The volume overload of the left ventricle raises the systolic pressure, and the rapid runoff of blood from the aorta to the pulmonary artery lowers the diastolic pressure. The jugular venous pressure increases if right-ventricular failure occurs, and prominent a waves appear if right-ventricular compliance decreases significantly as a result of the pressure overload. Whether the left- or right-ventricle is the more prominent on palpation is a function of the particular hemodynamic state associated with the defect. If the pulmonary vascular resistance is normal, then the left ventricle will be more prominent.

The murmur of a patent ductus arteriosus is best heard in the first and second left intercostal spaces, with either the bell or the diaphragm. With a left-to-right shunt, the murmur is continuous, that is, it continues uninterrupted through the second heart sound, and it peaks at that point. The murmur associated with a small shunt is usually soft and high-pitched, while the larger shunts result in the classical noisy "machinery murmur." As pulmonary hypertension develops, the pulmonary diastolic pressure approaches systemic levels, so that the diastolic portion of the murmur disappears. The patient is left with only a holosystolic murmur. Eventually, as the pulmonary hypertension increases, even the systolic murmur will shorten and eventually disappear. By this time, the findings of severe pulmonary hypertension can be elicited.

As in ventricular septal defect, the EKG can be normal or can show evidence of enlargement of the left or right ventricle, or of both, depending upon the hemodynamic characteristics of the shunt. The chest film is similar to that seen with a ventricular septal defect, with a comparable shunt. A significant difference, however, is that with a patent ductus arteriosus and a left-to-right shunt, there is dilatation of the ascending aorta. In older patients, calcification of a portion of the ductus can often be seen on the chest film. Cardiac catheterization reveals a left-to-right shunt in the pulmonary artery. Left-ventricular or aortic-root angiography results in prompt appearance of the dye in the pulmonary artery. In patients with a left-to-right shunt without severe pulmonary vascular disease, surgical closure of the patent ductus arteriosus should be carried out. The risk of surgery is minimal, and ligation of the ductus is curative.

COARCTATION OF THE AORTA

Coarctation of the aorta usually consists of a discrete narrowing of the aorta just distal to the left subclavian artery. It is commonly associated with other congenital cardiac abnormalities, most notably a biscuspid aortic valve. The coarctation results in hypertension in the upper portions of the body, with a decreased arterial pressure and delay in transmission of the arterial pulse to the legs. The left ventricle is subject to an increased afterload, because of the obstruction in the aorta. If the coarctation coexists with a bicuspid aortic valve, the valve may be stenotic or insufficient, producing an additional burden on the left ventricle.

Coarctation of the aorta is seen more commonly in men than in women. However, women with Turner's syndrome have an increased incidence of the abnormality. Patients with aortic coarctation usually first become symptomatic either early in infancy or during the third decade of life. The clinical course is determined by the severity of the narrowing, as well as by any associated abnormalities. Left-ventricular failure is the common manifestation of coarctation. Similarly, patients with coarctation are at a markedly increased risk for dissecting aortic aneurysm, which may occur either proximal or distal to the coarctation. Uncommonly, perforation of the aorta may occur at the site of poststenotic dilatation, with bleeding into the esophagus. Bacterial infections are an additional complication of coarctation of the aorta and may occur more commonly on the associated bicuspid aortic valve and less frequently distal to the coarctation. Finally, there is an incidence of intracranial aneurysms which may lead to a subarachnoid hemorrhage; this is most likely to occur in adolescents or young adults.

Physical examination reveals a higher systolic pressure in the arms than in the legs. In rare patients, in whom the coarctation actually involves the origin of the left subclavian artery, the right arm may be hypertensive and the left arm normotensive. Simultaneous palpation of the brachial and femoral arteries reveals a delay in the transmission of the pulse to the femoral arteries. The presence of significant aortic stenosis may lower the pressure in the arms, but the disparity between upper and lower extremities will still be noted. If left-ventricular enlargement results from the coarctation, a sustained, vigorous apical impulse is present. Aortic pulsations can often be detected in the second and third right intercostal space, and a suprasternal thrill is a frequent finding.

Systolic murmurs are common in aortic coarctation, and may arise in the coarctation itself, in a bicuspid aortic valve, or from flow through the collateral channels that have developed to bypass the obstruction. The systolic murmurs are ejection in type and usually loudest along the upper left sternal border or in the suprasternal notch and along the course of the collateral vessels. In addition, the coarctations may result in the murmur over the region of the thoracic spine, heard best in the back. Since, as already mentioned, many patients with coarctation will have an associated bicuspid aortic valve, a murmur of aortic stenosis or aortic insufficiency may be heard.

The electrocardiogram may be normal, or it may show left-ventricular enlargement. The classical pathognomonic chest-film finding of coarctation is notching of the inferior surface of the posterior ribs, caused by dilated collateral channels. Additional findings include dilatation of the ascending or descending aorta, sometimes with an aneurysm. Dilatation of the first portion of the left subclavian artery is often apparent on the chest film. At times in the chest film, a pattern in the shape of a "(3)" will be seen, with one convexity representing the large left subclavian artery, the narrowing being due to the coarctation, and a second convexity which represents dilatation of the aorta distal to the coarctation (poststenotic enlargement). Nonspecific abnormalities shown on the chest film include left-atrial and a ventricular enlargement and evidence of pulmonary congestion if the patient is in failure.

Cardiac catheterization reveals a pressure gradient across the coarctation. The narrowing can be seen at aortography, which is very helpful to the surgeon, since he is able to identify where the large collaterals occur and can thus avoid them at the time of operation.

It must be stressed that the only therapy for coarctation is surgical correction, which should be performed as soon as the condition is detected. Delay may result in the patient's not having his blood pressure returned to normal after surgery. In addition, because the technique was not perfected in former years, many children who were operated upon years ago have become hypertensive again and will have to have new surgery. For this reason, all patients who have had surgery for coarctations should be followed closely.

PULMONIC STENOSIS

Obstruction to the outflow of blood from the right ventricle may occur at the valvular, subvalvular, or supravalvular levels. Because the valvular type of pulmonic stenosis is the one most commonly seen in adults, the present discussion will be confined to this entity. The consequences of the lesion are in direct proportion to the severity of the obstruction. The major clinical manifestation is right-ventricular failure, resulting from pressure overload in that chamber.

Valvular pulmonic stenosis is equally common in men and women. Many survive into adulthood, partly because the area of the pulmonic valve tends to increase as the remainder of the body grows. Conversely, pathological changes, including calcification, may actually decrease the size of the pulmonic orifice as the individual ages. In such patients, hemodynamic deterioration may occur rapidly. The most common initial symptoms are dyspnea and fatigue, secondary to the low cardiac output. Because of the limitation in cardiac output imposed by the stenotic valve, exercise-induced syncope may occur. Patients with pulmonic stenosis are at increased risk for bacterial endocarditis.

Cyanosis may be seen in the extremities of patients with isolated severe pulmonic stenosis. This, however, is usually acrocyanosis caused by a low cardiac output, rather than central cyanosis from a right-to-left shunt. It should be emphasized that patients with central cyanosis will have discoloration of the mucous membrane as well as the extremities. However, in some patients with pulmonic stenosis, there may be a right-to-left shunt through a patent foramen ovale. With failure of the right ventricle, as in the other lesions, peripheral edema and hepatomegaly may occur.

One of the classical physical findings of pulmonic stenosis is increased prominence of the a wave in the jugular venous pulse. This reflects the necessity for a vigorous right-atrial contraction to adequately fill the hypertrophied right ventricle. If right-ventricular dilatation occurs, prominent v waves may occur in the venous pulses because of tricuspid-valve insufficiency. Palpation reveals a right-ventricular impulse which may vary in prominence from a gentle tap to a sustained lift. A thrill may often be palpated in the second and third left interspaces. Palpable pulmonary-arterial pulsations are characteristically absent. The first heart sound is normal. The intensity of the pulmonic component decreases with the severity of the stenosis, and the width of the splitting of the second heart sound increases. As in normal subjects, the width of the splitting of the second sound increases with inspiration. Because of diminished right-ventricular compliance, a right-sided S_4 sound is common in severe pulmonic stenosis. In the presence of right-ventricular failure, an S_3 sound may be heard.

The systolic murmur of pulmonic stenosis is of the crescendo-decrescendo ejection type and is preceded by a pulmonic ejection click early in systole. As the severity of the stenosis increases, the interval between the S_1 sound and the click decreases, and the murmur becomes longer and peaks later in systole.

The electrocardiogram often shows evidence of right-atrial and right-ventricular enlargement. As the severity of the pulmonic stenosis increases, there tends to be an increase in the amplitude of the R waves in lead V_1. The chest film typically shows dilatation of the main and left pulmonary arteries. Because the jet across the stenotic valve is directed towards the left pulmonary artery, there is often disproportionate enlargement of the left pulmonary artery. The right atrium and ventricle usually do not become significantly enlarged unless heart failure is present. In severe stenosis with a low cardiac output, there may be oligemic peripheral lung fields.

Cardiac catheterization reveals a gradient across the pulmonic valve. Right-ventricular angiography shows the characteristic upper doming of the leaflets of the pulmonic valve. It had been hoped that the echocardiogram would help in the diagnosis of pulmonic stenosis, and it does show the a wave and, of course, right-ventricular enlargement. However, it is not as helpful as had originally been hoped in adults. Adult patients with significant pulmonic stenosis will have at least a grade IV systolic murmur, and right-ventricular enlargement by EKG. If these are absent, the gradient across the pulmonic valve will, in general, not be significant and the patient will not require surgery. If there is a question, the patient should certainly be catheterized, and if the right-ventricular pressure exceeds 70 mmHg, most physicians would recommend surgery.

CYANOTIC CONGENITAL HEART DISEASE

Turning now to cyanotic congenital heart disease, we will cover three types which may be seen in adults: tetralogy of Fallot, Ebstein's anomaly which may be cyanotic, and transposition. In addition, of course, atrial and ventricular septal defects and patent ductus arteriosus may also develop cyanosis late in their course, when pulmonary hypertension leads to shunt reversal.

FALLOT'S TETRALOGY

By far, the most common type of cyanotic heart disease in patients who survive to adult life is Fallot's tetralogy. This is best described as a combination of ventricular septal defect and pulmonic stenosis. If the ventricular septal defect and the pulmonic stenosis is mild, there will be no cyanosis (the "acyanotic" Fallot's tetralogy). If the ventricular septal defect is small and the pulmonic stenosis severe, the disease will behave like simple pulmonic stenosis. However, if the ventricular septal defect is large and the pulmonic stenosis severe, the result will be the classic cyanotic Fallot's tetralogy, the subject of our discussion.

In cyanotic Fallot's tetralogy, the pulmonic stenosis may be infundibular or valvular, but usually the two are combined. The history is of cyanosis developing by 3 to 6 months after birth. The patient as a child was small, and had complaints of dyspnea. Patients also have a history of squatting frequently, an unusual symptom but quite classical for the tetralogy of Fallot. Squatting brings prompt relief of the dyspnea, and the patients discover this for themselves.

On physical examination, the patient is small, and there is central cyanosis, which increases with exercise. A thrill may be felt in the third left interspace. No specific chamber enlargement can be felt. The murmur is midsystolic, and the length varies: the second sound is single, since the pulmonic component of the second sound is inaudible.

The echocardiogram may show overriding of the aorta and will also show right-ventricular enlargement. The chest film is extremely valuable and is quite characteristic for Fallot' tetralogy. The lung vasculature is decreased, the pulmonary artery segment is absent or reduced, and the aortic arch is increased and may lie to the right. This combination produces the characteristic boot-shaped heart. As the patient reaches adult life, he will very often become polycythemic to an extreme degree.

In general, surgery is recommended for patients with a tetralogy of Fallot in adult life. Total correction can be achieved, with the ventricular septal defect patched and the pulmonic stenosis relieved, and the results are good.

EBSTEIN'S ANOMALY

Ebstein's anomaly of the tricuspid valve, while uncommon, may well be seen in adults. The basic defect is displacement of the abnormal tricuspid valve into the right ventricle. Some patients become cyanotic, owing to a right-to-left shunt at the atrial level, which occurs in about 20%; however, cyanosis is not usually a part of uncomplicated Ebstein's anomaly. The precordium is quiet, and palpation does not detect either classical right- or left-ventricular enlargement. The first sound is split, the second is reduced, and often S_3 and S_4 sounds are present. The murmur is that of tricuspid regurgitation. The electrocardiogram shows Wolff-Parkinson-White syndrome in 25% of the cases, and there is an even more frequent history of atrial arrhythmias. The QRS pattern is quite classical, with a QR and inverted T waves in leads V_1 through V_4. The chest film demonstrates clear lungs and a globular heart silhouette, reflecting the large right atrium. The echocardiogram has proved especially useful in this defect, confirming the abnormal and displaced tricuspid valve.

TRANSPOSITION OF THE GREAT VESSELS

The subject of transposition of the great vessels is far beyond the scope of this discussion. Involved in this are not only the transpositions of the great vessels but cardiac malpositions. However, to our astonishment, patients with congenitally corrected transposition reach adult life and may be asymptomatic, coming to the physician's attention for a murmur or some abnormality on the EKG. In transposition, the great arteries are arranged so that while the anatomic left ventricle pumps blood into the pulmonary artery, it is venous blood from the right atrium; therefore the patients are not cyanotic when the transposition is congenitally corrected. However, most patients have associated defects, such as a ventricular septal defect, disease of the left-sided atrioventricular valve, or obstruction to the outflow of the right ventricle, and they may become cyanotic if the ventricular septal defect produces pulmonary hypertension and shunt reversal. Very interestingly, about 75% of them will have abnormalities of atrioventricular conduction on the electrocardiogram, which, as we have said, is often the thing that brings them to medical attention. The electrocardiogram will also show Q waves in lead 3 and a QS in lead V_1. The chest film is quite helpful, showing abnormalities in the aortic arch and pulmonary artery. The left side of the cardiac silhouette at the base consists of the aortic knuckle, rather than the pulmonary trunk. In corrected transposition, the left upper border is formed by the ascending aorta, and the pulmonary trunk does not form the left border, so that an experienced cardiac or radiologist can usually make the diagnosis of this abnormality.

Catheterization is indicated, if in doubt, and if the associated defects are hemodynamically significant, they may be corrected by surgery.

THE FUNCTIONAL MURMUR

Finally, no discussion of congenital heart disease would be complete without briefly mentioning the problem of the functional murmur. This was discussed in Chapter 2, but let us again emphasize certain key points. Most children have functional murmurs, which are most often heard along the left sternal border but may be heard in the base and the apex. The murmurs characteristically vary in intensity from time to time, are very seldom over grade II, occur classically in the early part of systole, and are not heard in the later part of systole. Diastolic murmurs are usually significant, with the exception of the diastolic murmur heard in febrile children, called a Carey-Coomb's murmur. The rule that has proved invaluable to us is to say very little to the family or the patient if the murmur is heard; if in doubt, listen again; and, if still in doubt, use chest film, EKG, and echocardiogram for further evaluation of the murmur. With a normal chest film, EKG, and echocardiogram, one can certainly follow such patients for long periods of time without being concerned about the need for immediate treatment.

NUCLEAR CARDIOLOGY

F. Deaver Thomas

19

Of the diagnostic methods using radionuclides in the evaluation of cardiac disease, many are useful as research tools only; we will limit our discussion to three studies of particular clinical importance: *1*) myocardial perfusion imaging; *2*) myocardial imaging with infarction-seeking agents; *3*) radionuclide ventriculography.

The radiation detection equipment and radioactive agents will be briefly discussed to provide an appreciation of the advantages and limitations inherent in their use.

SCINTILLATION CAMERA SYSTEMS

The fundamental radiation detector in nuclear medicine is the sodium iodide crystal. This crystal has the property of producing light (a "scintillation") from its interaction with the electromagnetic radiation (gamma rays) emitted from radioactive materials. The radioactive materials (**radiopharmaceuticals**) are injected into the patient intravenously and distributed in the body according to their physical and chemical properties. To provide an image of the gamma-ray emitter in the body, a device known as a **collimator** (from the Latin "to make parallel") is interposed between the patient and the detector. This produces (like the lens on a camera) an image in the crystal representing the distribution of radioactivity emitted by the patient. The gamma rays interact with the crystal, producing light, which, after conversion to electrons by a photocathode surface and subsequent current multiplication by a photomultiplier tube, is used to produce corresponding light on a cathode ray tube for photographic purposes. This entire system is called a **scintillation camera.**

Since the amount of radioactivity injected is limited by considerations of radiation exposure to the patient, the number of gamma rays actually available to produce this image is small. A typical photograph taken with a conventional light camera might contain 10^9 recorded photons; a gamma-ray image typically contains only 10^4 to 10^5 recorded photons, each photon representing a separate gamma-ray interaction. Since each gamma-ray interaction is a discrete event in the detector, its occurrence and relative position may be encoded by digital circuits into an image in a magnetic core or other digital storage device. Ultimately, this digital image may be manipulated to produce useful quantitative information about the distribution of radioactivity in the patient (see Fig. 19-1).

MYOCARDIAL PERFUSION IMAGES

The pattern of myocardial perfusion is of great clinical interest, since any interruption in it produces ischemia, angina, and, frequently, infarction, of heart muscle. To delineate myocardial blood flow, the radiopharmaceutical must be readily taken up by the myocardium, retained for a reasonable period of time, and simultaneously cleared rapidly from the vascular pool in the body, so as not to obscure the myocardium. The need for rapid blood clearance is apparent when one considers the problem of dealing with radioactive tracer in the intracardiac blood pool (that is, within the chambers of the ventricles or atria), when only myocardial concentration is desired.

Of the various agents which can delineate the blood-flow patterns in the heart muscle, the one most compatible with the physiology of the body would be potassium, the basic intracellular cation. The radionuclide ^{43}K and analogues of potassium in Group I of the Periodic Table (cesium, in the form of ^{129}Cs and rubidium, in the form of ^{81}Rb) have been tried as radioactive markers, but the most successful to date has been the radionuclide of thallium, ^{201}Tl, in the form of univalent thallous ion. The rationale for the ^{201}Tl study, then, is to establish which areas of myocardium receive normal blood flow, as revealed by normal radiotracer concentration, while regions of ischemia or infarction (reduced or absent blood flow) are seen as diminished or absent radiotracer concentration.

In these studies, exercise by the patient is useful to produce stress on the myocardium, enhancing myocardial blood flow, increasing thallium concentration, and improving image quality. More important, however, this increased workload will also produce ischemia in the areas of coronary artery disease. Thus the exercise load will produce greater contrast between normal and abnormal areas of myocardial perfusion, since uptake will *increase* in normally perfused muscle and *decrease* in poorly perfused muscle.

These effects of exercise are short-lived (like the angina it produces), and the perfusion in ischemic areas will return to normal after a period of rest. Therefore, the ^{201}Tl is injected at the peak of exercise, and the imaging study is performed immediately thereafter. Later, after a 1- or 2-hour rest period, the

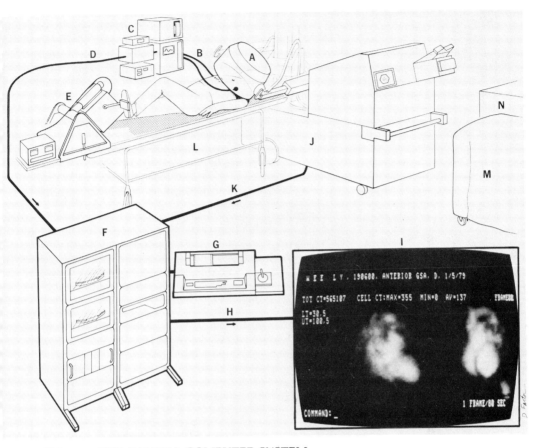

FIG. 19-1. THE CAMERA-COMPUTER SYSTEM.

Patient under study lies in supine position on stretcher (**L**). Scintillation camera detector (**A**) is placed in approximation to anterior chest wall at 45° angle in left-anterior oblique view (LAO 45°). ECG leads are attached to chest (**B**); these signals are sent to ECG monitor and signal processor (**C**); R-wave pulses are sent over a control line (**D**) to computer (**F**). Scintillation events within detector head (**A**) are processed by camera electronics (**J**), and this information is also sent to computer over data line (**K**). Operator controls computer's acquisition and processing of these data through keyboard (**G**). The images produced in computer are then displayed on television screen (**I**). If patient is to be studied during exercise, bicycle ergometer (**E**) attached to foot of stretcher is utilized. This provides a control of workload imposed during exercise. Emergency drugs and resuscitation devices are kept nearby (**M**), as well as cardiac defibrillator (**N**).

images are repeated, and the ischemic areas are seen to "fill in" with radioactivity as the ^{201}Tl is redistributed. However, if an area of infarction (scar) is present in the myocardium, the thallium study will then show a defect in concentration at the site of scarring, both in the exercise and resting portions of the study (see Fig. 19-2).

A normal study both during exercise and at rest would tend to exclude a sizable area of transmural myocardial ischemia or infarction. A study which showed a defect both at rest and at exercise would confirm the diagnosis of a previous myocardial infarction. A study which showed exercise-induced defects which disappeared with rest would support the diagnosis of ischemia resulting from coronary artery disease.

What are the limitations of this procedure? A *positive* study is very good evidence of coronary artery disease. However, a *negative* study does not exclude that diagnosis, since abnormal areas may be obscured by overlying normal tissue. Although transmural involvement is usually detected, subendocardial lesions are frequently missed.

Since only 3% to 5% of the administered dose of ^{201}Tl localizes in the myocardium, the quality of the images obtained is frequently suboptimal, further complicating interpretation. If the patient is unable to exercise, owing to severe coronary disease or other debilitating factors, the quality of the images will be further compromised by diminished uptake in the myocardium. Competing uptake of the ^{201}Tl in the liver and adjacent organs will then overlie portions of the heart, thereby obscuring real lesions.

Despite these limitations, the procedure is valuable in the evaluation of the patient with coronary artery disease and in lessening the likelihood of that

FIG. 19-2. THALLIUM STUDIES.

Computer-enhanced images of three patient studies. Two views illustrated are anterior and LAO 45° projections. First pair of images in each row is made immediately after exercise and second pair after period of 2 hours of rest.

First row (1) demonstrates a normal study with reasonably homogeneous distribution seen on both anterior and LAO views at exercise and rest. Note normal thinning of activity at apex, especially well seen in anterior view. There is relatively little change in the resting study.

Second row (2) represents images from patient with coronary artery disease in which a large area of diminished uptake is noted in inferior and apical portions of left ventricle, best seen on anterior view. Rest images show some redistribution in this region, although it has not returned entirely to normal. This redistribution is consistent with ischemia induced by exercise, which recovers with time. Background activity seen below heart in resting study is thallium uptake in stomach, a normal finding.

The third row of images (3) demonstrates large area of diminished uptake, best seen in LAO views in region of posterolateral wall. There is very little change on resting study, suggesting that this large scar resulted from a prior myocardial infarction.

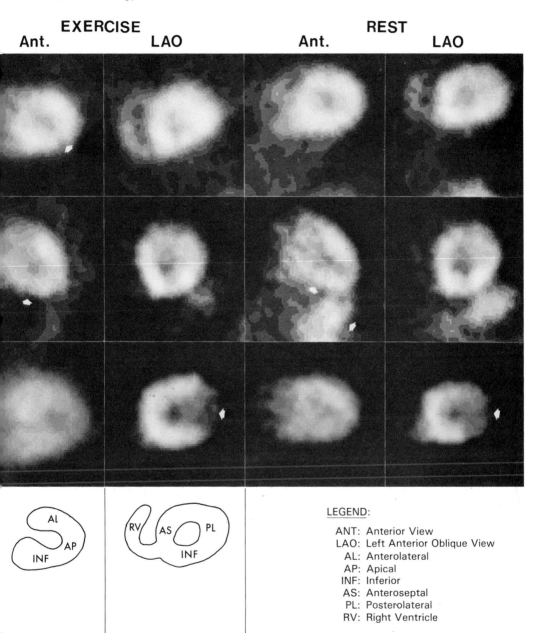

EXERCISE
Ant.   LAO

REST
Ant.   LAO

LEGEND:

ANT: Anterior View
LAO: Left Anterior Oblique View
AL: Anterolateral
AP: Apical
INF: Inferior
AS: Anteroseptal
PL: Posterolateral
RV: Right Ventricle

diagnosis in patients with atypical non-coronary chest pain. The technique may also reveal areas of acute infarction, especially when EKG changes and enzyme studies are inconclusive; however, distinguishing old from new infarctions is not feasible with this method.

One additional disadvantage of ^{201}Tl is its relatively high cost, since it is cyclotron-produced. Because of its relatively short physical half-life of 73 hours, it must be shipped individually for each study, limiting its availability.

MYOCARDIAL IMAGING WITH INFARCTION-SEEKING AGENTS

In 1974, it was discovered that the radiopharmaceuticals developed for imaging the skeletal system, the phosphates and the phosphonates labeled with ^{99m}Tc, would localize in areas of acute myocardial ischemia and infarction. Since then, they have been widely used for demonstrating acute myocardial infarctions within 2 weeks of onset, and sensitivities of 70% to 90% have been reported. The mechanism for this localization is apparently related to the influx of calcium ions into injured myocardial cells, since these agents tend to concentrate in areas of active calcium metabolism.

Most patients with acute myocardial infarction can be diagnosed with more conventional techniques, such as historical and physical findings, EKG changes, and serum enzyme elevations. However, this imaging procedure is useful when the diagnosis is uncertain because of equivocal chemical or EKG changes.

The imaging technique requires the intravenous injection of a ^{99m}Tc-labeled phosphate or phosphonate compound, followed by imaging 1 to 2 hours later. An area of myocardial infarction appears as an area of *increased* uptake. This positive uptake is seen 12 hours or later after infarction, peaks at 3 to 5 days, and generally persists for 7 to 10 days (but occasionally longer). Serial studies are frequently helpful in documenting these events or in clarifying minimal findings in the early stages of infarction.

Unfortunately, this technique is not specific for acute myocardial infarction, and increased uptake has been noted in other conditions, including calcification of the aortic and mitral valves, traumatic contusion of the myocardium, unstable angina, cardiomyopathies, pericarditis, post-electrical cardioversion, ventricular aneurysms, and myocardial amyloidosis. False negative studies have been encountered in subendocardial infarction and even in small transmural infarction, if the quantity of the tissue involved is less than 3 g (see Fig. 19-3).

Thus, while not an absolute indicator of acute infarction, a negative study is strong evidence against a recent, substantial transmural infarction. The procedure can be very useful in: 1) patients with typical histories of infarction but ambiguous laboratory determinations; 2) patients with infarction following cardiac surgery, where both enzyme elevations and EKG abnormalities are expected; and 3) patients with recurrent myocardial infarctions when EKG changes from older infarctions may obscure the diagnosis.

RADIONUCLIDE VENTRICULOGRAPHY

In the two techniques described above, the radiopharmaceuticals concentrate *within the myocardium.* In radionuclide ventriculography, the blood pool *within the ventricular cavities* is imaged to assess the function of the heart as a pump.

Conventional radiographic ventriculography requires direct catheterization of the ventricular cavities through the arterial or venous circulation, followed by injection of a radiopaque contrast agent; this invasive technique is technically difficult at best, and dangerous at worst. In any given patient, the study may be performed infrequently because of the trauma and risk involved.

On the other hand, radionuclide ventriculography requires only a single intravenous injection of a radiopharmaceutical which remains in the intravascular blood pool and is virtually without risk, except for a small radiation dose (a fraction of that required for the radiographic procedure). This procedure may be repeated often, if necessary, and may be conveniently performed at rest, during exercise, or with various pharmacological interventions. It is the best noninvasive method currently available for evaluating left-ventricular function. Since quantitative functional information is needed, a simple imaging procedure alone will not suffice. Hence, parallel image processing by a computer is essential.

Two basic techniques must be distinguished: the so-called *first-pass technique* and the *gated-blood pool technique.* In the *first-pass technique,* the sequential passage of an intravenous radiopharmaceutical bolus is recorded as it traverses the heart and great vessels during the first circulation by rapid acquisition of scintillation camera data, with both conventional film techniques and computer storage. Films are usually obtained at the rate of one or more frames per sec; the computer-stored data may be replayed later at various operator-controlled rates. The entire first-pass technique usually requires only 30 sec of data-acquisition, during which the radiopharmaceutical passes through the right heart, lungs, left heart, and the peripheral arterial, capillary, and venous circulation.

Almost any radiopharmaceutical may be used for this first-transit study, since little diffusion out of the vascular space occurs during this short interval. The most commonly used radiopharmaceutical is ^{99m}Tc in the form of pertechnetate, TcO_4-, although ^{99m}Tc-labeled albumin or red blood cells are frequently used if a gated blood-pool study is to follow the first-pass procedure.

From the sequential images, one can assess transit times between the various portions of the heart, chamber size, and abnormal pathways (such as right-to-left or left-to-right shunts). The computer can provide additional numerical data on the quantity of radioactivity in a given cardiac chamber, from which one can determine the efficiency of the heart as a pump. Since the radioactivity

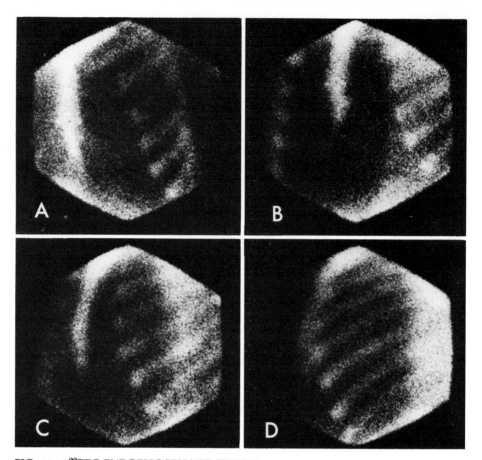

FIG. 19-3. ^{99m}TC PYROPHOSPHATE STUDY.
Case No. 1. Four views represented are anterior (**A**), 45° LAO (**B**), 60° LAO (**C**), and
left lateral (**D**), obtained 3 hours after injection of 15 mCi of ^{99m}Tc MDP. This normal
study shows uptake in ribs and sternum but no evidence of abnormal uptake in
region of heart. (*Continued on opposite page*)

is proportional to the actual volume of blood present, changes in radioactivity
reflect chamber volume changes (see Fig, 19-4).

Therefore, if one measures the radioactivity (proportionate to volume) in
the left ventricle at end-diastole and end-systole, the difference (end-diastolic
volume minus end-systolic volume) is proportional to *stroke volume*. From this
one can obtain a normalized value (a percentage), by dividing the stroke volume
by the end-diastolic volume. This expression is called the *ejection fraction* and
represents the percentage of the left-ventricular volume ejected with each systolic contraction. Mathematically,

$$\text{Ejection fraction} = \frac{\text{EDV} - \text{ESV}}{\text{EDV}}$$

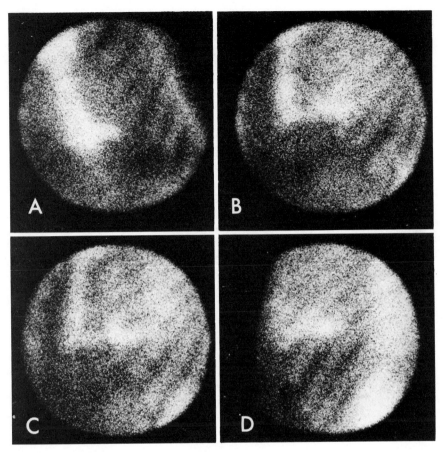

FIG. 19-3. (*Continued*)
Case No. 2. Same four views are obtained and show area of intense uptake just
to left of sternum at level of inferior wall of left ventricle. This patient had
sustained an inferior-wall infarction three days prior to this study. Intense uptake
of the radiopharmaceutical is seen in region of recent infarction owing to influx
of MDP into myocardial cells damaged by ischemia.

Normally, the left ventricle ejects more than 50% of its end-diastolic volume
with each systolic contraction.

The *gated blood-pool technique* requires the intravenous injection of a radiopharmaceutical, usually ^{99m}Tc-labeled red blood cells or serum albumin, which
remains in the intravascular space during the procedure. Unlike the first-pass
technique, the heart is imaged during multiple cardiac cycles, rather than only
during the first transit of the radioactive material through the heart. Again, the
combined scintillation camera-computer system is used, and the data acquisition is basically similar to that described above, with one important exception:
the cardiac cycle is divided into multiple segments, and images of each segment

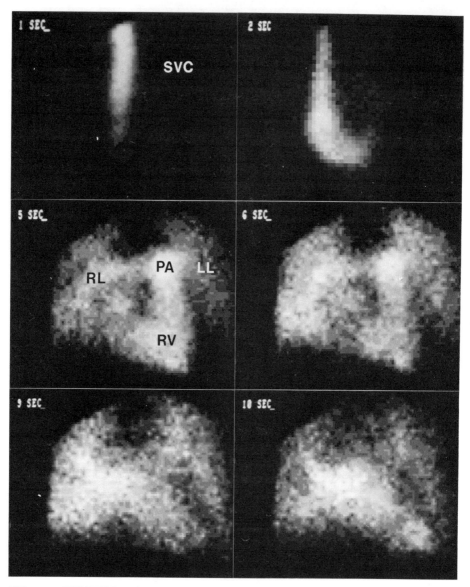

FIG. 19-4. VENTRICULOGRAPHY.
SVC, superior vena cava; RA, right atrium; RV, right ventricle; LL, left lung; PA, pulmonary artery; RL, right lung; LA, left atrium; LV, left ventricle; AO, aorta. (*Continued on opposite page*)

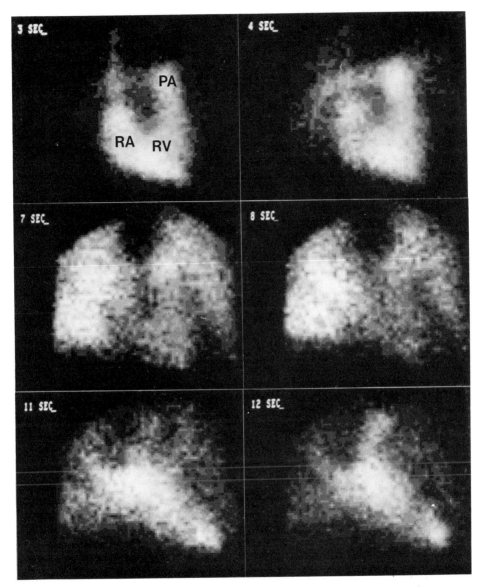

FIG. 19-4. (*Continued*)
First-pass radionuclide ventriculography. Series of 1-sec images obtained immediately
after injection of bolus of 15 mCi of red blood cells labeled with ^{99m}Tc shows
sequential passage of radioactivity through right side of heart, lungs, left side of heart,
and into systemic circulation. Time intervals begin as bolus appears in superior vena
cava. Second image shows activity filling right atrium and just beginning to fill right
ventricle. Third image shows main pulmonary artery and small amount of
radioactivity beginning to appear in right pulmonary artery. Lung (*Continued*)

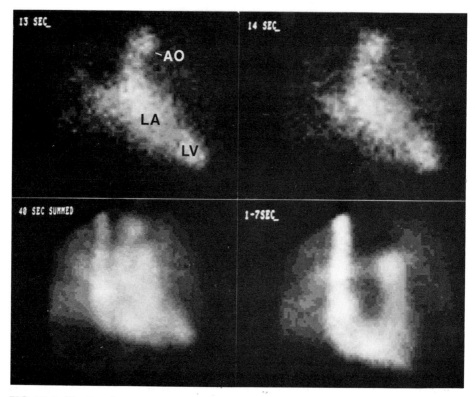

FIG. 19-4. (*Continued*)
fields are beginning to appear at 4 sec and are much more obvious in 5-sec image.
Lung activity persists through 8 sec as activity in right atrium and right ventricle
fades. At 9 sec, pulmonary veins are draining into left atrium; at 10 sec, left ventricle
appears. At 12 sec, aortic arch is visible; by 13 sec, lungs have almost completely
cleared. Bottom row of images shows first entire 40 sec of study summed together; it
is very difficult to separate the anatomical features of the heart. Next image summed
over the first 7 sec shows excellent anatomical delineation of right heart and
(*Continued on opposite page*)

are separately and repeatedly recorded. This method is necessary because the
radiopharmaceutical is distributed throughout the body blood pool, and the
amount contained within the blood volume of the cardiac chambers is relatively
small; if an image of the heart in motion is to be generated, the data from a large
series of cardiac cycles must be registered over a period of 5 to 10 min, in order
that sufficient numbers of gamma-scintillations are recorded to produce a valid
image. To accomplish this, an EKG signal from the patient's heart is used by the
computer system as a "gate" to signal the beginning and end of each cardiac
cycle (hence the term "gated" blood pool). If the cardiac cycle is then divided
into time segments spanning the interval between successive R waves, the com-

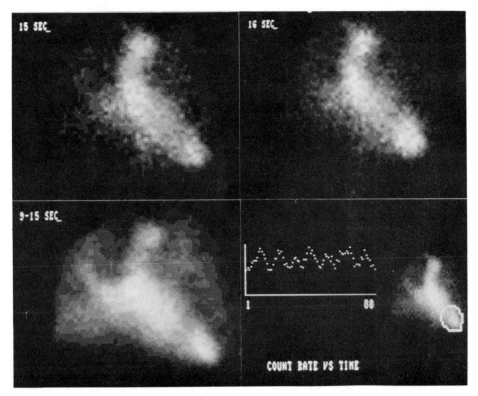

FIG. 19-4. (*Continued*)
pulmonary artery. Images summed between 9 and 15 sec show predominantly left
side of heart. Last frame shows region of interest placed around left ventricle and
resulting histogram of activity in relation to time; these data points are samples
obtained at a rate of 10 per sec, so that volume changes of left ventricle may be seen.
Peaks in histogram represent end-diastole, valleys end-systole. By subtracting valleys
from peaks, one obtains stroke volume, which can then be divided by peak amplitude
to obtain ejection fraction. (*Concluded*)

puter may record the incoming data in relation to its occurrence in the cardiac
cycle. Once these frames of data are accumulated, they may be played back in
movielike ("cine") fashion to provide a visual display of the motion of the heart
(see Fig. 19-5).

Since the data from which the images are constructed are proportionate to
the quantity of blood within a cardiac chamber, the amplitude of radioactivity
in a chamber may be plotted against time, producing a ventricular volume
curve. By applying the formula described above to this curve, an ejection fraction may be calculated. The view of the heart used to calculate the ejection
fraction is the left anterior oblique at a 45° angle from the straight anterior view

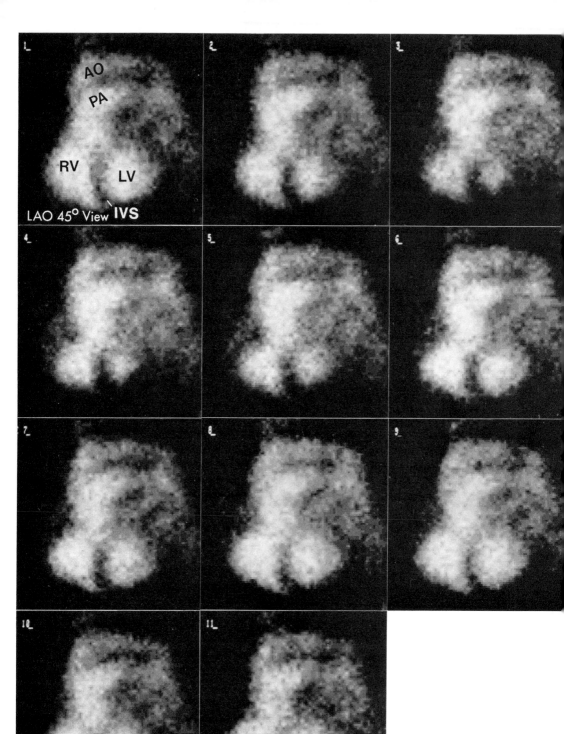

AO

PA

RV   LV

LAO 45° View **IVS**

2.

3.

4.

5.

6.

7.

8.

9.

10.

11.

◀FIG. 19-5. ECG-GATED CARDIAC IMAGES.
AO, aorta; PA, pulmonary artery; RV, right ventricle; LV, left ventricle; IVS, interventricular septum. ECG-gated cardiac images. These eleven images were produced in reference to R wave from ECG; this wave signals end of diastole and beginning of systolic contraction. Each image represents approximately 0.1 sec during average cardiac cycle, obtained in LAO 45° view. Major anatomical structures are indicated. Note change in shape of left and right ventricles between frames 1 and 4, as ventricles contract. Diastole begins at frame 5 and contains through frame 11, as ventricles become progressively larger. Each image represents same period in time over average cardiac cycle and is summation of some 600 cardiac cycles over 10-minute acquisition time. The eleven images, viewed in rapid sequence, constitute the cine playback.

(LAO 45°). This view generally provides the best separation of the right and left ventricles, since the camera view is along the axis of the ventricular septum dividing the two chambers (see Fig. 19-6).

By viewing the cine images, one may also appreciate abnormalities of wall motion, chamber enlargement, and other morphological characteristics of the heart. A similar sort of analysis can also be done using the data from first-pass technique to produce a movie-film display of the passage of the radioactivity through the chambers of the heart on its first transit. From the observations of ventricular-wall motion, abnormalities of contraction (**dyssynergy**) may be noted as areas of reduced motion (**hypokinesis**), absent motion (**akinesis**), or paradoxical motion (**dyskinesis**).

The major advantage of the first-pass technique is that the radioactivity is confined to the cardiac blood pool itself, resulting in very low background radioactivity and good delineation of the edges of the ventricular chambers. Its basic disadvantage is that very little time is available for the acquisition of the data, and thus the image quality suffers somewhat by comparison to the gated-pool technique. In general, this technique is also limited to a single projection of the heart, so that multiple views are not available for analysis.

The gated blood-pool technique has the advantages of generating multiple views and giving good statistical image quality but has the disadvantages of a much higher background radioactivity from the general distribution of the radiopharmaceutical and hence poorer image delineation of the ventricular walls.

The ejection-fraction calculation described above is based on the reasonable assumption that the radioactivity in the ventricle under observation is proportional to the ventricular volume; therefore no geometric assumptions are made regarding the actual shape of the ventricular cavities. This constitutes a major advantage over the radiographic technique, which requires the assumption of an ellipsoidal shape to the left ventricle. The ejection fraction is derived from radiographic studies by a measurement of the major and minor axes of the ellipsoid at end systole and end diastole and the substitution of these into an equation for the volume of an ellipsoid. This technique works well for a nor-

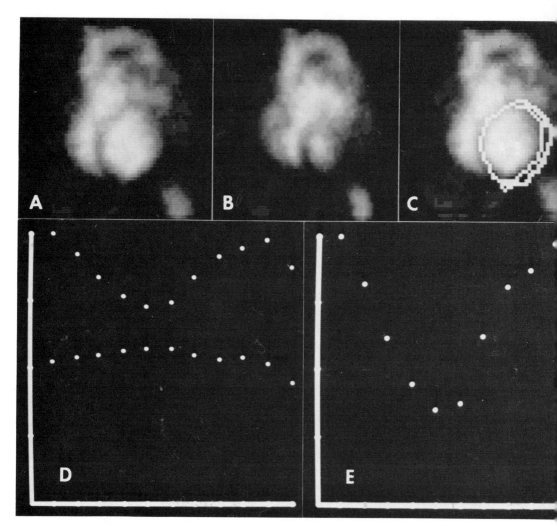

FIG. 19-6. REGIONS OF INTEREST OVER LEFT VENTRICLE AND BACKGROUND, AND RESULTANT VOLUME CURVES.
(A) Heart viewed from LAO 45° view at end-diastole; (B) Same view at end systole. (C) Region of interest placed around borders of left ventricle and background region of interest surrounding posterior aspect of left ventricle. (D) Note left-ventricular volume curve above and background curve below. Subtracting background curve from ventricular-volume curve results in E, net left-ventricular-volume curve. This is a normal study showing ejection fraction of 65%, obtained by subtracting the fifth point (end systole) from the first point (end diastole) of net left-ventricular volume curve and dividing result by the first point.

mally contracting heart which maintains a regular shape. However, it frequently errs when applied to the irregularly contracting heart damaged by coronary artery disease.

One of the more useful adaptations of the radionuclide ventriculogram has been the evaluation of the cardiac response to exercise and to the effects of drugs which may alter cardiac performance, such as nitroglycerin. A patient with coronary artery disease may have relatively good left-ventricular contraction while resting, but during exercise reduced left-ventricular function may become obvious. This results from the inadequacy of the coronary circulation to meet the demands of the added workload. Normally, of course, the left ventricle increases its contractility (and the ejection fraction) in proportion to the workload imposed, a moderate workload increasing the ejection fraction by 10% to 15%. In the patient with significant coronary artery disease, however, either no increase will occur, or an actual decrease of 10% or 20% or more may be seen; new areas of dyskinesis may also develop. A similar response may occur in patients with valvular disease such as aortic stenosis or insufficiency. On the other hand, a reduced resting ejection fraction may return towards normal if a coronary vasodilator is given.

The exercise device frequently used during the imaging study is a bicycle ergometer—simply a device to maintain a known, but variable workload. The patient may be supine, with the ergometer mounted at the end of the imaging stretcher (see Fig. 19-1, E), or he may be seated over the pedals, facing the camera placed against his chest. Other forms of stress (hand grips, peripheral vasodilators) have also been used. The patient using the bicycle ergometer is exercised initially to allow familiarization with the procedure and to gain information on the maximum workload that he can sustain before fatigue or angina supervenes. During the actual imaging exercise study, the patient works against this predetermined load until the pulse rate stabilizes, and data are collected for 2 to 3 min. The ejection fraction estimate is made and compared to the resting study. Thus, this technique objectively examines myocardial dysfunction secondary to significant coronary artery disease and the effects of medical and surgical therapy which may produce an improvement in response during workload (see Fig. 19-7).

The technique of radionuclide ventriculography therefore represents a substantial addition to the diagnostic armamentarium and is undergoing rapid development. The regional wall-motion analysis and the ejection-fraction measurement are both very important indicators of pump performance and are very difficult to obtain by other techniques.

In the analysis of gated blood-pool images, it is useful to produce a functional image, or a two-dimensional display of wall motion. This frequently produces a more obvious and sensitive assessment of wall motion-abnormalities which might be overlooked in viewing the cine images. It also provides a means of recording, in a single photograph, the essence of the cine study. This functional image may be constructed in a number of ways, but we have found the

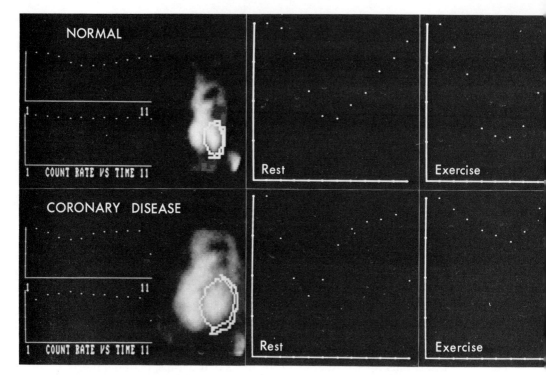

FIG. 19-7. LEFT-VENTRICULAR VOLUME CURVES DURING REST AND EXERCISE.
Curves are shown at rest and exercise in normal individual (*top*) and in patient with significant coronary artery disease (*bottom*). In normal patient, resting ejection fraction is 62%, with pronounced increase to 73% during exercise. In contrast, patient with coronary artery disease shows normal resting ejection fraction of 60% but during exercise this drops to 27%. Note that one cannot distinguish these two patients on basis of resting study alone. The stress of exercise clearly demonstrates the abnormal myocardial function that results from coronary artery disease.

ejection-fraction image most descriptive. This is produced in a fashion analogous to the global (or overall ventricular) ejection-fraction measurement.

The image which represents end-systole is subtracted from the end-diastolic image. The result is a functional image of the *stroke volume*. Since the background radioactivity is the same in both the end-diastolic and end-systolic images, the subtraction cancels out the background contribution. To produce the ejection-fraction image, the stroke-volume image is divided by an end-diastolic image which has been corrected for background radiation. The numerical values in this image are proportional to the ejection fraction (and ventricular-wall motion), on a point-by-point basis, for the left and right ventricles. If ejection-fraction images are produced from both the anterior and LAO 45° views, most of the ventricular wall is visualized. Segmental and global abnormalities stand out vividly in such a display, and areas of hypokinesis or akinesis are seen as regions of lesser intensity than the normal image. Such regions can be represented using a grey scale or a color scale. The latter is more readily appreciated, and we use a color scale ranging from white (at maximum intensity), through orange and red, to black (minimum intensity).

If either akinesis or dyskinesis is present, the intensity level will be black. To distinguish these two, an image representing dyskinesis can be constructed: if an area of the heart is actually dyskinetic, it appears to increase in activity during systole rather than decrease (that is, there is paradoxical motion). Therefore, if one reverses the sequence and subtracts the diastolic image from the systolic image, those areas which are paradoxical will be shown as regions of greater intensity (positive values). This dyskinesis image is useful in detecting subtle regions of dyskinesis not readily apparent by other means. Note that other regions which normally increase in size during ventricular systole, such as the atria and major vessels, will also be displayed as regions of greater intensity on the color scale (see Fig. 19-8).

Radionuclide ventriculography is especially useful in making the following determinations:

In *coronary artery disease:*

1. The differential diagnosis between atypical angina and non-coronary chest pain
2. The clarification of false negative EKG stress tests in patients with typical angina or positive EKG stress tests in asymptomatic patients
3. The documentation of prior myocardial infarctions in patients with equivocal EKG findings
4. The detection of ventricular aneurysms or pseudoaneurysms
5. The assessment of ventricular function before and after surgery in patients undergoing coronary-vein graft procedures
6. The evaluation of the effects of drug therapy (vasodilators, digitalis, and cardiotoxic chemotherapeutic agents)

In *valvular heart disease:*

1. Preoperative assessment of ventricular reserve and surgical risk
2. Postoperative evaluation of changes in left-ventricular function after valve surgery

The basic limitations of radionuclide ventriculography, as opposed to contrast ventriculography, are the result of the limited spatial resolution of the scintillation camera. The fine morphological resolution of contrast radiography is lacking, and accurate delineation of such structures as valve leaflets or coronary artery architecture is impossible.

Therefore the radionuclide technique should not be looked upon as a replacement for contrast ventriculography, but rather as an adjunct to it. It is an extremely useful screening test to determine if sufficient ventricular function remains to warrant more invasive diagnostic procedures. As with most nuclear medicine techniques, this procedure should be looked upon as a functional assessment, rather than an anatomical one.

My thanks to my colleagues, Drs. John McAfee, Zachary Grossman, and Amolak Singh, for their many suggestions and careful reviews; to Carol Westfall and Frederica Partridge, for manuscript preparation; and to Julia Hammack, David Foster, and John Hodgson, for illustrative materials.

FIG. 19-8A. EJECTION FRACTION IMAGES.

First row (anterior images): from study of 55-year-old manual laborer with angina. *Frame 1*, end-diastole; *frame 2*, end-systole; subtracting frame 2 from frame 1 results in *stroke-volume image, frame 3*. Dividing this image by end-diastolic image (frame 1), *ejection fraction image* in *frame 4* results. Similarly, **second row** shows end-diastolic and end-systolic images in LAO 45° view in same patient and resultant stroke-volume and ejection-fraction images. This is normal study with ejection fractions of approximately 80%. Same patient had substantial drop in ejection fraction to 69% during exercise and was subsequently found to have three-vessel coronary artery disease.

Third row: images from patient with advanced coronary artery disease and history of inferior-wall and anterolateral-wall infarctions. *Frame 1:* anterior view of heart; compare to frame 4 above. There is large defect in contraction of heart involving anterolateral, apical, and inferior portions of left ventricle. *Frame 2:* dyskinesis image shows significant activity in right- and left-atrial areas and small region of increased activity near apex; latter is region of dyskinesis, confirming presence of ventricular aneurysm. *Frame 3:* LAO 45° view, showing large defect in inferior wall which may be better oriented on *frame 4*, where systolic outline of heart is superimposed. Resting ejection fractions were 27% in anterior view and 23% in LAO 45° view. Since ejection fractions are below 30%, this patient would not be likely surgical candidate for coronary artery bypass. (*Continued on overleaf*)

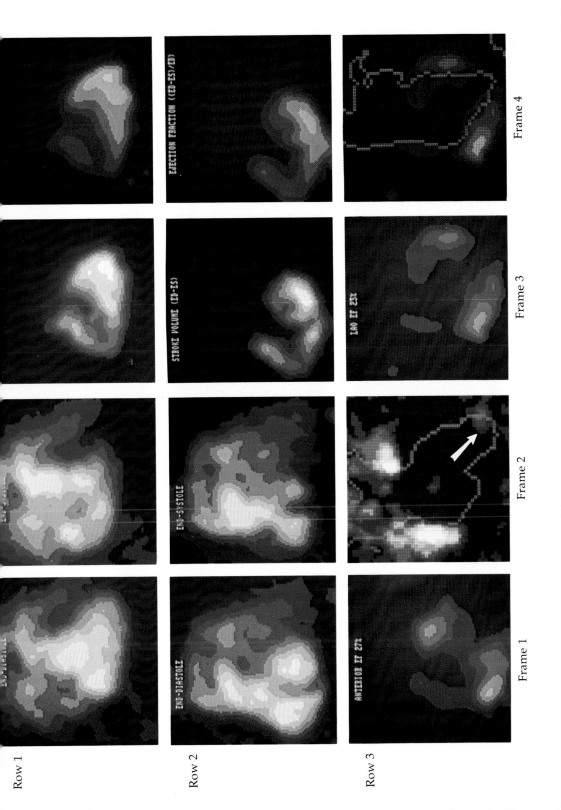

Row 1

Row 2

Row 3

Frame 1   Frame 2   Frame 3   Frame 4

Fig. 19-8. **A**

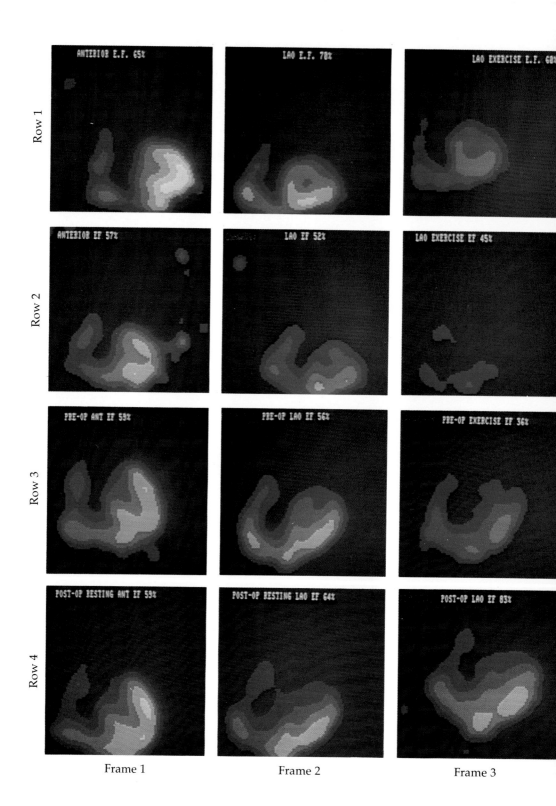

Row 1

ANTERIOR E.F. 65%   LAO E.F. 78%   LAO EXERCISE E.F. 68%

Row 2

ANTERIOR EF 57%   LAO EF 52%   LAO EXERCISE EF 45%

Row 3

PRE-OP ANT EF 59%   PRE-OP LAO EF 56%   PRE-OP EXERCISE EF 36%

Row 4

POST-OP RESTING ANT EF 59%   POST-OP RESTING LAO EF 64%   POST-OP LAO EF 85%

Frame 1   Frame 2   Frame 3

Fig. 19-8. **B**

♦FIG. 19-8B. EJECTION FRACTION IMAGES. (*Continued*)
First row: images from 69-year-old man with calcific aortic stenosis and symptoms of fatigue. *Frame 1:* anterior ejection fraction image with calculated ejection fraction of 65%; LAO 45° ejection-fraction image seen in *frame 2* was accompanied by measured ejection fraction of 70%. During exercise, *frame 3* shows marked drop in intensity generally and ejection fraction was calculated to be 60%. This drop of 10% between resting and exercise LAO views indicates need for surgery in patient with aortic valve disease.

    Second row: images from patient with aortic regurgitation shows normal ejection fractions in anterior and LAO views, of 57% and 52%, respectively. However, there is marked drop in ejection fraction during exercise to 45%, accompanied by obvious reduction in intensity on ejection-fraction image, again suggesting early decompensation and need for corrective surgery.

    Third row: images from 56-year-old male with substernal chest pain is preoperative study showing normal ejection fractions in anterior and LAO 45° views of 59% and 56%, respectively. However, marked drop during exercise in ejection fraction to 36%. Cardiac catheterization studies also showed normal resting ejection fraction and significant lesion (90% stenosis) of left anterior descending coronary artery.

    Fourth row: postoperative studies from same patient, again showing normal resting values of 59% and 64%, respectively, in anterior and LAO views and value of 83% during exercise—marked improvement over preoperative values above.

SUGGESTED READING

General

Parisi AF, Tow DE (eds): Noninvasive Approaches to Cardiovascular Diagnosis. New York, Appleton-Century-Crofts, 1979
Parkey RW, Bonte FJ, Buja LM, Willerson JT (eds): Clinical Nuclear Cardiology. New York, Appleton-Century-Crofts, 1979
Strauss HW, Pitt B, James AE (eds): Cardiovascular Nuclear Medicine. St. Louis, C.V. Mosby, 1974
Willerson JT (ed): Nuclear Cardiology. Cardiovascular Clinics, Vol. 10, No. 2. Philadelphia, F.A. Davis, 1979

Myocardial Perfusion

Bodenheimer MB, Banka VS, Fooshee CM, et al: Extent and severity of coronary heart disease. Arch Int Med 139:630–634, June 1979
Botvinick EH, Taradach MR, Shames DM, et al: Thallium 201 myocardial perfusion scintigraphy for the clinical clarification of normal, abnormal, and equivocal electrocardiographic stress tests. Am J Cardiol 41:43–51, 1978
Bulkley BH, Rouleu J, Strauss HW, et al: Idiopathic hypertrophic subaortic stenosis: Detection by thallium-201 myocardial perfusion imaging. N Engl J Med 293:1113–1116, 1975

Gewirtz H, Beller GA, Strauss HW, et al: Transient defects of resting thallium scans in patients with coronary artery disease. Circulation 59(4):707–713, April 1979

Ritchie J, Zaret B, Strauss W, et al: Myocardial imaging with thallium-201 at rest and exercise—a multicenter study. Circulation 56(Suppl III):230, 1977

Wackers FJT, van der Schoot JB, Sokole EB, et al: Noninvasive visualization of acute myocardial infarction in man with thallium-201. Br Heart J 37:741, 1975

Wackers FJT, Sokole EB, Samson G, et al: Value and limitations of thallium-201 scintigraphy in the acute phase of myocardial infarction. N Engl J Med 295(1):1–5, 1976

INFARCT-AVID IMAGING

Berger HJ, Gottschalk A, Zaret BL: Dual radionuclide study of acute myocardial infarction. Ann Int Med 88:145–154, 1978

Berman DS, Amersterdam EA, Hines HH, et al: New approach to interpretation of technetium-99m pyrophosphate scintigraphy in detection of acute myocardial infarction. Am J Cardiol 39:341–346, 1977

Bonte FJ, Parkey RW, Graham LD, et al: A new method for radionuclide imaging of myocardial infarcts. Radiology 110:473–474, 1974

Cowley MJ, Mantle JA, Rogers WJ, et al: Technetium-99m stannous pyrophosphate myocardial scintigraphy—reliability and assessment of acute myocardial infarction. Circulation 56:192, 1977

Holman BL, Lesch M, Alpert JS: Myocardial scintigraphy with technetium-99m pyrophosphate during the early phase of acute infarction. Am J Cardiol 41:39–42, 1978

Walsh WF, Karunaratne HB, Resnekov L, et al: Assessment of diagnostic value of technetium-99m pyrophosphate myocardial scintigraphy in 80 patients with possible acute myocardial infarction. Br Heart J 39:974–981, 1977

Willerson JT, Parkey RW, Bonte FJ, et al: Acute subendocardial myocardial infarction in patients. Circulation 51:436–441, 1975

Wynne J, Holman BL, Lesch M: Myocardial scintigraphy by infarct-avid radiotracers. Prog Cardiovasc Dis 20:243, 1978

RADIONUCLIDE VENTRICULOGRAPHY

First-pass Technique

Alexander J, Dainiak N, Berger HJ, et al: Serial assessment of doxorubicin cardiotoxicity with quantitative radionuclide angiocardiography. N Engl J Med 300(6): 278–283, 1979

Berger HJ, Reduto LA, Johnstone DE, et al: Global and regional left ventricular response to bicycle exercise in coronary artery disease. Am J Med 66:13–21, 1979

Marshall RC, Berger HJ, Reduto LA, et al: Assessment of cardiac performance with quantitative radionuclide angiocardiography. Circulation 56(5):808–814, 1978

Marshall RC, Berger HJ, Reduto LA, et al: Variability in sequential measures of left ventricular performance assessed with radionuclide angiocardiography. Am J Cardiol 41:531–536, 1978

Gated Technique

Borer JS, Bacharach SL, Green MV, et al: Real-time radionuclide cineangiography in the noninvasive evaluation of global and regional left ventricular function at rest and during exercise in patients with coronary-artery disease. N Engl J Med 296(15):839–844, 1977

Borer JS, Kent KM, Bacharach SL, et al: Sensitivity, specificity, and predictive accuracy of radionuclide cineangiography during exercise in patients with coronary artery disease. Circulation 60(3):572–580, September 1979

Green MV, Bailey JJ, Ostrow HG, et al: Computerized EKG-gated radionuclide angiocardiography. Computers in Cardiology, Proc. IEEE Computer Society, 137–141, 1975

Hopkins GB, Kan MK, and Salel AF: Scintigraphic assessment of left ventricular aneurysms. JAMA 240(20):2162–2165, 1978

Kent KM, Borer JS, Green MV, et al: Effects of coronary-artery bypass on global and regional left ventricular function during exercise. N Engl J Med 298(26):1434–1439, 1978

O'Toole JD, Gerson EA, Reddy PS, et al: Effect of preoperative ejection fraction on survival and hemodynamic improvement following aortic valve replacement. Circulation 58:1175, 1978

Rigo P, Alderson PO, Robertson RM, et al: Measurement of aortic and mitral regurgitation by gated cardiac blood pool scans. Circulation 60:306–312, 1979

Salel AF, Berman DS, DeNardo GL, et al: Radionuclide assessment of nitroglycerin influence on abnormal left ventricular segmental contraction in patients with coronary heart disease. Circulation 53(6):975–982, 1976

COR PULMONALE

Robert Warner and Harold Smulyan

20

ACUTE COR PULMONALE

Cor pulmonale is defined as an abnormality of the structure and/or function of the right ventricle resulting from diseases of the pulmonary parenchyma or vasculature. The definition specifically excludes congenital heart disease as well as diseases which affect the left ventricle. The most common cause of acute cor pulmonale is sudden pulmonary embolism. At autopsy, a high incidence of unsuspected pulmonary emboli has been found. This has led to the teaching that pulmonary embolism and its most common antecedent, deep vein thrombosis of the legs, is clinically underdiagnosed. Since it is well known that anticoagulation has a salutary effect on both disorders, many patients in whom the diagnosis of either deep vein thrombosis or pulmonary embolism was clinically not well substantiated have been anticoagulated. More recently, the techniques for the diagnosis of both disorders have been improved and more patients spared the risks of unnecessary anticoagulation.

Clots which embolize to the pulmonary artery may originate anywhere in the systemic venous system. A few come from pelvic veins, arm veins, other systemic veins, and the right atrium. But more than 90% arise from the iliac veins and below. Therefore, an understanding of acute pulmonary embolism must begin with its most frequent antecedent, that of deep vein thrombosis of the legs.

DEEP VEIN THROMBOSIS OF THE LEGS

Most patients with massive pulmonary embolism have no antecedent symptoms referable to the legs and completely normal physical examinations. This indicates the difficulty in the clinical diagnosis of deep vein thrombosis.

Those patients at high risk for deep vein thrombosis can, however, be readily identified. This is a population characterized by low blood flow or stasis in the legs and hypercoagulability of the blood. Such individuals include the obese, the bedridden, the edematous, the pregnant, and those who have just had surgery, most especially those subjected to orthopedic procedures on a leg. Those at risk from hypercoagulability include pregnant women, women taking birth control pills, and patients with certain malignancies, particularly adenocarcinomas of the pancreas, stomach, and ovaries.

The physical examination in deep vein thrombosis may be negative or misleading. Homan's sign and the presence of peripheral edema are particularly unreliable indications, since they also occur in other disorders. Disturbances which may lead to a false positive diagnosis of deep vein thrombosis include cellulitis, chronic venous disease, arthritis, and hematomata of the leg, traumatic or otherwise. A palpable venous cord is obviously a useful sign, making superficial thrombophlebitis easier to diagnose, particularly when pain is referred to the tender inflamed superficial vein. Superficial thrombophlebitis alone is rarely related to pulmonary embolism, but it may extend to involve deep veins and thereby result in pulmonary embolism. The diagnostic dilemma in patients with obvious superficial thrombophlebitis is to decide whether or not there is associated deep vein phlebitis.

To improve accuracy in the diagnosis of deep vein thrombosis, a variety of laboratory techniques are used. These can be conveniently subdivided into three groups: 1) methods which measure a decrease in blood flow through occluded or partly occluded veins; 2) methods to identify the clots themselves by labeling with radioactive fibrinogen, and 3) radiopaque venography.

Laboratory Techniques

Flow studies to detect deep vein thrombosis. *Ultrasound devices (Doppler).* A Doppler flowmeter utilizes the shift of an emitted ultrasound frequency by the moving blood as the means of detecting blood flow. Most Doppler flow probes emit continuous (some models use pulsed) ultrasound from one crystal while a second crystal receives the back-scattered (echo) sound. Ultrasound reflected from moving objects, such as the red cells in a flowing column of blood, has a higher or lower frequency than the emitted sound, depending on the flow direction. The difference between the emitted and received frequencies is presented as audible sound, and the circuitry of these devices is arranged so that high-velocity flow is depicted as higher-pitched noise and low-velocity flow as lower-pitched noise, all played through a small speaker or earphones.

In practice, flow signals are sought from the femoral, popliteal, and posterior tibial veins. The flow probe is first placed on the skin overlying the femoral artery, whose double-peaked flow signals are readily identified. The probe is then moved slightly medially to overlie the femoral vein. These flow signals sound like a windstorm and vary with spontaneous respiration. Flow is faster during expiration than inspiration, because of the related changes in intraabdominal pressure resulting from movement of the diaphragm. Light compression or squeezing of the thigh produces an augmentation of flow velocity. Popliteal venous flow signals are similarly studied, with the patient prone and the knees flexed to approximately 30 degrees. The popliteal vein is usually positioned just medial to the popliteal artery, and venous flow augmentation is achieved by compression of the calf. With the patient supine, the posterior tibial vein is located just below the posterior tibial artery. Spontaneous flow in this vein is not usually detectable, but patency of the vein can be established when flow is augmented by squeezing the foot.

Inability to detect venous flow signals suggests that the vein is occluded. High-velocity flow sounds without respiratory variations or failure of distal compression to augment the flow suggests partial venous occlusion or the detection of collateral venous flow.

False positive results, that is diminished or absent flow signals without deep vein thrombosis, are most often the result of poor technique and inexperience. Excessive pressure with the flow probe may occlude the vein, or there may be anatomical distortion resulting from previous surgery. Slow flow rates may also be present from congestive heart failure, hepatic cirrhosis with ascites, or old venous occlusions. Such occlusions could arise from large lymph nodes, tumors, or previous venous disease.

False negative results are less frequent. Small clots, or those in the process of formation, could go undetected, and flow signals from venous collaterals secondary to longstanding venous occlusions could be confused with normal venous flow.

The method has been criticized for its many disadvantages. It is less accurate in the calf veins than in the femoral vein and useless for detection of iliac vein thrombosis. In the femoral vein, experienced observers have found a sensitivity of 76% and specificity of 91% when compared with the radiopaque venogram. A negative Doppler study, therefore, has a high likelihood of excluding femoral deep vein thrombosis. Although not as accurate as the other methods to be described, it is cheap, safe, and readily available. It is most valuable when used as a supplement to the physical examination.

Impedence Plethysmography. This method requires special equipment and cannot be considered an extension of the physical examination. The device senses changes in calf volume during inflation and following deflation of a venous occlusion cuff about the thigh. The method is not calibrated, and absolute volumes are not obtained. The cuff is inflated for 45 sec to 2 min, and the percentage of reduction in volume after cuff deflation is plotted against time. Inflow into the leg is unimpeded in the presence of proximal deep vein thrombosis, but the rate of outflow is slowed because of the venous obstruction.

False positive results may be caused by reduced inflow from arterial obstructive disease or reduced outflow from the high venous pressures of congestive heart failure or ascites. False negatives could result from well-developed collateral circulation or newly formed clots which are not yet fully obstructive.

By comparison, the method appears to be more accurate than the Doppler flow studies, and it is also completely noninvasive, but it does require a small amount of laboratory equipment. It is sensitive to femoral and iliac obstructions but not to deep vein thrombosis below the knee. It shares with the Doppler method the inability to separate venous clots from other forms of venous obstruction.

Isotopic Clot Labeling. This method is based on the incorporation of fibrinogen labelled with a radioactive isotope (usually ^{125}I) into forming clots and is therefore useful for the diagnosis of actively occurring thrombi, rather than the detection of previously formed clots. The technique has made possible several important epidemiologic studies of the prevalence and prophylaxis of deep vein thrombosis in patients at high risk for the disorder. The method is most accurate in the calf and thigh regions and is less so for the iliac veins, in which clot radioactivity is difficult to separate from radioactive urine in the bladder and blood in large blood vessels. False positive results may occur from postoperative inflammation or hematomata (postoperative inguinal herniorrhaphy, hip replacements and so forth). False negative results may be caused by clots which formed before radioactive fibrinogen injection or those formed after its dissipation. Its major advantage is the detection of small, forming, but as yet nonocclusive venous thrombi and its ability to separate them from obstructions other than blood clots. A theoretical risk is the development of transmitted hepatitis, but this has been minimized by the use of screened donors.

Radiopaque Venograms. This method is the standard against which all the other methods are measured. It also is the costliest, requires the most expertise and equipment, and is the most difficult for the patient. With the patient in the vertical or semivertical position, 75 to 100 ml of radiopaque dye are injected slowly into a foot vein, and serial radiographs of the leg are taken as the veins fill. Despite the difficulties and expense of this test, it is our opinion that using the test to establish the diagnosis is preferable to anticoagulation of patients in whom the diagnosis of deep vein thrombosis is questionable.

Prophylaxis

Using the ^{125}I fibrinogen method for the detection of deep-vein thrombosis, it has been found in the International Multi-center Trial that approximately 25% of patients undergoing routine types of abdominal surgery develop deep vein thrombosis. These clots often begin to form during the day of operation and the first postoperative day. It has been shown that when thrombi remain in the calf vein, there is little risk of pulmonary embolism. Twenty percent of calf thrombi, however, propagate to veins above the knee, and 40% to 50% of ileo-femoral thrombi embolize to the lung. The results also showed that low doses of heparin significantly reduced the incidence of deep vein thrombosis, of all pulmonary emboli, and of fatal pulmonary embolism. The low-dose heparin regimen used was 5000 u given subcutaneously 2 hours prior to surgery and 5000 u given every 12 hours after surgery for 7 days. This program does not require the use of clotting times or partial thromboplastin times. Higher heparin doses increase both the protection against clots and the transfusion requirements after surgery. Oral anticoagulants are probably equally effective in preventing deep-vein thrombosis but also increase postoperative bleeding problems.

This low-dose heparin regimen was, however, ineffective in preventing deep-vein thrombosis among patients who had received hip replacements. Effective prophylaxis in these patients may be achieved with higher doses of heparin (5000 u every 8 hours) or the use of low-molecular-weight dextran or aspirin to reduce platelet aggregability. Other methods to reduce the incidence of deep vein thrombosis include measures directed toward the elimination of circulatory stasis. Electrical stimulation of the calf muscles, pneumatic compression of the calves, and mechanical passive plantar flexion and dorsiflexion of the foot offer some protection. The use of compressive legwear appears to be of no value in preventing deep vein thrombosis.

Although most studies demonstrating a salutary effect of low doses of heparin have been carried out in postoperative patients, there is similar information on smaller groups of patients recovering from myocardial infarction. The risk of deep vein thrombosis in this disease has also been reduced by the trend toward earlier patient ambulation. Presumably, the low-dose heparin regimen would protect most patients with any illness requiring bed rest for at least several days.

Treatment

The mainstay of therapy is anticoagulation to prevent extension of the clotting process, during which time normal body mechanisms induce clot lysis. Since anticoagulation carries serious risks, it should not be instituted unless the diagnosis of deep-vein thrombosis is well established, preferably by radiopaque venography. Although thrombi in deep calf veins do not usually embolize, patients with this disorder should also be anticoagulated, since these clots may propagate proximally and then embolize. Adequate anticoagulation in patients with deep leg vein thrombosis significantly reduces the incidence of pulmonary embolism to less than 5% and makes fatalities rare.

Heparin should be used first. It can be given by intermittent intravenous injections, but our preference is for constant intravenous infusions, controlled by automatic flow-adjusting devices. The approximate loading dose is 5000 u, then 1000 u per hour, with modifications based on either the clotting time (2–2½ times normal) or the partial thromboplastin time (2 times normal).

After intravenous heparinization and satisfactory anticoagulation has been achieved for a time, oral anticoagulation with warfarin sodium crystalline (Coumadin) can be started. The determination of the duration of heparin therapy is somewhat arbitrary, but it should be continued for a week or 10 days. On oral anticoagulants, the prothrombin time should remain at 2 to 2.5 times control. There is also controversy regarding the total duration of oral anticoagulant therapy. It is our belief that it should be carried on for at least 3 months or longer, if the stimulus to deep-vein thrombosis persists.

Other forms of medical therapy have shown little advantage over the anticoagulant programs described above. Surgical venous interruption is usually unnecessary except when anticoagulation has clearly failed to prevent clot propagation or where anticoagulants are contraindicated.

Superficial thrombophlebitis alone rarely results in pulmonary embolism and does not require anticoagulants. However, superficial venous clot may be associated with deep vein thrombosis. Where this can de demonstrated, the anticoagulation program outlined above should be carried out. As a rule, if superficial thrombophlebitis is restricted to the veins below the knee, anticoagulants are usually not necessary. When the superficial thrombophlebitis occurs in the thigh, anticoagulation is probably justified, since extension into the deep-venous system is common.

PULMONARY EMBOLISM

Pulmonary thromboembolism is a disorder which varies in severity from lung filtration of trivial clots, on the one hand, to massive fatal obstruction of the pulmonary circulation, on the other. Between these extremes are many nonfatal pulmonary emboli in patients with a variety of associated diseases. Therefore, the clinical features vary widely. This spectrum of differences in severity and clinical presentation make pulmonary embolism a difficult diagnosis to establish and equally difficult to exclude with certainty.

Pathophysiology

The pulmonary circulation is a vascular bed with low resistance and high compliance. Pulmonary blood flow can triple (for example, during exercise) without a rise in pulmonary artery pressure, indicating that a normal threefold reduction in pulmonary vascular resistance has occurred. When flow to any segment of the pulmonary vasculature increases more than two to three times normal, however, it exceeds the ability of the peripheral pulmonary circulation to dilate. A pulmonary embolism blocking part of the pulmonary circulation forces the entire cardiac output through the remaining unoccluded pulmonary circulation, thus reducing the vascular resistance in these segments. This mechanism compensates for the high resistance induced by the clots and operates to keep the pulmonary artery pressure normal.

Therefore, pulmonary emboli involving less than half of both lungs usually result in no increase in pulmonary artery pressure. With progressively greater degrees of occlusion, however, the pulmonary artery pressure must rise if blood is to pass through maximally dilated unoccluded vessels. The right ventricle, not previously stimulated to hypertrophy, cannot generate systolic pressures higher than 50 or 60 torr. In order to achieve even these levels, the right-ventricular filling pressure rises, which accounts for the associated elevation of right-atrial and systemic venous pressure. Further pulmonary occlusion results in a fall in cardiac output since even the maximally stressed right ventricle cannot maintain adequate flow in the presence of such a marked elevation of pulmo-vascular resistance.

The bronchial arteries from the aorta and upper intercostal arteries also deliver blood to the lungs but at systemic arterial pressure. This flow normally nourishes the airways only down to the level of the respiratory bronchiole. There are extensive anastomotic channels between branches of the pulmonary and bronchial arterioles and pulmonary and systemic venules. These channels allow the blood from the bronchial arteries to irrigate the lung parenchyma when the pulmonary circulation is obstructed, thus tending to prevent pulmonary infarction. Pulmonary infarction may occur, however, if pulmonary arteries of small size (approximately 2 mm in diameter) are occluded. If the bronchial circulation is impaired because of systemic hypotension or congestive heart failure (which raises the systemic venous pressure), then occlusion of larger pulmonary arteries will also produce pulmonary infarction.

The mechanism explaining the hypoxemia usually found in pulmonary embolism is far less clear. Loss of alveolar surfactant, bronchoconstriction caused by serotonin release from platelets, or simple local hypoxia could cause alveolar collapse or atelectasis. Pulmonary blood flow to atelectatic or under-ventilated areas outside the area of pulmonary vascular occlusion would shunt unoxygenated blood to the arterial side of the circulation. Other possible explanations for the hypoxemia include the opening of arteriovenous shunts by the high pulmonary arterial pressure and by impaired diffusion of oxygen across edematous alveolar membranes.

Immediately on lodging in a major pulmonary artery, the clot may be gradually penetrated by the blood under higher than normal pressure. This oozing of blood through the clot represents the earliest form of recanalization. Recanalization breaks up the clot so that fragments move into more distal vessels. Clot dissolution then occurs gradually as the result of the action of normal plasma fibrinolysins.

Left-ventricular failure has frequently been attributed to bouts of pulmonary embolism. It is always difficult to determine whether pulmonary embolism has occurred in a patient with heart failure or whether the heart failure was a consequence of the pulmonary embolism. A large, carefully documented series of patients with pulmonary embolism producing left heart failure has not been described, yet it is conventional clinical wisdom that this sequence occurs. It probably only happens in individuals with predisposing heart disease and may relate to left-ventricular dysfunction induced by hypoxemia and low blood flow. Therefore patients with coronary artery disease might be prone to this complication.

Although the elevation of pulmonary arterial pressure correlates fairly well with the amount of the vascular bed occluded, it is possible that humoral or neurogenic mechanisms contribute to the increased vascular resistance to flow. These reflexes may account for some of the pulmonary hypertension unexplained by the magnitude of obstruction.

Clinical Presentation

Patients with acute pulmonary embolization are most frequently those with some predisposition for this disease. They usually are, or have recently been, bedridden because of recent surgery, pregnancy, or congestive heart failure, or have been immobilized for orthopedic procedures. Obesity and previous lower extremity venous disease add to the predisposition. Their presenting complaint is usually shortness of breath without an obvious explanation. This dyspnea may be constant, but is frequently and inexplicably episodic. Less often, pulmonary embolism may present with dizziness or syncope, and, occasionally, crushing substernal chest pain may make it difficult to separate from acute myocardial infarction. Most patients with pulmonary embolism are acutely apprehensive and aware that a major internal calamity has occurred.

Some patients present in shock. These individuals are hypotensive, apprehensive, sweaty, and oliguric. They are often fighting for air and present as an obvious medical catastrophe.

The physical examination may be entirely negative, and the combination of normal physical findings, severe shortness of breath, and apprehension should alert the examiner to the possibility of acute pulmonary embolism. If pulmonary hypertension accompanies the embolism, signs of right heart failure and a paradoxical pulse may be present. Neck vein distension and hepatic enlargement indicates systemic venous hypertension. The lungs are usually clear. Examination of the heart reveals a rapid rate and the presence of a right-ventricular lift or thrust, just to the left of the sternum. Auscultation may reveal an S_3 or S_4 gallop sound originating from the right ventricle and best heard along the left sternal border. The pulmonic component of the second heart sound is often accentuated and more widely separated than usual from the aortic component.

The electrocardiogram is not a reliable confirmatory tool in this disorder. More often than not it is abnormal, but the abnormalities are frequently nonspecific, consisting of ST-segment and T-wave variations, usually in the inferior and right precordial leads. Changes in the electrocardiogram strongly suggestive of the diagnosis occur in a minority of instances, usually when the embolization is massive. These changes include tall, peaked P waves in the inferior leads (P pulmonale), frontal-plane QRS-axis shift toward the right, deep S waves in leads I, II, and III, with incomplete or complete right bundle-branch block. Sometimes transient, deep Q waves in the inferior leads may be indistinguishable from those present in acute inferior-wall myocardial infarction. Atrial tachyarrhythmias, such as atrial flutter and atrial fibrillation, occasionally accompany acute pulmonary embolism.

The chest film is often normal. If the pulmonary artery pressure is elevated, the main pulmonary arteries may appear somewhat enlarged, and areas of reduced vascularity may be apparent in the embolectomized segments. Occasionally, atelectasis is the only radiographic manifestation of pulmonary embolism. The chest film and ECG findings, when present, are often evanescent and can resolve in 24 to 48 hours.

In more than 90% of patients with this disorder, the arterial Pa_{O_2} is less than 80 torr when the patient breathes room air. Although a normal arterial oxygen tension is good evidence against the diagnosis, arterial hypoxemia occurs in many pulmonary and cardiac disorders, so that the diagnosis cannot be made on this basis alone. The tachypnea associated with acute pulmonary embolism results in a reduction of the Pa_{CO_2}. There may be superimposed metabolic acidosis if the cardiac output is low.

Elevation of the activity of lactic acid dehydrogenase enzyme is typical of acute pulmonary embolism, especially in association with normal activity of serum glutamic oxaloacetic transaminase and creatine phosphokinase. Small amounts of creatine phosphokinase are present in the lung normally, and mild elevations of this enzyme may occur. These enzyme changes, as well as elevation of the serum bilirubin, have been previously described in this disorder but are so nonspecific that they add little to the diagnosis.

Lung perfusion scanning is widely used in the study of patients with suspected acute pulmonary embolism. Albumin particles of appropriate size and number, when injected intravenously, lodge in a small minority of the pulmonary capillaries. When the particles are labeled with 99m Tc and the lungs are scanned for radioactivity, the distribution of pulmonary blood flow is apparent. The test is highly sensitive, since a normal examination virtually excludes the diagnosis. Positive lung scans, however, are found in nearly all other lung diseases and in congestive heart failure. They are also common in the elderly without specific pulmonary disease. Pulmonary embolism may be suspected when markedly abnormal perfusion lung scans occur in patients with relatively normal chest films. Comparison of the abnormal perfusion scan with a ventilation scan obtained by having the patient breathe radioactive xenon is often helpful, since pulmonary embolism causes a greater abnormality in the perfusion than in the ventilation scan. When the perfusion scan is markedly abnormal and the chest film and ventilation scan minimally so, the diagnosis is in little doubt.

The most reliable means for establishing the diagnosis of acute pulmonary embolism is the contrast pulmonary angiogram. Although it is most specific and sensitive for large clots, smaller emboli in smaller branches of the pulmonary artery are less easily recognized. Unfortunately, the method is also the most difficult, the most expensive, and (especially in seriously ill patients) the most hazardous. It involves the injection of radiopaque dye into the pulmonary artery through a cardiac catheter and the exposure of rapid-sequence roentgenographs. The clots can be seen as partially or completely occluded pulmonary arteries proximal to avascular segments of the lung. In desperately ill patients, this examination must be carried out by an experienced team, in order to mini-mize the risk of shock, atrial and ventricular arrhythmias, and worsening hy-poxemia. Nonetheless, when crucial therapeutic decisions must be made, an ac-curate diagnosis is mandatory, and pulmonary angiography is indicated.

When pulmonary infarction complicates acute pulmonary embolism, a number of findings may be added to the above clinical description. Low-grade fever is common. Although septic pulmonary emboli is also associated with fever, pulmonary infarction by a bland thrombus is far more often the cause. In addition, there is usually pleuritic pain and cough, with or without hemoptysis. Hemoptysis can occur with pulmonary congestion from left-ventricular failure or mitral stenosis, but when it coexists with shortness of breath and clear lung fields by auscultation, pulmonary infarction must be added to the differential diagnosis. On physical examination, the findings of pleural fluid and/or pleural friction rub may be present. The ECG would be no different in the presence of a pulmonary infarction, but the chest film of most patients with this disorder will show a pulmonary infiltrate. Only in occasional cases is the chest film entirely normal. All other findings would be similar to those previously described for pulmonary embolism.

Prognosis

Since some patients with pulmonary emboli go undiagnosed, the overall mor-tality is difficult to ascertain. Among patients with clinically obvious pulmonary emboli, the overall mortality ranges from 20% to 35%. Many patients die imme-diately on lodgement of the emboli in the pulmonary vasculature. Some survive the first insult only to succumb in the next hour or so. The remainder who sur-vive the first 2 hours following acute pulmonary embolism have a good prog-nosis, provided that further embolization can be prevented. Natural dissolution of the clots usually is completed in several weeks, as shown by the return to normal of the pulmonary lung perfusion scan and angiogram. In most individu-als, little residual lung disease persists following pulmonary embolism, but in occasional patients varying degrees of pulmonary hypertension remain. Rarely, multiple pulmonary embolism is associated with steadily progressive pulmo-nary hypertension and produces a disease clinically indistinguishable from pri-mary pulmonary hypertension.

Therapy

The major goal of treatment is the prevention of further embolism. Those pa-tients who survive the first few hours after the initial insult will usually survive the illness, if additional emboli can be prevented. Anticoagulation is the most important means used to prevent recurrence of embolization, and, given intra-venously, heparin therapy provides the fastest and most effective means by which to accomplish this goal. In addition, heparin may have some effect on re-ducing the bronchospasm to which some of the hypoxemia is attributed.

Intermittent intravenous heparin produces peaks and troughs of anticoagulation. Steady intravenous heparin administration using automatic intravenous flow-regulators eliminates these fluctuations. Patients with massive pulmonary embolism may be initially resistant to anticoagulation and may require large priming doses of heparin. As much as 12,000 to 15,000 u may be necessary to achieve clotting times of 2 to 2½ times control values. The dose of intravenous heparin can then be adjusted downward to approximately 1,000 u per hour or less, as indicated by the appropriate clotting studies. If the patient improves, the anticoagulants can be switched to warfarin sodium crystalline (Coumadin) in 7 or 10 days and thereafter maintained for as long as is necessary.

The duration of chronic anticoagulation therapy after an acute pulmonary embolism is the subject of debate. It certainly should be continued as long as the stimulus to clotting and subsequent embolism persists. If there is no evidence for continued predisposition for embolism, anticoagulation could be discontinued in 2 or 3 months. In patients with recurrent pulmonary embolism, anticoagulation should be continued for longer periods, and occasionally for life.

Where recurrent pulmonary embolism develops despite adequate anticoagulation, or in those patients in whom the risk of hemorrhage is great, surgical interruption of the inferior vena cava below the renal veins is performed. This prevents propagation of clot to the lungs. Complete inferior vena cava ligation has given way to either clipping of the inferior vena cava (applying a device which subdivides the vena cava into numerous smaller channels) or inserting an inferior vena cava umbrella filter. This last procedure avoids the need for abdominal surgery, since the umbrella filter, mounted on a cardiac catheter, is inserted through a neck vein and advanced to the inferior vena cava under fluoroscopic control. When the correct position is obtained below the renal veins, the umbrella is opened, protrusions along its perimeter engage the wall of the vena cava to prevent its migration, and the catheter is unscrewed and withdrawn.

All three methods have advantages and disadvantages. Complete ligation and the application of a clip require general anesthesia, a hazard among desperately ill patients. Inferior vena caval ligation clearly prevents further embolization from the veins distal to the ligature but can be associated with the development of clot above the ligature from stagnant flow. Developing collateral venous circulation around the ligature can also carry recurrent emboli to the lungs. Furthermore, inferior vena caval ligation is associated with a high incidence of disabling venous insufficiency of the legs, following recovery from the pulmonary embolism. Inferior vena caval clipping avoids some of these difficulties by allowing blood, and only small clots, through the multiple channels. This method also requires an abdominal operation using general anesthesia but is effective in preventing recurrent emboli, while minimizing disabling postoperative venous disease. The inferior vena caval umbrella filter eliminates the need for general anesthesia or abdominal surgery, but its accurate placement requires an experienced team. Incorrect placement and migration of the device have both been described. Although the umbrella's fenestration permits blood flow initially, the device often becomes completely occluded later, so that lower-extremity venous insufficiency develops. Vena caval occlusive surgery is reserved for those patients in whom anticoagulants have failed to prevent recurrent embolization or in whom anticoagulation cannot be used.

There are a few patients in whom, despite all attempts to prevent it, recurrent pulmonary embolization recurs and shock develops. Initially, these cases can be managed by attempting to increase the blood flow through the lungs by augmenting the fluid intake (at a risk of worsening right heart failure) and stimulating the depressed myocardium with pressor amines, such as dopamine or dobutamine. If these measures fail to improve the patient, efforts are then directed toward artificial dissolution, or mechanical removal, of the thrombi. In 1973, the results of the Urokinase Pulmonary Embolism Trial were published. These results indicated that a 12-hour infusion of urokinase increased the rate of dissolution of clots during the first few days of the illness. The most frequent side effect was bleeding from cut-down sites, previous needle-puncture sites, and so forth. There was no difference in overall mortality between those treated with heparin and those given urokinase. It is possible that actual differences in mortality may have been obscured by the small number of deaths in both groups. The results suggest, however, that in patients whose survival depends on faster clot dissolution than might occur normally, urokinase may have a clinical role to play.

Otherwise, the only course of action remaining is the formidable surgical procedure of pulmonary embolectomy. This requires not only general anesthesia but cardiopulmonary bypass, incision of the pulmonary artery, and extraction of the clots from within. Since this operation is only done in the most desperate situations, it is not surprising that the mortality is high. There are also some striking successes. Since the need for pulmonary embolectomy is uncommon, no single group or hospital has accumulated a large experience with it. It seems possible that with improved anesthesia and surgical techniques, the procedure might be applied in the future to patients before their clinical deterioration raises the surgical risks to its present level.

Recently, a transvenous pulmonary embolectomy catheter has been described. Experience with this device thus far is limited, but it could be an important advance in management.

It should be obvious that procedures such as vena caval interruption, urokinase administration, or pulmonary embolectomy should not be carried out without absolute assurance of the diagnosis. Any of these techniques could be lethal when applied to a patient with a disease other than pulmonary embolism. Therefore, pulmonary angiography has generally been carried out before any of these procedures are undertaken. More recently, we have been able to avoid the risk of pulmonary angiography in desperately ill patients in whom the diagnosis seemed secure on clinical grounds, supported by a markedly abnormal perfusion lung scan.

In summary, any patient who survives the first few hours after acute pulmonary embolism will usually survive the illness, if further embolism can be prevented. Usually this is accomplished with anticoagulants, but, rarely, incomplete interruption of the inferior vena cava is necessary. Among that small group in whom massive pulmonary embolism threatens survival, medical therapy is used to support the circulation and to increase the rate of clot dissolution. When these fail, removal of the emboli at surgery or by catheter is the only recourse.

CHRONIC COR PULMONALE

Chronic cor pulmonale can result from a variety of intrinsic lung diseases, abnormalities of the thoracic cage, and impaired ventilatory drive. The right-ventricular enlargement associated with cor pulmonale may consist of dilatation, hypertrophy, or both. Whether one or the other predominates in a given patient largely depends upon the severity and duration of the pulmonary hypertension responsible for the disorder. Hypertrophy occurs earlier in the course of pulmonary hypertension and dilation is superimposed later. The presence of heart failure is not implicit in the definition of cor pulmonale but is a frequent complication of the condition. The presence of pulmonary hypertension, however, is a requirement for the development of cor pulmonale, and the increased afterload imposed on the right ventricle by the elevation of pulmonary arterial blood pressure is responsible for the characteristic functional and anatomical abnormalities of cor pulmonale.

In order to understand the disease and its treatment, a grasp of the factors which control the pulmonary artery pressure is essential. In normal individuals, the pulmonary systolic pressure is determined mainly by the vigor of contraction of the right ventricle and the pulmonary diastolic pressure largely by the compliance of the left ventricle. The reason for this is that during diastole, the right-ventricular stroke volume runs off through the lungs, as the pulmonary artery pressure falls to equal that of the left atrium. Normally, left-atrial and left-ventricular end diastolic pressures play a minor role, but when concomitant left heart disease is present, elevation of these filling pressures will raise the pulmonary artery pressure as well. The paucity of muscle in the pulmonary precapillaries and the large size and distensibility of the pulmonary arterioles permit a threefold increase in pulmonary blood flow with little change in pulmonary arterial pressure. This is easily shown by the fact that normal pulmonary artery pressure is maintained even when there has been significant reduction in the size of the pulmonary vascular bed, such as occurs with pulmonary embolism or pneumonectomy. Neither neural stimulation nor the hormones of the renin-angiotensin system have an appreciable effect on pulmonary vasomotor tone. On the other hand, alveolar hypoxia and acidemia are powerful stimuli for increasing pulmonary vascular resistance. Because of this, pulmonary disorders resulting in alveolar hypoventilation and the resultant combination of hypoxia and respiratory acidosis are especially likely to result in pulmonary hypertension followed by cor pulmonale. Hypercapnia, per se, has no direct effect on pulmonary vascular resistance but may exacerbate alveolar hypoventilation by interfering with ventilatory drive. Since not all patients with significant chronic alveolar hypoxia and respiratory acidemia develop cor pulmonale, there are individual differences in the degree of susceptibility to the disorder. Such variability may be partially the result of genetically determined differences in pulmonary vascular reactivity.

Poiseuille's law describes the relationships among resistance, pressure, flow, radius, length, and viscosity in a given hydraulic system. The increases in vascular tone due to Pao_2 and pH changes which alter vascular radius and increase resistance and pressure have already been described. In addition, persistent pulmonary hypertension itself tends to result in anatomical changes in the walls of the pulmonary vessels which cause further narrowing of the vascular lumen and higher vascular resistance. In this way, pulmonary hypertension tends to perpetuate itself. Pressure is determined by the product of flow and resistance. Therefore, besides the factors that cause pulmonary hypertension from an increased resistance, conditions such as exercise, fever, or hypoxemia, which are associated with an elevation of the cardiac output, raise the pulmonary arterial pressure even higher. This helps to explain why patients with chronic cor pulmonale commonly experience further deterioration of right-ventricular function when they acquire infections. Few other diseases produce significant changes in the viscosity of the blood. But patients with lung disease are often hypoxemic—a setting in which polycythemia and high blood viscosity occur. In such individuals, the high viscosity also contributes to pulmonary hypertension.

Many patients with chronic cor pulmonale also have evidence of associated left-ventricular dysfunction. Considerable controversy exists as to whether the left-ventricular abnormality results from the cor pulmonale itself (because of abnormalities of oxygenation and acid-base balance) or whether it is caused by concurrent diseases such as systemic hypertension and coronary artery disease. Regardless of the etiology, the presence of left-ventricular failure in patients with chronic cor pulmonale tends to accelerate the progression of the pulmonary hypertension. As discussed above, the higher left-ventricular filling pressures associated with failure of this chamber are transmitted back to the left atrium, pulmonary veins, and capillaries. Pulmonary arterial pressure must therefore also rise, in order to drive blood through the pulmonary circuit. In addition, the increased blood volume in the pulmonary circulation associated with left-ventricular failure tends to increase the pressure in the pulmonary vessels still further. This effect is magnified by the presence of interstitial pulmonary edema, which reduces pulmonary vascular distensibility. Finally, pulmonary edema from left-ventricular failure exacerbates alveolar hypoxia, which in turn elevates the pulmonary vascular resistance.

A wide variety of respiratory diseases can result in cor pulmonale, but the most common of these is chronic obstructive airway disease. About 40% of patients who die from this condition are found to have evidence of cor pulmonale at autopsy. Among patients with chronic obstructive airway disease, those that have chronic bronchitis are more likely to develop cor pulmonale than those without, since these patients tend to have more severe hypoxemia and respiratory acidosis than the others. Not only do these stimuli directly increase pulmonary vascular resistance, but the low oxygen content of the arterial blood produces polycythemia and a relatively high cardiac output, to maintain adequate oxygenation of the peripheral tissues. These factors, as described above, result in higher pulmonary arterial pressure. In the earliest phase of the pathogenesis of cor pulmonale, both normal right-sided filling pressure and a normal cardiac output are present at rest and during exercise. Later, the cardiac output is augmented to meet increased circulatory demands, but only by elevating the right-ventricular filling pressures to abnormal levels. When right-ventricular failure develops as a complication of cor pulmonale, the right ventricle cannot raise the cardiac output enough to meet increased circulatory demands, despite elevation of right-ventricular filling pressure. In some patients with chronic right heart failure caused by cor pulmonale, tricuspid or pulmonic insufficiency occurs and further reduces the forward cardiac output.

CLINICAL PRESENTATION

The clinical recognition of cor pulmonale unassociated with cardiac failure depends upon the ability to detect right-ventricular enlargement. This may be manifested on the physical examination by an abnormal parasternal cardiac impulse. Elevation of right-atrial pressure can be both detected and quantified by inspection of the jugular veins. On the chest film, enlargement of the right atrium, vena cava, and pulmonary arteries, as well as of the right ventricle, may be seen. The electrocardiogram often shows evidence of right-atrial and/or right-ventricular enlargement. In addition, a variety of supraventricular arrhythmias, such as atrial flutter and multifocal atrial tachycardia, may be noted. The echocardiogram is useful for demonstrating dilatation of the cavity of the right ventricle. If right-ventricular failure supervenes, the physical findings then include peripheral edema, hepatomegaly, and occasionally the manifestations of tricuspid and pulmonic insufficiency.

It should be emphasized that in patients in whom cor pulmonale occurs as a consequence of chronic obstructive airway disease, the physical and laboratory findings of right-ventricular enlargement are often modified by the stigmata of the pulmonary disease. For example, the increased anteroposterior diameter of the thorax commonly present in chronic obstructive airway disease may prevent palpation of the right-ventricular impulse, obscure the diagnosis of chamber enlargement by chest film, lower the amplitude of QRS complexes on the ECG, and greatly increase the difficulty of obtaining a satisfactory echocardiogram. The high intrapleural pressure associated with chronic obstructive airway disease may produce distension of the neck veins, even when right-atrial pressure is not elevated. Finally, the lowered diaphragm that results from hyperinflation of the lungs may displace the liver inferiorly and thus give a false impression of hepatomegaly.

THERAPY

The therapy of cor pulmonale is directed toward the amelioration of the pulmonary hypertension. Ideally, this should be achieved by relieving the alveolar hypoxia and acidemia responsible for the elevated pressures. Unfortunately, the majority of respiratory diseases that lead to chronic cor pulmonale are not readily reversible. Nevertheless, measures to improve pulmonary function, such as the use of expectorants, postural drainage, and the prompt treatment of respiratory infections should be employed. The administration of oxygen has been used to help reduce the pulmonary vascular resistance in patients with cor pulmonale. However, the long-term use of oxygen is often inconvenient, particularly for ambulatory patients, and the risks of carbon dioxide narcosis and oxygen toxicity also limit its applicability. Diuretics may improve gas exchange in the lungs by helping to relieve interstitial pulmonary edema. However, hypovolemia produced by these agents may dangerously lower the cardiac output and increase the viscosity of the blood by raising the hematocrit levels. Furthermore, hypokalemic alkalosis, another potential complication of diuretic therapy, diminishes the responsiveness of the medullary respiratory center to hypercapnia. Phlebotomy to reduce the blood's viscosity has been suggested, but reduction in the patient's red cell mass can critically lower his capacity to transport oxygen.

If congestive heart failure accompanies cor pulmonale, digitalis may be used with benefit. However, a number of precautions should be taken when digitalis is given to these patients. The dosage of the drug may be difficult to regulate, since hypoxia as well as heart failure may produce tachycardia. Optimal digitalization then may not lower the heart rate to normal. Digitalis may interact with hypoxia, hypokalemia, and concomitantly administered bronchodilators to produce serious arrhythmias. In contrast to its effect on the systemic circuit, digitalis does not reduce right-ventricular afterload by a reflex reduction of sympathetic tone. In fact, the drug's ability to augment the cardiac output through its inotropic effect tends to increase pulmonary artery pressure and right-ventricular afterload. Therefore, although digitalis may improve cardiac function in heart failure due to cor pulmonale, it is not likely to be as beneficial in this disorder as it is in heart failure due to other diseases. Nitrates and other vasodilators may be employed to reduce the pulmonary vascular resistance, but their propensity to produce systemic hypotension limits their usefulness.

SUGGESTED READING

DEEP VEIN THROMBOSIS

Hull R, Taylor DW, Hirsh J, Sackett DL, Powers P, Turpie AGG, Walker I: Impedance plethysmography: the relationship between venous filling and sensitivity and specificity for proximal vein thrombosis. Circulation 58:898–902, 1978

Kakkar VV: Deep vein thrombosis. Detection and prevention. Circulation 51:8–19, 1975

Prevention of fatal postoperative pulmonary embolism by low doses of heparin. An international multicenter trial. Lancet 2:45–51, 1975

Sigel B, Felix WR Jr, Popky GL, Ipsen J: Diagnosis of lower limb venous thrombosis by Doppler ultrasound technique. Arch Surg 104:174–179, 1972

Strandness DE, Sumner DS: Ultrasonic velocity detector in the diagnosis of thrombophlebitis. Arch Surg 104:180–183, 1972

Wray R, Maurer B, Shillingford J: Prophylactic anticoagulant therapy in the prevention of calf-vein thrombosis after myocardial infarction. N Engl J Med 288:815–817, 1973

PULMONARY EMBOLISM

Alpert JS, Smith R, Carlson CJ, Ockene IS, Dexter L, Dalen JE: Mortality in patients treated for pulmonary embolism. JAMA 236:1477–1480, 1976

Bell WR, Simon TL, De Mets DL: The clinical features of submassive and massive pulmonary emboli. Am J Med 62:355–360, 1977

Dalen JE, Haffajee CI, Alpert JS, Howe JP III, Ockene IS, Paraskos JA: Pulmonary embolism, pulmonary hemorrhage and pulmonary infarction. N Engl J Med 296:1431–1435, 1977

McIntyre KM, Sasahara AA: The hemodynamic response to pulmonary embolism in patients without prior cardiopulmonary disease. Am J Cardiol 28:288–294, 1971

Miller GAH, Hall RJC, Paneth M: Pulmonary embolectomy, heparin and streptokinase: their places in the treatment of acute massive pulmonary embolism. Am Heart J 93:568–574, 1977

Paraskos JA, Adelstein SJ, Smith RE, Rickman FD, Grossman W, Dexter L, Dalen JE: Late prognosis of acute pulmonary embolism. N Engl J Med 289:55–58, 1973

The Urokinase Pulmonary Embolism Trial, National Cooperative Study. Circulation [Suppl] 47(2):1–108, 1973

Wilson JE III, Pierce AK, Johnson RL Jr, Winga ER, Harrell WR, Curry GC, Mullins CM: Hypoxemia in pulmonary embolism, a clinical study. J Clin Invest 50:481–491, 1971

CHRONIC COR PULMONALE

Baum GL, Schwartz A, Llamas R, et al: Left ventricular function in chronic obstructive lung disease. N Engl J Med, 285:361, 1971

Burrows B, Kettel LJ, Niden AH, et al: Pattern of cardiovascular dysfunction in chronic obstructive lung disease. N Engl J Med 286:912, 1972

Gottlieb LS, Balchum OJ: Course of chronic obstructive pulmonary disease following the first onset of respiratory failure. Chest 63:5, 1973

Lindsay DA: Pulmonary vascular responsiveness in the prognosis of chronic obstructive lung disease. Am Rev Respir Dis 105:242, 1972

Renzetti AD, McClement JH, Litt BD, et al: The VA Cooperative Study of Pulmonary Function. Am J Med 41:115, 1966

SYNCOPE

Robert H. Eich

21

We have included this brief chapter on syncope because the problem can be caused by a number of cardiac conditions, including arrhythmias and aortic valve disease, and can be extremely perplexing. Therefore we felt it important to summarize the subject in a single chapter.

Syncope is defined as a brief episode of loss of consciousness. The duration is not rigidly defined, but implicit in the diagnosis of syncope is that the patient recovers. By the time he or she is seen in the emergency room or the office, after consciousness has returned, there may be no clue as to the actual cause of the syncope. In addition, the patient may not actually lose consciousness but may be presyncopal and complain only of an episode of giddiness or lightheadedness. Unfortunately, symptoms of lightheadedness, dizziness or giddiness also occur with patients who are not presyncopal, but who have vertebral-basilar artery cerebrovascular disease, disorders of the middle ear, or even cervical arthritis, which may not lead to syncope.

For the patient with syncope, the etiology is either circulatory, neurophysiologic, or metabolic. Circulatory problems can lead to a decreased cerebral blood flow and syncope on the basis of cerebral ischemia. The circulatory abnormalities can be either extracardiac and intracardiac. The accompanying list, devised by Samet, shows the various causes of syncope, and I will follow his classification in this chapter.

Causes of Syncope

I. *Circulatory causes*
   A. Extracardiac abnormalities
      1. Common faint, or vasodepressor syncope
      2. Orthostatic hypotension

3. Cerebrovascular occlusive disease
4. Carotid sinus syncope
5. Tussive syncope
6. Postmicturation syncope
B. Intracardiac abnormalies
  1. Intracardiac obstruction to blood flow
    a) Aortic stenosis
    b) Pulmonic stenosis
    c) Primary pulmonary hypertension
    d) Atrial myxoma
    e) Ball-valve thrombosis
  2. Arrhythmias
    a) Bradyarrhythmias
    b) Tachyarrhythmias
II. *Syncope of neurophysiologic origin*
  A. Epilepsy
  B. Brain tumors
  C. Migrainous syncope
  D. Hysteria
III. *Syncope of metabolic origin*
  A. Hypoxia
  B. Hypoglycemia
  C. Hyperventilation

(Samet P: Syncope of circulatory origin. Primary Cardiology 6:114, 1980)

In the approach to the patient with syncope, the history may be of considerable value. The known circumstances which precipitated the event are extremely important. If the patient cannot recall the precipitating events, any witness to the episode should be carefully questioned. Syncope caused by decreased cerebral blood flow usually is not instantaneous. The patient will have some warning, starting with a period of lightheadedness preceding the syncope. Most circulatory syncope occurs in the upright position, but the patient remains conscious long enough to lower himself. While unconscious, the patient with circulatory syncope may make some abnormal movements, but tonic and clonic seizures are uncommon. The syncope of aortic stenosis often occurs after exertion, while that resulting from tachycardia and bradycardia occurs more often at rest. Orthostatic syncope follows assumption of the upright position.

With syncope resulting from seizure disorders, the loss of consciousness is practically instantaneous, with only a very brief aura. The patient will often be unable to protect himself when he falls and will be injured by the fall. The seizure disorders have true tonic and clonic movements, associated with incontinence. Finally, there is a period of post-ictal confusion which is not seen in circulatory syncope.

A gradual development of symptoms suggests hypoglycemia or hyperventilation.

We will deal with each of the types of syncope in some detail, starting first with syncope with an extracardiac circulatory origin.

SYNCOPE WITH A CIRCULATORY CAUSE

EXTRACARDIAC CAUSES

Fainting, or Vasodepressor Syncope

The most common type of syncope from an extracardiac cause is the common faint, or **vasodepressor syncope.** This has been referred to in the past as **vasovagal syncope,** but the term is no longer widely used. With vasodepressor syncope, the history is often quite helpful. This form of syncope is frequently associated with some kind of frightening experience, such as having blood drawn, or spending the first few minutes in the operating room, or receiving an injection. The patient is almost always upright; vasodepressor syncope seldom occurs in the supine position.

The pathophysiology has been extensively studied, and there appear to be two hemodynamic abnormalities. One is a severe sinus bradycardia due to high vagal tone, and the other is decreased vasomotor tone, which results in venous pooling and a fall in arteriolar resistance. Cardiac output and blood pressure fall, from the combination of the slow rate and the venous pooling and lack of arteriolar vasoconstriction. Atropine, while it will reverse the bradycardia, will not affect the venous pooling and the arteriolar vasodilatation.

There are fairly classical premonitory symptoms before the patient actually loses consciousness. He will be seen to yawn and will complain of epigastric distress and nausea. This is followed by hyperventilation and then, unless the patient is placed flat, syncope will occur. The patient will appear cold, clammy, and pale and will look ill; however, he will have a slow, rather than a fast, pulse.

The treatment consists of putting the patient flat and elevating the feet. Atropine is useful to increase the heart rate, but this alone may not return the blood pressure, and the feet have to be elevated to improve venous return. With a classical history, typical physical findings, and a prompt return of the blood pressure when the patient is flat, no further study is necessary for this kind of syncope. The patient can be reassured and warned to avoid situations where this might occur.

Orthostatic Syncope

In orthostatic syncope, orthostatic hypotension occurs when the patient assumes the upright position. The basic mechanism for this is a fall in cardiac output and blood pressure caused by abnormal venous pooling. The abnormal venous pooling is usually the result of loss of compensatory venous constriction owing to a defect in the autonomic nervous system. However, a decreased blood volume can result in orthostatic hypotension or syncope purely because the blood volume is not adequate to maintain cardiac output. In addition, an occasional patient will have orthostatic syncope from varicose veins and the pooling of blood in the large, dilated veins. When assuming the erect position, the blood pressure falls and the patient becomes lightheaded or faint. The symptoms may be more severe if the patient also has cerebrovascular disease. In this case, cerebral blood flow decreases out of proportion to the fall in blood pressure, because of significant narrowing in the cerebral vessels, and the patient develops lightheadedness or syncope. If the defect is in the compensatory mechanism for venoconstriction, this may either be idiopathic or may be caused by diseases which involve the sympathetic nervous system, such as diabetes, a peripheral neuropathy, or an alcoholic neuropathy. In addition, drugs used in the treatment of hypertension notoriously may produce orthostatic hypotension. The drugs which block out the sympathetic nervous sytem are especially likely to do this. Finally, prolonged bed rest may result in orthostatic hypotension, owing to some loss of the necessary vasoconstriction reflexes.

Diagnosis involves measuring the blood pressure when the patient is supine and when he is standing. The patient should have the blood pressure measured first when he is supine and then after he has stood up rapidly. A fall of more than 10 mmHg in the systolic blood pressure when the patient stands is considered significant, but more important is that it falls below 100. In addition, there may be signs of a peripheral neuropathy, such as bladder dysfunction, impotence, or loss of sweating in the lower extremities.

Treatment consists of elastic stockings to prevent venous pooling. The blood volume can also be increased if it is safe to do this by increasing the sodium in the diet and using a sodium-retaining steroid. People who are hypovolemic should obviously have that condition corrected. Patients on antihypertensive medication should be alerted to the possibility of orthostatic hypotension and instructed to get up slowly after they have been sitting. Interestingly, some patients not only have venous pooling resulting from loss of the autonomic nervous system, but their heart rate may fail to increase as well when standing.

Syncope from Cerebrovascular Occlusive Disease

Syncope of circulatory origin owing to cerebrovascular occlusive disease is one of the most difficult kinds to recognize. First, as we have said, cerebrovascular disease may produce giddiness, lightheadedness, or dizziness which is not presyncopal. Second, the presence of the cerebrovascular disease may occur with, and exaggerate, an orthostatic defect. Even if the autonomic system is adequate, cerebrovascular disease may lead to dizziness or vertigo on assuming the upright position in this case, because even the slightest fall in blood pressure may impair cerebral blood flow. Third, some of the symptoms of carotid sinus syncope may be in part the result of cerebrovascular disease. However, cerebrovascular disease of the carotid vertebral-basilar artery system can rarely result in a true syncopal attack, a "drop attack" in which the patient falls from the upright position with no premonitory symptoms whatsoever. Usually the patients only complain of some lightheadedness, dizziness, or blurred vision, but do not have true syncope. In addition, transient ischemic attacks or strokes seldom result in syncope.

One should always suspect cerebrovascular disease in older people with symptoms of dizziness or lightheadedness, and routinely examine the carotids for bruits. However, one should be very careful about carotid compression in older people and especially in older people with bruits. Recently, it has been demonstrated that carotid flow can be measured with the Doppler flowmeter, and this may be a useful adjunct in evaluating the extent of a patient's cerebrovascular disease. Vertebral-basilar artery disease is, of course, impossible to evaluate on the physical examination other than by reproducing the symptoms by having the patient extend his head or turn it from side to side.

Carotid Sinus Syncope

Carotid sinus syncope is a fascinating entity produced by a hypersensitive carotid sinus. Maneuvers such as turning the head or shaving the neck stimulate the carotid baroreceptors and syncope then occurs as a result of a reflex fall in arteriolar resistance and heart rate. The patient may not be aware that his syncope is related to turning his head or shaving, and one may not be able to obtain this from the history.

Three types of carotid sinus syncope were originally described; **cardioinhibitory,** in which the carotid sinus stimulation slows the heart rate and the blood pressure falls; **vasodepressor,** in which stimulation of the carotid sinus results in vasodilatation and a fall in blood pressure, without slowing the heart rate; and finally a third kind which is called **cerebral.** The cerebral type is probably caused simply by carotid artery disease. In the vasodepressor type, we have even seen an occasional case in which the heart rate was controlled with a transvenous pacemaker but carotid sinus stimulation by pressing on the carotid sinus still resulted in syncope.

The diagnosis in all types is established by using carotid massage to reproduce the symptoms. One should listen over the carotid artery first, and should remember not to press if there is a bruit. In any case, carotid pressure must be only unilateral, never for more than 15 to 20 sec, and always accompanied by electrocardiogram and blood pressure monitoring.

Cardioinhibitory carotid sinus syncope can be treated by a pacemaker, but the vasodepressor type is best treated by denervation of carotid sinus.

Tussive Syncope

Tussive syncope, or **cough syncope,** is not uncommon, and the history is classical. It is more common in men, than in women, probably because men cough harder. It almost always occurs in a patient who has been a heavy smoker for years and who has a chronic cough. He may have had a drink or two prior to the episode or syncope. Typically, the patient begins coughing very hard, cannot stop, and then suddenly loses consciousness. Recovery is prompt, and the patient will often be able to resume conversation as soon as the syncope has cleared.

In the past, cough syncope was believed to be caused by a Valsalva maneuver secondary to the long-sustained paroxysm of coughing. It was felt that cough syncope was quite similar to the old "schoolboy trick" of hyperventilating and then, by Valsalva maneuver, producing syncope. However, in a variant called **cough concussion syncope,** occasional patients may faint with just a single cough. Here syncope is actually produced by concussion resulting from the tremendous rise in cerebrospinal fluid pressure produced by the cough. The treatment of the cough syncope is actually quite simple and requires only pointing out to the patient that coughing so hard is what made him lose consciousness; he will seldom cough that hard again. Obviously, he should be encouraged to stop smoking, since the smoking plays a major role in the cough.

Postmicturation Syncope

Postmicturation syncope is a combination of orthostatic hypotension augmented by a Valsalva maneuver. It usually occurs in older men who awaken at night to urinate and, while straining, develop syncope. Treatment is to recommend urination in the sitting position.

INTRACARDIAC CAUSES

Turning to the intracardiac abnormalities which produce syncope of circulatory origin, these may be either intracardiac obstruction to blood flow or arrhythmias.

INTRACARDIAC OBSTRUCTION TO FLOW

The intracardiac obstruction is most commonly aortic stenosis or the more recently identified subaortic stenosis. Syncope resulting from aortic stenosis may be exertional. The postulated mechanism here is that the patient exerts, this produces vasodilatation, the blood pressure falls, but because of the fixed aortic stenosis cardiac output cannot rise to compensate for the fall in blood pressure; therefore the patient loses consciousness. Classically, with syncope of aortic stenosis the patient experiences some lightheadedness with the exertion and then, if he continues to exert, loses consciousness. Usually the patient will recognize this and stop his exertion short of syncope.

Other postulated mechanisms for syncope in the presence of aortic stenosis are: 1) acute failure of the left ventricle, which can result in a vasodepressor reflex or 2) either tachyarrhythmias or bradyarrhythmias. Aortic stenosis does involve calcification or the conducting system and the patient may have bradyarrhythmias or tachyarrhythmias.

The diagnosis of aortic stenosis would be confirmed by the characteristic murmur, and an echocardiogram should be obtained to evaluate both the aortic valve and the subaortic area. Similarly, we have found the use of fluoroscopy to identify calcification in the aortic valve to be extremely useful. If the echocardiogram is normal and there is no calcification in the aortic valve, then one can assume that the syncope is not caused by aortic stenosis, even though the murmur is present.

Both pulmonic stenosis and primary pulmonary hypertension may cause exertional syncope in much the same way, either as a result of a fixed cardiac output or as a reflex set off by ventricular failure. Again, the physical examination would be most helpful in pulmonic stenosis, confirmed by the echocardiogram and chest film.

Primary pulmonary hypertension may be a very difficult diagnosis to make. It is most common in women in their 20s and 30s. The patients complain bitterly of fatigue and shortness of breath, and they may have syncope. The EKG is helpful and will show enlargement of the right ventricle. The chest film does not show the typical findings of aortic or pulmonic stenosis. However, cardiac catheterization may be necessary to establish the diagnosis.

Atrial myxoma again may be extremely puzzling but can certainly cause syncope. The variable murmur, new murmur, and the presence of an embolic event should make one suspect it, and it can be absolutely diagnosed by obtaining the echocardiogram, which is really pathognomonic for an atrial myxoma.

As for ball-valve thrombosis, again one would suspect this in someone with rheumatic heart disease and mitral disease, and again this could be confirmed by the echocardiogram.

ARRHYTHMIAS

Cardiac arrhythmias as a cause of syncope are a very complicated subject. Both tachyarrhythmias and bradyarrhythmias may cause syncope. The responsible tachyarrhythmias are generally ventricular in origin and occur with a ventricular rate over 150. However, there are well-documented cases of brief syncopal episodes resulting from ventricular fibrillation which reverts spontaneously. Atrial arrhythmias seldom produce syncope except in the Wolff-Parkinson-White syndrome, in which the ventricular rat may be well over 200 in atrial fibrillation. The bradyarrhythmias are much more commonly causes of syncope.

Patients with syncope or lightheadedness resulting from tachyarrhythmias will usually be aware of the rapid heart rate and have some warning before they actually lose consciousness.

As mentioned, the bradyarrhythmias are a common cause of syncope. The two types of bradyarrhythmias that cause syncope are second- and third-degree heart block and the sick sinus syndrome. We have already shown how brady-cardia plays a role in the common faint and in carotid sinus syncope; however, that is a temporary sinus bradycardia. Similarly, syncope may develop in the acute phase of a myocardial infarction from sinus bradycardia or sinus arrest, and syncope may be the presenting symptom of an acute pulmonary embolism. However, these are acute episodes and will not be treated in this discussion. The bradyarrhythmias which we are concerned with are chronic ones, caused by degenerative changes in the sinus node, the atrioventricular node and the cardiac conducting system. These degenerative changes may be caused by fi-brosis or ischemia. The name **Stokes-Adams syndrome** has been applied in the past to syncope resulting from heart block, but it is seldom used at present and is confusing, since it is used in different ways by different clinicians; we prefer to avoid it. In general, atrioventricular block does not cause syncope unless there is a high degree of second- or third-degree block.

The **sick sinus syndrome** is better described by the term **tachycardia-bra-dycardia syndrome,** since it is characterized by both supraventricular tachyar-rhythmias, usually atrial fibrillation or atrial flutter, and episodes of sinus arrest and sinus bradycardia. The patient usually develops syncope when the tachyar-rhythmia breaks and the sinus node does not take over or during periods of ex-treme sinus bradycardia.

With the bradyarrhythmias, the history is often helpful. The patient with chronic heart block usually has had multiple episodes of lightheadedness be-fore the first episode of true syncope. He often complains of fatigue and de-creased exercise tolerance. Some patients are aware of the slow heart rate and occasional patients will actually be aware that their heart rate is slower prior to lightheadedness or actual syncope. The sick sinus syndrome, or tachycardia-bradycardia syndrome, is characterized by episodes of supraventricular tachy-cardia, which the patient usually has been aware of, and episodes of sinus bra-dycardia with sinus pauses; again, the patient may be aware of the slow rate and may associate this with his episodes of lightheadedness.

The electrocardiograph may be helpful in evaluating the bradyarrhyth-mias. Heart block will often be shown on the electrocardiogram, including vari-ous combinations of second- or third-degree heart block, although in some cases there may be evidence of bilateral bundle-branch block, commonly right bundle-branch block, and left-axis deviation. Patients who show symptoms of sick sinus syndrome probably at least have sinus bradycardia.

Holter monitoring has been invaluable in aiding the diagnosis in the case of both tachyarrhythmias and bradyarrhythmias, if the diagnosis cannot be made by the standard EKG. As we have mentioned in an earlier chapter, Holter monitoring consists of a 24-hour electrocardiogram, made by a machine that can be worn by the patient. The 24-hour tape is then scanned by machine at a rapid rate to detect either tachyarrhythmias or bradyarrhythmias. There are four possible outcomes of the Holter monitoring: *1)* the patient experiences symptoms and the recording indicates the presence of arrhythmias, resulting in a diagnosis of symptomatic tachyarrhythmia or bradyarrhythmia. *2)* The patient has symptoms during the 24 hours, but the recording shows no arrhythmias whatsoever, which excludes arrhythmias as a basis for his symptoms. *3)* The patient has no symptoms during the monitoring period, and the recording shows no arrhythmias; in this case the best program is to repeat the Holter monitoring. We have been quite successful in continuing the Holter monitoring until the patient has symptoms; several tries may be needed in order to confirm the diagnosis. *4)* Finally, the most difficult of the possibilities is the development of arrhythmias on a Holter monitor in the absence of symptoms. The best course here is to assume that there is some disturbance at a subclinical level that would have produced symptoms if it had been, more severe, and that therefore proper treatment should be started for the arrhythmias.

If repeated Holter monitorings are unsuccessful in establishing the diagnosis of bradyarrhythmias, special studies may be carried out. For atrioventricular conduction defects, these consist of measurement of the conduction time in the bundle of Hiss; for the sick sinus syndrome, they consist of measurement of conduction time from sinus node to atrium and of the sinus node recovery time. While such sophisticated electrophysiological studies have certainly proved valuable in assessing the disease in general, we have not found it particularly helpful in making decisions about the need for a permanent pacer in people who have bradyarrhythmias.

The correct treatment for the symptomatic bradyarrhythmias is the insertion of a permanent pacemaker. Currently, with the lithium iodide battery, there are several brands of pacemakers with a good battery life. The major concern is over the system of leads. We always try to attach the pacer to the ventricle by way of a transvenous lead in the right ventricle first. If that is unsuccessful, we then use epicardial leads, either subxyphoid, or, if that does not work, through a thoracotomy on the left ventricle. This is discussed further in the chapter on bradyarrhythmias.

SYNCOPE OF NEUROPHYSIOLOGIC ORIGIN

Syncope in this category is most commonly caused by epilepsy or a brain tumor. However, rarely, migraine can produce syncope, or it can be caused by hysteria.

The history, in epilepsy, is usually helpful. The patient loses consciousness instantly. There are tonic and clonic seizures, incontinence and, a confused state after recovery. We have found that if the diagnosis of the cause of syncope is not clear, an electroencephalogram and a brain scan are extremely valuable. The brain scan usually will rule brain tumors in and out, whether they are metastatic or primary. The electroencephalogram will establish the diagnosis for epilepsy and seizure disorders. Syncope from migraine is uncommon, and the symptoms of syncope are rarely if ever, encountered in the ordinary types of migraine. However, rarely, especially if the basal artery system is involved, the premonitory aura of the migraine may terminate in a period of unconsciousness.

Hysterical fainting is a fascinating entity which seems to have become less fashionable as the years go on. The episode usually occurs in the presence of an audience, and the patient slumps gently and gracefully to the floor without injury. There are no abnormalities in hemodynamics, and the patient appears calm and comfortable. Likewise, assuming the recumbent position does not alter the symptoms.

SYNCOPE OF METABOLIC ORIGIN

Hypoglycemia clearly can produce syncope. This is usually of gradual onset and is ordinarily caused by an islet cell tumor or, rarely, by reactive hypoglycemia. As the symptoms develop, the patient will complain of inward trembling and a shaky feeling; he becomes sweaty and then loses consciousness. A glucose tolerance test is the obvious way to diagnose this, and we have seen an occasional patient with hypoglycemia who actually faints during the test.

Obviously, severe hypoxia can produce syncope. In the healthy adult, the hypoxia is more likely to be related to high altitudes than any other entity.

Finally, hyperventilation can produce syncope. This is the basis of the schoolboy trick mentioned earlier in which the subject hyperventilates and then stands up suddenly or performs a Valsalva maneuver and loses consciousness. The hyperventilation decreases the venomotor tone and the arteriolar tone, so that performing the Valsalva maneuver or abruptly assuming the upright position will produce syncope because of reduced cerebral blood flow. Similarly, in the simple faint, hyperventilation plays a major role in the loss of the appropriate vasoconstriction.

Patients with dyspnea on exertion may occasionally get lightheaded and should be warned that when they climb stairs, they should move away from the top of the stairs before they stop, because standing motionless after hyperventilation can produce syncope.

INDEX

Acrocyanosis, 14
Action potential, 44
Afterload, 104
Age as risk factor, 120–121
Ambulation and myocardial infarction,
    131
Angina
    Prinzmetal's, 137, 139
    unstable, 138
Angina pectoris, 134–144
    Diagnosis of, 136–141
        coronary angiography in, 141
        ECG in, 139–140
        exercise testing in, 140
        history in, 136–139
        reduction of, 113
            cold and, 137
            mornings and, 137
            pain and, 136
            pain pattern in, 138
            physical activity and, 137
            risk factors and, 138–139
            stress and, 136
        physical examination in, 139
        radionuclear studies in, 140
    history taking and, 3–4
    incidence of, 134
    myocardial infarction and, 122
    normal coronary arteries in, 4
    pathophysiology of, 134–136
        epicardial arteries in, 136
        oxygen delivery in, 135
        oxygen demand in, 135
        resistence in, 135–136
    patient description of, 4
    special features of, 4
    treatment of, 141–144
        beta adrenergic blocking agents
            and, 142

Angina pectoris, treatment (*continued*)
        exercise training and, 142–143
        hospitalization in, 143
        nitroglycerin in, 141–142
        smoking and, 142
        surgery in, 143–144
Angiography, 100–103
    angina pectoris and, 141
    coronary artery anatomy and,
        100–101
    indications for, 102
    left ventricular function and, 101–102
    valvular insufficiency and, 102
Angiotensin, 182–183
Aorta
    coarctation of, 273–274
Aortic dissection, 5
Aortic insufficiency, 255–258
    catheterization in, 257–258
    causes of, 255
    diagnosis of, 256
    lab data in, 257
    murmur in, 256, 257
    physical examination in, 256–257
    symptoms of, 256
    treatment of, 257–258
Aortic stenosis, 253–255
    angina in, 255
    carotid pulse in, 254
    catheterization in, 95
    clinical studies in, 254–255
    murmur in, 254
    physical examination in, 254
    surgery in, 255
    symptoms in, 253–254
Aortic valve
    cusp separation in, 76–77, 77
    dissection of, 77